GABA and Benzodiazepine Receptors

Advances in Biochemical Psychopharmacology
Volume 26

Advances in Biochemical Psychopharmacology

Series Editors:

E. Costa, M.D.

Chief, Laboratory of Preclinical Pharmacology
National Institute of Mental Health
Washington, D.C.

Paul Greengard, Ph.D

Professor of Pharmacology
Yale University School of Medicine
New Haven, Connecticut

GABA and Benzodiazepine Receptors

Advances in Biochemical Psychopharmacology
Volume 26

Volume Editors

E. Costa, M.D.
Chief, Laboratory of Preclinical Pharmacology
National Institute of Mental Health—Saint Elizabeths Hospital
Washington, D.C.

Gaetano Di Chiara, M.D.
Institute of Pharmacology
University of Cagliari School of Medicine
Cagliari, Italy

G.L. Gessa, M.D.
Institute of Pharmacology
University of Cagliari School of Medicine
Cagliari, Italy

Raven Press ■ New York

Raven Press, 1140 Avenue of the Americas, New York, New York 10036

Made in the United States of America

International Standard Book Number 0-89004-530-5
Library of Congress Catalog Card Number 80-24-660

Preface

The synaptic mechanism whereby low doses of benzodiazepines selectively attenuate anxiety, frustration, and fear has puzzled the neuropharmacologist, the neurochemist, and the neurophysiologist for the twenty years that the drugs have been best sellers throughout the world. An important break-through in the elucidation of the mechanism of action of the benzodiazepines has been the realization that the primary action of the benzodiazepines occurs at GABA-ergic synapses where they maximize GABA transmission. This realization originated from independent seminal observations made at Hoffman-LaRoche Laboratories in Basel and at the Laboratory of Preclinical Pharmacology, National Institute of Mental Health, in Washington, D.C. Both observations were published in Volume 14 of *Advances in Biochemical Psychopharmacology*, (1975). At that time, this was only a timid working hypothesis; five years hence, this working hypothesis has been confirmed and this volume represents an evaluation of that hypothesis. It is clear that today there is almost a total validation of GABAs participation in the action of benzodiazepines. This validation was made at a symposium organized by the editors of this volume in Porto Cervo (Sardegna), Italy.

This volume represents the results of research activities carried out in laboratories in various countries including Austria, Canada, Denmark, Switzerland, and the USA. These efforts have been highlighted by important discoveries such as the identificaiton of high-affinity binding sites for benzodiazepines, and the photoactiviation labeling of flunitrazepam, which showed at the electronmicroscopic level, that the high-affinity binding site for the benzodiazepines is located in the postsynaptic membrane facing axon terminal buttons that synthesize GABA. Moreover, the volume documents that biochemically, physiologically, and pharmacologically the benzodiazepines appear to act via a GABAergic mechanism.

But, a message that is not clearly spelled out but one that permeates almost every paper goes beyond the revelation that GABA is operative in the action of the benzodiazepines. The message singles out a new avenue of research in neuropharmacology that may lead to the discovery of new beneficial drugs for the mentally ill. These new drugs, similarly to benzodiazepines, may be devoid of side effects, and may maximize or minimize primary transmitter responsiveness in various types of synapses. This discovery is possible, because the lesson learned from benzodiazepines is one of general significance in the regulation of synaptic transmission. Now, evidence is accumulating showing that more than one neuromodulator coexists in an axon terminal, and now there is reason to believe that both are secreted extraneuronally. Perhaps one acts as the primary transmitter, which, like GABA, transacts the exchange of information, and the other acts on a membrane molecule that works as a fine tuning device for the receptor of the primary transmitter. In this paradigm, the benzodiazepine binding sites can be viewed as the site of action for a cotransmitter that we suspect is stored in the GABAergic terminals and modulates the GABA receptors. In fact, this cotransmitter may restrict the receptor resonse to GABA by facilitating the action of GABA-modulin, a protein that allosterically limits the expression of high affinity binding sites for GABA. The benzodiazepines, by displacing GABA-modulin maximize responses to endogenously released GABA. This explanation implies that the endogenous agonist of the benzodiazepine receptor, by facilitating the action of GABA-modulin, minimizes the GABA responses. One could then speculate that this co-transmitter of GABA synapses might be responsible for the increments in anxiety, fear, and frustration experienced in coping with daily events. It remains to be seen whether other synapses have their own transmitters. By knowing the structure of these cotransmitters (and some, such as cholecystokinin and VIP, are already known), and their mode of action, we can hope that in the not too distant future we may be able to design drugs that act on cotransmitter receptors, and thereby maximize or minimize at will the responses to many other transmitters.

I hope that this book will provide the necessary stimulation to search for the reason the benzodiazepines cause so few side effects, whereas drugs that block receptors for primary transmitters usually elicit severe side effects. Perhaps, the blocker of the receptor for the primary transmitter plays havoc with rhythms of neuronal firing and this disruption triggers responses in collateral neuronal loops that, in turn, cause the side effects. Conversely, drugs that affect co-transmitter receptors leave the neuronal firing rhythm intact and either minimize or maximize the response to primary transmitter. This may be a dream, but in research, the realities of tomorrow are the dreams of today. The ancient Greeks used to believe that dreams occurring in the early morning hours were the truthful ones... let us hope that the "cotransmitter dream" is an early morning dream.

E. Costa
Washington D.C.

Acknowledgments

The symposium was organized under the auspices of FIDIA S.p.A., Abano Terme, Italy. We are thankful to FIDIA S.p.A. for their generous support, and to the participants for their contributions which made the symposium an historical success in the field of psychopharmacology.

Contents

Contributors

L.F. Agnati
Department of Human Physiology
University of Modena
Bologna, Italy

M. Aguera
INSERM U 171
Groupe de Neurochimie Fonctionnelle
Université Claude Bernard
Faculté de Médecine
69008 Lyon, France

C. Aldinio
FIDIA Research Laboratories
35031 Abano Terme, Italy

B.E. Alger
Departments of Pharmacology and Physiology
University of California
San Francisco, California 94143

K. Andersson
Department of Histology
Karolinska Institutet
S-104 01 Stockholm, Sweden

J. Apud
Institute of Pharmacology and Pharmacognosy
University of Milan
Milan 20129, Italy

M. Balzano
FIDIA Research Laboratories
35031 Abano Terme, Italy

J. Bancaud
Unite 97
INSERM
Paris, France

J.C. Baron
Service Hospitalier F. Joliot
Department of Biology
CEA-Saclay
91190 Gif-sur-Yvette, France

M.G. Belin
INSERM U 171
Groupe de Neurochimie Fonctionnelle
Université Claud Bernard
Faculté de Médecine
69008 Lyon, France

G. Berger
Service Hospitalier F. Joliot
Department of Biology
CEA-Saclay
91190 Gif-sur-Yvette, France

L. Bossi
Research Department
Synthélabo-LERS
Paris 75013, France

Claus Braestrup
Research Laboratories
A/S Ferrosan
DK-2860 Soeborg, Denmark

M.J.W. Brennan
Brain Research Group
Department of Medical Biochemistry
School of Pathology
University of Witwatersrand, and
South African Institute for Medical Research
Johannesburg 2001, South Africa

Nereo Bresolin
Departments of Pharmacology and Psychiatry
University of Arizona Health Sciences Center
Tucson, Arizona 85724

M. Brownstein
Laboratory of Clinical Science
National Institute of Mental Health
National Institute of Health
Bethesda, Maryland 20205

I.J. Butler
Departments of Pharmacology, Neurobiology, Anatomy, and Neurology
University of Texas Medical School at Houston
Houston, Texas 77025

R.C. Cantrill
Brain Research Group
Department of Medical Biochemistry
School of Pathology
University of the Witwatersrand; and
South African Institute for Medical Research
Johannesburg 2001, South Africa

F. Casanueva
Department of Pharmacology
University of Milan
Milan 20129, Italy

C. Cepeda
Département de Neurophysiologie Appliquée
Laboratoire de Physiologie Nerveuse
C.N.R.S.
91190 Gif-sur-Yvette, France

C. Civati
Institute of Pharmacology and Pharmacognosy
University of Milan
Milan 20129, Italy

D. Cocchi
Department of Pharmacology
University of Milan
Milan 20129, Italy

D. Comar
Service Hospitalier F. Joliot
Department of Biology
CEA-Saclay
91190 Gif-sur-Yvette, France

E. Costa
Laboratory of Preclinical Pharmacology
National Institute of Mental Health
Saint Elizabeths Hospital
Washington, D.C. 20032

Pushpa P. Deshmukh
Department of Pharmacology and Psychiatry
University of Arizona Health Sciences Center
Tucson, Arizona 85724

H.M. Emrich
Max-Planck-Institut für Psychiatrie
D-8000 München 40, Germany

P. Eneroth
Hormone Laboratory
Department of Obstetrics and Gynaecology
Karolinska Hospital
S-104 01 Stockholm, Sweden

S.J. Enna
Departments of Pharmacology, Neurobiology, Anatomy, and Neurology
University of Texas Medical School at Houston
Houston, Texas 77025

J.W. Ferkany
Departments of Pharmacology, Neurobiology, Anatomy, and Neurology
University of Texas Medical School at Houston
Houston, Texas 77025

K. Fuxe
Department of Histology
Karolinska Institute
S-104 01 of Stockholm, Sweden

Dorothy W. Gallager
Section on Biochemistry and Pharmacology
Biological Psychiatry Branch
National Institute of Mental Health
Bethesda, Maryland 20205

J.M. Godot
Service Hospitalier F. Joliot
Department of Biology
CEA-Saclay
91190 Gif-sur-Yvette, France

Lindsey Grandison
Department of Physiology and Biophysics
College of Medicine and Dentistry of New Jersey
Rutgers Medical School
Piscataway, New Jersey 08854

Ole Gredal
St. Hans Mental Hospital
DK-4000 Roskilde, Denmark

A. Guidotti
Laboratory of Preclinical Pharmacology
National Institute of Mental Health
Saint Elizabeths Hospital
Washington, D.C. 20032

C.E. Jahr
Departments of Pharmacology and Physiology
University of California
San Francisco, California 94143

G.A.R. Johnston
Department of Pharmacology
University of Sydney
New South Wales, 2006, Australia; and
Department of Pharmacology
Australian National University
Canberra City, ACT, 2601, Australia

M. Karobath
Department of Experimental Psychiatry
Psychiatrische Universitätsklinik
University of Vienna
A-1090 Vienna, Austria

G. Kirschner
FIDIA Research Laboratories
35031 Abano Terme, Italy

W. Kissling
Max-Planck-Institut für Psychiatrie
D-8000 München 40, Germany

C. Köhler
Astra Läkemedel AB
S-151 85 Södertälje, Sweden

I.J. Kopin
Laboratory of Clinical Science
National Institute of Health
Bethesda, Maryland 20205

K. Krnjević
Departments of Anaesthesia Research and Physiology
McGill University
Montreal PQ Canada H3G 1Y6

P. Krogsgaard-Larsen
Department of Chemistry, BC
Royal Danish School of Pharmacy
Universitetsparken
DI-2100 Copenhagen, Denmark

Michael J. Kuhar
Departments of Pharmacology and Experimental Therapeutics, and Psychiatry and the Behavioral Sciences
Johns Hopkins University School of Medicine
Baltimore, Maryland 21205

Fredrick Leeb-Lundberg
Division of Biomedical Sciences and Department of Biochemistry
University of California
Riverside, California 92521

A. Leon
FIDIA Research Laboratories
35031 Abano Terme, Italy

K.G. Lloyd
Research Department
Synthélabo-LERS
Paris 75013 France

V. Locatelli
Department of Pharmacology
University of Milan
Milan 20129, Italy

Pierre Mallorga
Section on Biochemistry and Pharmacology
Biological Psychiatry Branch
National Institute of Mental Health
Bethesda, Maryland 20205

P. Marangos
Clinical Psychobiology Branch
National Institute of Health
Bethesda, Maryland 20205

A. Martinez-Campos
Department of Pharmacology
University of Milan
Milan 20129, Italy

M. Massotti
Laboratory of Preclinical Pharmacology
National Institute of Mental health
Saint Elizabeths Hospital
Washington, D.C. 20032;
and
FDA
Bureau of Drugs
Division of Drug Biology
Federal Drug Administration
Washington, D.C. 20204

M. Mazière
Sevice Hospitalier F. Joliot
Department of Biology
CEA-Saclay
91190 Gif-sur-Yvette, France

S. Mazzari
Laboratory of Preclinical Pharmacology
National Institute of Mental Health
Saint Elizabeths Hospital
Washington, D.C. 20032

S.M. McCann
Department of Physiology
University of Texas Health Science Center at Dallas
Dallas, Texas 75235

Brian Meldrum
Department of Neurology
Institute of Psychiatry
London SE5 8AF, United Kingdom

M. Memo
Institutes of Pharmacology and Pharmacognosy
Universities of Cagliari and Milan
Cagliari 09100 and Milan 20129, Italy

Ch. Menini
Département de Neurophysiologie Appliquée
Laboratoire de Physiologie Nerveuse
C.N.R.S.
91190 Gif-sur-Yvette, France

Takashi Mimaki
Department of Pharmacology and Psychiatry
University of Arizona Health Sciences Center
Tucson, Arizona 85724

H. Möhler
Pharmaceutical Research Department
Hoffman-La Roche
CH-4002 Basle, Switzerland

H.-J. Möller
Max-Plank-Institut für Psychiatrie
D-8000 München 40, Germany

P.L. Morselli
Research Department
Synthélabo-LERS
Paris 75013, France

E.E. Müller
Institute of Pharmacology and Pharmacognosy
University of Cagliari
Cagliari 09100, Italy

C. Munari
Unite 97
INSERM
Paris, France

R. Naquet
Département de Neurophysiologie Appliquée
Laboratoire de Physiologie Nerveuse
C.N.R.S.
91190 Gif-sur-Yvette, France

A. Negro-Vilar
Department of Physiology
University of Texas Health Science Center at Dallas
Dallas, Texas 75235

R.A. Nicoll
Departments of Pharmacology and Physiology
University of California
San Francisco, California 94143

Mogens Nielsen
St. Hans Mental Hospital
DK-4000 Roskilde, Denmark

G. Nisticò
Institute of Pharmacology
University of Messina
Messina, Italy

W.H. Oertel
Laboratory of Clinical Science
National Institute of Health
Bethesda, Maryland 20205

S.O. Ögren
Astra Läkermedel AB
S-151 85 Sodertälje, Sweden

Richard W. Olsen
Division of Biomedical Sciences and
Department of Biochemistry
University of California
Riverside, California 92521

Jose M. Palacios
Departments of Pharmacology and Experimental Therapeutics, and Psychiatry and the Behavioral Sciences
Johns Hopkins University School of Medicine
Baltimore, Maryland 21205

S. Paul
Clinical Psychobiology Branch
National Institute of Health
Bethesda, Maryland 20205

M. Pérez de la Mora
Centro de Investigaciones en Fisiologica Celular
Universidad Nacional Autõnoma de México
Apartado Postal 70-600, México 20, D.F.

P. Placheta
Institute of Pharmacology
A-1090 Vienna, Austria

J.F. Pujol
INSERM U 171
Groupe de Neurochimie Fonctionnelle
Université Claude Bernard
Faculté de Médecine
69008 Lyon, France

G. Racagni
Institute of Pharmacology and Pharmacognosy
University of Milan
Milan 20129, Italy

F. Riccardi
Institutes of Pharmacology and Pharmacognosy
Universities of Cagliari and Milan
Cagliari 09100 and Milan 20129, Italy

J.G. Richards
Pharmaceutical Reserach Department
Hoffman-La Roche
CH-4002 Basle, Switzerland

D.E. Schmechel
Laboratory of Clinical Science
National Institute of Health
Bethesda, Maryland 20205

W. Sieghart
Psychiatrische Universitätsklinik
A-1090 Vienna, Austria

P. Skolnick
Laboratory of Bioorganic Chemistry
NIAMDD, National Institute of Health
Bethesda, Maryland 20205

Hanne Skovbjerg
Panum Institute
Biochemical Department C,
3 Blegdamsvej
DK-200 Copenhagen, Denmark

P.F. Spano
Institutes of Pharmacology and Pharmacognosy
Universities of Cagliari and Milan
Cagliari 09100 and Milan 20129, Italy

Robert C. Speth
Department of Pharmacology and Psychiatry
University of Arizona Health Sciences Center
Tucson, Arizona 85724

Richard F. Squires
Rockland Research Institute
Orangeburg, New York 10962

P. Supavilai
Psychiatrische Universitätsklinik
A-1090 Vienna, Austria

J. Talairach
Service de Neurochirurgie Fonctionnelle
Hôpital Ste. Anne
Paris, France

John F. Tallman
Section on Biochemistry and Pharmacology
Biological Psychiatry Branch
National Institute of Mental Health
Bethesda, Maryland 20205

M.L. Tappaz
INSERM U 171
Groupe de Neurochimie Fonctionnelle
Université Claude Bernard
Faculté de Médecine
69008 Lyon, France

John W. Thomas
Section on Biochemistry and Pharmacology
Biological Psychiatry Branch
National Institute of Mental Health
Bethesda, Maryland 20205

G. Toffano
FIDIA Reasearch Laboratories
35031 Abano Terme, Italy

M. Trabucchi
Institutes of Pharmacology and Pharmacognosy
Universities of Cagliari and Milan
Cagliari 09100 and Milan 20129, Italy

James R. Unnerstall
Departments of Pharmacology and Experimental Therapuetics, and Psychiatry and the Behavioral Sciences
Johns Hopkins University School of Medicine
Baltimore, Maryland 21205

D. v. Zerssen
Max-Planck-Institut für Psychiatrie
D-8000 München 40, Germany

E. Vijayan
Department of Physiology
University of Texas Health Science Center at Dallas
Dallas, Texas 75235

M. Willow
Department of Pharmacology
University of Sydney
New South Wales, 2006, Australia; and
Department of Pharmacology
Australian National University
Canberra City, ACT, 2601, Australia

P. Worms
Research Department
Synthélabo-LERS
Paris 75013, France

J.-Y. Wu
Department of Cell Biology
Baylor College of Medicine
Houston, Texas 77020

Henry I. Yamamura
Department of Pharmacology and Psychiatry
University of Arizona Health Sciences Center
Tucson, Arizona 85724

W. Scott Young, III
Departments of Pharmacology and Experimental Therapeutics, and Psychiatry and the Behavioral Sciences
Johns Hopkins University School of Medicine
Baltimore, Maryland 21205

GABA and Benzodiazepine Receptors,
edited by E. Costa et al.
Raven Press, New York © 1981.

GABA Receptors as Supramolecular Units

S. Mazzari, M. Massotti, A. Guidotti, and E. Costa

Laboratory of Preclinical Pharmacology, National Institute of Mental Health, Saint Elizabeths Hospital, Washington, D.C. 20032

The biochemical study of postsynaptic GABA receptors started several years ago in Dr. Snyder's laboratory (6,7) as an attempt to characterize the processes whereby GABA binds to crude synaptic membranes prepared from various areas of mammalian brain. During these studies, it became clear that the binding of GABA to specific recognition sites was a process regulated by other membrane proteins that participate in GABA receptor function (5,9,18). This finding generated in several laboratories attempts to characterize these proteins; we became interested in a protein (GABA-modulin) that modulates the availability of high affinity GABA recognition sites (1). During these studies, additional complexities in the organization of GABA receptors were uncovered; the most intriguing was the evidence that the high affinity binding sites for benzodiazepines (13,16) probably regulate GABA receptor function (5) and that GABA receptors can regulate the affinity of specific binding sites for benzodiazepines (10). Such complexities are not unusual in studies of postsynaptic receptors because the function of most of the postsynaptic receptors for neurotransmitters depends on interactions of specific regulatory proteins with the transmitter recognition proteins and with the processes that couple the transmitter recognition proteins with specific ion channels or effector enzymes. Thus, receptor studies bear similarities to enzymatic studies: in both cases, an understanding of their function involves the isolation and purification of constituent subunits which are then recombined into a functional unit. From this dissection and recombination one learns which processes are essential for receptor function, and thus can plan a strategy to synthesize and study pharmacological agents that maximize or minimize receptor responses without acting on the transmitter recognition site. In fact, current experience shows that occupancy of the recognition sites for transmitters by drugs leads to the development of receptor super or subsensitivity which in turn, determines a number of untoward side effects of the various receptor blockers.

This presentation is a progress report of our efforts to dissect the GABA receptors. We believe that GABA receptors include the following components: 1) recognition protein; 2) GABA-modulin; 3) Cl^- ion channel; 4) a protein that couples GABA recognition protein with ion channels; and 5) a benzodiazepine binding protein.

Since the latter unit has grown in complexity and includes its own recognition site and modulator, it will be discussed in a separate chapter of this volume.

Evidence has accumulated indicating that benzodiazepines function as antagonists for an endogenous receptor site whose natural agonist still defies detection (2). A number of observations (1, 4,10) still support the view that the protein that recognizes benzodiazepines is part of the GABA receptor and, perhaps, is a regulatory subunit of this receptor. The benzodiazepine binding protein may function as a molecular device that couples the protein that recognizes GABA with the specific Cl- channel. This connection may be the molecular mechanism whereby the benzodiazepines maximize GABA receptor responses (3). However, we are not sure whether the benzodiazepine binding protein is part of every GABA receptor or of a subpopulation of these receptors (8).

2. The GABA Recognition Protein

When one begins to study the recognition sites for a neurotransmitter, one often discovers that brain contains several populations of binding sites which differ from each other in regard to their affinity for the natural ligand. When confronted with this heterogeneity of receptors, one is attracted instinctively to give a functional value to the high affinity recognition site as if this were the most important process for the function of the neurotransmitter. When GABA binding studies were initiated using brain membranes the presence of two populations of recognition sites was detected (7): one population appeared to have an affinity constant (Kd) of about 150 nM, the second population had a Kd of about 20 nM (8,9,18). Soon afterwards, it was reported that the latter receptor population was regulated by a mechanism that is disabled by a number of procedures (5,9,11,18). The following procedures can unmask the high affinity binding for GABA in crude synaptic membranes: 1) freezing, thawing, and extensive washing with buffer; 2) freezing and thawing followed by incubation in Tris buffer (Cl-, 50 nM, pH 7.1) at 37° C for 30 minutes; 3) the efficiency of the latter procedure can be increased by adding to the buffer 0.05% Triton X-100; 4) an incubation with phospholipase also appears to unmask high affinity binding sites. It is important to know the exact molecular mechanism that is affected by these procedures. Indeed, this is not an easy task because these procedures cause several modifications of the membrane components. For one thing, successive washes remove GABA, the amounts of GABA present in crude synaptic membrane (CSM) preparations are so great that they may dilute the ^{3}H-GABA used to measure the affinity constant of the binding of this amino acid to the membranes and the number of such binding sites (14). However, washing procedures and treatments with Triton X-100 or with phospholipase do not exclusively accomplish the removal of GABA (17). Proteic and lipidic membrane components are also removed and these components may have an intrinsic value in receptor regulation. Dr. Toffano and co-workers (17) in another presentation to this meeting have discussed the importance of membrane delipidation with regard to GABA receptor function. They concluded that membrane delipidation accounts for some facilitation of GABA binding but it does not appear to have a specific role in unmasking those sites that bind GABA with high affinity.

In order to evaluate the intrinsic value that these various components have in the regulation of the membrane protein that binds GABA with high affinity, it is essential to purify the GABA binding protein and then study in vitro how the other membrane components will affect its function. When we began these studies, our immediate goal was to ascertain whether or not the protein that binds GABA is different from the protein that binds benzodiazepines. Using a variety of detergents, working conditions and various Triton X-100 concentrations, etc., we gradually became aware that the recognition sites for GABA and for benzodiazepines are located in two different molecules; each molecule probably has a different relationship with the membrane lipid as can be inferred from the different conditions that facilitate its extraction. As an example, we report in Table 1 the extent of fluidification of these two specific membrane proteins following a Triton X-100 (1%) extraction of crude synaptic membranes at 4 and 37°C.

Table 1: Fluidification of binding sites for muscimol and diazepam from crude synaptic membranes extracted with with 1% Triton X-100 (w/v)

Incubation with Triton X-100		pmol/bound g of cortex	
Temperature	Time	^{3}H-Muscimol	^{3}H-Diazepam
4°	30 min	30	10
37°	30 min	n.d.	14

^{3}H-Diazepam and ^{3}H-muscimol binding were measured in the 10^5 x g supernatant. The reactions were terminated by applying the incubation mixture on G-25 columns according to Penefsky (12,15). The concentration of ^{3}H-ligand was 10 nM for ^{3}H-muscimol and 24 nM for ^{3}H-diazepam. The total amount of GABA and diazepam binding sites in 1 gram of cortex was approximately 80 and 50 pmoles, respectively. n.d. = not detected

The data of Table 1 indicate that the protein which binds ^{3}H-muscimol with high affinity is destroyed when the membranes are incubated at 37° with 1% Triton X-100 but this protein can be extracted from these membranes when they are incubated at 4° with 1% Triton X-100. In contrast, the amount of benzodiazepine binding protein extracted is about the same under both conditions (incubation at 37° and 4°) reported in Table 1. However, when GABA or muscimol binding capacity extracted at 4° from CSM prepared from 1 g of brain is compared with the starting GABA binding capacity, one finds that about 40% and 28% of the GABA and benzodiazepine binding capacity are extracted, respectively (Table 1).

The data also reveal a possible difference in the stability and physical characteristics of the proteins that contain the binding sites for GABA and for benzodiazepines. When the experiments of Table 1 were repeated using brain homogenates rather than crude synaptic membranes as starting material, it was possible to obtain a better separation of the two proteins that bind GABA and benzodiazepines. Presumably, the amounts of GABA contained in brain homogenate are higher than those present in washed CSM and GABA may function as a stabilizing element of the recognition site during the extraction. This stabilizing action might explain the differences in the data of Tables 1 and 2.

Table 2: Distribution of ^{3}H-GABA and ^{3}H-diazepam binding sites in supernatant and pellet following incubation of brain cortex homogenates with 1% Triton X-100

Tissue Preparation	pmoles/g cortex	
	^{3}H-GABA	^{3}H-Diazepam
Homogenate	80±9	53±5
10^5x g supernatant	68±6	7±0.9
Pellet	10±2	45±5

The homogenate was prepared with 20 vol of 50 mM Tris-citrate buffer containing 1% Triton X-100, 1% beta-mercaptoethanol, soybean trypsin inhibitor 100 g, N-ethylameimide 2.5 mg, TLCK 10 μg, leupeptin 20 μg, in 1 ml. Incubation was carried out at 4° for 30 min. Binding was measured using 40 nM ^{3}H-GABA and 24 nM of ^{3}H-diazepam. Binding in the supernatant was determined by the procedure described in Table 1. Binding in pellet was measured by the method of Toffano et al. (18).

Table 2 shows that an incubation at 4° for 30 min with 1% Triton X-100 in Tris buffer solution extracts only 12% of the benzodiazepine binding capacity of the starting material; in contrast, in the same conditions about 86% of the GABA binding capacity can be extracted. That the difference is real and that the benzodiazepine binding material was not lost during the extraction is confirmed by the measurements obtained from the pellet fraction. As expected, the pellet contains 12% of the total GABA binding capacity and about 86% of the total benzodiazepine binding capacity (Table 2). It is important to note that when the GABA binding capacity located in membranes is fluidified, it is more stable if this fluidification occurs in the presence of an excess of GABA. This stabilizing action of the receptor agonist is not unusual in the purification of the transmitter recognition sites. The binding of GABA to the fluidified receptor can be inhibited by adding GABA-modulin to the preparations; this protein per se fails to bind ^{3}H-GABA or ^{3}H-muscimol (Table 3). Actually, when the inhibitory potency displayed by a certain amount of GABA-modulin is measured by binding ^{3}H-GABA to either CSM or to the fluidified GABA recognition site, one finds that the inhibition is much better when the fluidified binding protein is used to bind GABA (Table 3).

Table 3

Inhibition of GABA binding by partially purified GABA-modulin: comparison of membrane bound receptors (CSM) and fluidified binding protein (B.P.)

Addition	Specific binding of GABA (pmol/mg protein)			
	CSM	Inhibition %	Fluidified B.P.	Inhibition %
None	0.72	0	1.15	0
GABA-modulin (50 μg)	0.55	23	0.52	54

20 nM ^{3}H-GABA was used in these experiments as the ligand.

3. GABA-modulin and other endogenous inhibitors of GABA binding

Several endogenous compounds have been shown to act as possible inhibitors of ^{3}H-GABA binding and, therefore, at least theoretically they could be considered as candidates for the endogenous regulation of GABA binding. These compounds include GABA itself, phospholipids, a polypeptide of about $1.4x10^{4}$ M.W. and metabolites of this peptide with M.W. of about $1.2x10^{3}$. We have termed the $1.4x10^{4}$ M.W. inhibitor GABA-modulin (1). The possibility that a specific inhibitor present in the CSM prepared from rat brain is operative in modulating GABA binding was suggested as a tentative explanation for the unmasking of high affinity GABA receptors which was obtained when the membranes were washed with Triton X-100 (0.05%) (5,9,18). Using gel filtration and polyacrylamide gel electrophoresis, GABA-modulin was purified from crude extracts of rat brain membrane (18). The compound is thermolabile and is quickly digested by endogenous brain proteinases (4). In both instances, GABA-modulin yields the formation of a lower molecular weight (about 1000 daltons)compounds which still can inhibit the binding of GABA to its recognition site. The contribution and possible physiological role of this inhibitory material for the regulation of GABA binding to its postsynaptic receptor sites has been investigated in our laboratory. The presence in brain of a large amount of GABA which is released or formed during homogenization procedure complicates the study and characterization of GABA-modulin. GABA competes with the binding of ^{3}H-GABA or ^{3}H-muscimol to CSM preparations and thereby interferes with the identification and characterization of endogenous inhibitory factors of GABA binding, such as GABA-modulin. To purify the GABA-modulin from GABA and from other contaminants, and to preserve its structure by avoiding degradation, we homogenized the tissue with the following mixture: soybean trypsin inhibitor (100 mg/1000 ml); N-α-p-Tosyl-L-Lysine Chloromethyl Ketone (TLCK) (1mM); N-ethyl-maleimide (10 mM) and dithiotreitol (1 mM). The solution was prepared in Tris buffer (50 mM), pH 7.1, containing 0.05% Triton. The homogenate was centrifuged at 100,000 x g for 1 hr, then the supernatant was condensed by lyophilization and filtered five times according to Penefsky (15) with Biogel P2 columns as described in Table 1. The filtrate was collected and chromatographed in Sephadex G-50 columns.

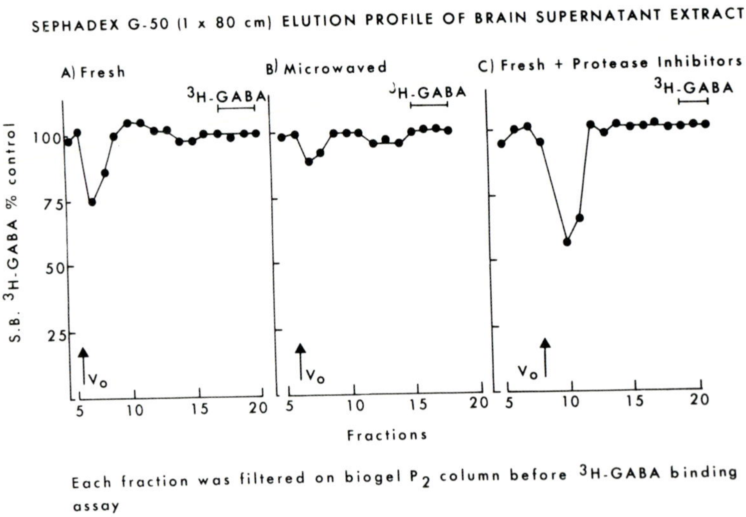

Figure 1
Sephadex G-50 column chromatography (1x80 cm) of the Biogel P2 filtrate (5-fold) of extracts prepared from fresh or microwaved brains: a) fresh brain extracted with Tris-citrate buffer containing 0.05% Triton X-100; b) microwaved brain extracted with Tris-citrate containing 0.05% Triton X-100; c) fresh brain extracted with Tris-citrate buffer containing 0.05% Triton X-100 and protease inhibitors. The column was equilibrated with the same buffer. An amount of extract corresponding to two rat brains was applied to the column, each elution fraction was 2 ml.

Figure 1 shows the inhibition of GABA binding caused by GABA-modulin present in Sephadex G-50 filtrates of various brain tissues.

The filtrate of Panel A is a supernatant of a brain homogenized with Tris buffer and 0.05% Triton X-100 without the antioxidant mixture (dithiotreitol) and the peptidase inhibitors. If the fractions were not filtered in Biogel P2 columns, in addition to the peak that emerges with the void volume (shown in the figure, (Panel A), there would be a peak of inhibition emerging in fractions No. 12 to 18. In Panel A of the figure, the amount of inhibitory material that elutes at the end of the void volume is much greater than that contained in a similar peak shown in Panel B. Since the same amount of starting material (2 brains) was used in both experiments and the only difference was the way in which the rats were killed (microwave in B versus decapitation in A), we conclude that the inhibitory material is thermolabile. Other indirect data suggest that GABA-modulin is thermolabile and that when exposed to high temperatures, it generates a low molecular weight material which still inhibits GABA binding but can be eliminated from the preparation with Biogel P2 filtration (12). Panel C of the figure represents a Sephadex G-50 filtrate prepared with the supernatant of fresh brain that was homogenized with the antioxidant mixture containing the protease inhibitors. The elution profile includes only one peak of GABA binding inhibitory activity corresponding to the void volume; this elution profile is typical for GABA-modulin. Using the material of the chromatographic peak of Panel C, the binding of GABA to CSM and to fluidified GABA receptors prepared as reported in Table 3 was inhibited.

Conclusions

The procedures whereby the GABA recognition protein and GABA-modulin can be isolated, stabilized and purified have been discussed. Preliminary recombination experiments show that GABA-modulin inhibits the binding of GABA to the fluidified GABA recognition sites. Since the fluidified GABA recognition site does not bind benzodiazepines and since benzodiazepines added to the fluidi fied GABA recogniton protein fail to modify the binding of GABA, it can be inferred that the benzodiazepine binding protein is not the protein that recognizes GABA. Since activation of the benzodiazepine recognition protein modifies GABA receptor function and since this differs from the protein which contains the GABA recognition site, it can be inferred that the GABA receptor includes at least four proteins: GABA-modulin, the protein that contains the GABA recogniton site, the protein that contains benzodiazepine recognition sites, and the Cl^- ion channel.

References

1. Baraldi, M., Guidotti, A., Schwartz, J.P. and Costa, E. (1979) Science 205: 821-823
2. Braestrup, C., Nielsen, M., and Olsen, C.E. (1980). Proc Natl. Acad. Sci. USA 77: 2288-2292

3. Cananzi, A.R., Costa, E. and Guidotti, A. (1980). Brain Research 200: in press
4. Costa, E., Guidotti, A., Massotti, M., and Mazzari, S. (1980) In: Proceedings of the EMBO Workshop, held in Jerusalem, February 1980, in press
5. Costa, E., Guidotti, A., and Toffano, G. (1978). Brit. J. Psychiatry 133: 239-248
6. Enna, S.J. and Snyder, S. H. (1975). Brain Research 100: 81-86
7. Enna, S. J. and Snyder, S. H. (1977). Molecular Pharmacol. 13: 442-450
8. Guidotti, A., Gale, K., Suria, A. and Toffano, G. (1979) Brain Research 172: 566-571
9. Guidotti, A., Toffano, G., and Costa, E. (1978). Nature 257: 533-555
10. Karobath, M., Placheta, P., Lippitseh, M. and Krogsgaard-Larsen, P. (1979). Nature 278: 749-759
11. Lloyd, K. G. and Davidson, L. (1979). Science 215: 1147-1149
12. Mazzari, S., Leon, A., Massotti, M., Guidotti, A. and Costa, E. (1980). In: Proceedings of a Conference on Psychopharmacology and Biochemistry of Neurotransmitter Receptors, held at Tucson, Arizona, in press
13. Mohler, H., and Okada, T. (1977). Science 198: 849-860
14. Olsen, R.W., Van Ness, P., Napias, C., Bergman, M. and Tourtellotte, W.W. (1980). Advances in Biochemical Psychopharmacology Vol. 21: 451-460
15. Penefsky, H.J. (1977). J. Biol. Chem. 252: 2891-2899
16. Squires, R.F. and Braestrup, G. (1977). Nature 266: 732-740
17. Toffano, G., Aldinio, C., Balzano, M., Leon, A. and Kirschner, G., this volume
18. Toffano, G., Guidotti, A., and Costa, E. (1978). Proc. Natl. Acad. Sci. USA 75: 4024-4028

GABA and Benzodiazepine Receptors,
edited by E. Costa et al.
Raven Press, New York © 1981.

Benzodiazepine Binding Sites: Properties and Modulation

John F. Tallman, Pierre Mallorga, John W. Thomas, and Dorothy W. Gallager

Section on Biochemistry and Pharmacology, Biological Psychiatry Branch, National Institute of Mental Health, Bethesda, Maryland, 20205

Ligand binding studies with radioactive benzodiazepines have provided rapid methods to study the ways in which the benzodiazepines elicit their characteristic pharmacological actions. The behavioral, electrophysiological, pharmacological and biochemical literature underlying our current knowledge about this widely-prescribed class of drugs was reviewed recently.[42] This paper is complementary to that review and focusses on recent investigations into the nature of changes in benzodiazepine binding elicited by pharmacological agents and the issue of multiple receptors. We also update information concerning the properties of the soluble receptor.

PROPERTIES OF BENZODIAZEPINE BINDING SITES

Peripheral vs. Central

The high affinity and stereospecific binding sites for benzodiazepines in brain seem to represent the places where benzodiazepines exert their pharmacological effects. This conclusion is based upon the high degree of correlation between the ability of an extensive series of benzodiazepines to displace binding of [^{3}H]diazepam from the high affinity sites in brain and their activity in a number of behavioral tests including conflict, muscle relaxant and anticonvulsant tests.[42] One of the most potent compounds observed is clonazepam, 5-(o-chlorophenyl)-1,3-dihydro-7-nitro-2H-1,4-benzodiazepine-2-one; in addition, clonazepam is a potent (<2 nM, K_i) displacer of [^{3}H]diazepam binding to brain specific sites.[4,6,28,29] At the other end of the spectrum of potency is RO5-4864, 7-chloro-1,3-dihydro-1-methyl-5-(p-chlorophenyl)-2H-1,4-benzodiazepine-2-one, which does not have central behavioral effects and is inactive (>100 μM, K_i)[4] in displacing [^{3}H]diazepam from the high affinity sites in brain.

The lack of potency of RO5-4864 is particularly striking because it is quite similar to diazepam, differing from diazepam only by possessing a p-chloro substituent.

Initial investigations of the binding of [^{3}H]diazepam indicated that specific high-affinity binding of [^{3}H]diazepam could be obtained not only to brain but also to several peripheral tissues including kidney.[4] The sites on the kidney cells, although possessing a high affinity for [^{3}H]diazepam, showed different pharmacological spectrum from the brain site. RO5-4864 is a rather potent (5 nM) displacer of [^{3}H]diazepam binding; in contrast, clonazepam is much weaker (>100 nM). Thus, although peripheral tissues possess high affinity sites for diazepam, they seem to be different from the central sites.

In addition to the kidney, the "peripheral sites" seem to be on cultured cells of various types, including those of presumptive neuronal origin.[20,40,41] Both rat astrocytoma[41] and neuroblastoma[8,20,40] cells possess a large number of these peripheral sites--they do not possess the clonazepam displaceable binding.

TABLE 1. Properties of [^{3}H]Diazepam Binding in Various Preparations

Concentration of [^{3}H]Diazepam	[^{3}H]Diazepam Bound (cpm/mg protein) Total	+ Clonazepam	+ RO5-4864
Adult Rat Brain (1 nM)	12,543 ±163	1,117 ±55	12,214 ±317
Adult Rat Kidney (2 nM)	21,473 ±351	21,098 ±768	2,867 ±432
C_6 (5 nM)	84,300 ±3530	79,840 ±1365	4,715 ±39
NB_2A (5 nM)	21,083 ±1377	17,406 ±93	7,512 ±477

Cells were cultured as described,[40] then scraped, pelleted and resuspended for assay. Binding of [^{3}H]diazepam was determined alone or in the presence of 10^{-7} M of the indicated drug.[40] Brain and kidney homogenates were assayed as described.

The nature and biological significance of this peripheral binding site is obscure; it is interesting to note that this site may activate phospholipid methylation either directly or indirectly.[40]

One of the early issues that investigators examined was the cellular localization of the central type of receptor. Although initial reports indicated a neuronal localization,[4,6,28,29] subsequent[7,21] reports supported a glial localization. These reports used kainic acid lesioning or tissue culture; in the case of the kainic acid lesioning experiments, it became clear that a sufficient degeneration period was necessary before neuronal membrane fractions containing sites from lesioned animals could be degraded. When such a period was observed, degeneration studies support a neuronal localization for the binding sites.[8]

Recently, a nuclear benzodiazepine binding site was described in brain.[3] This site has lower affinity for the benzodiazepine [^{3}H]flunitrazepam than the cell membrane binding site; however, clonazepam is far more potent in displacing binding than RO5-4864 (unpublished) indicating that the nuclear site has properties similar to the membrane binding site.

One possible interpretation of these pharmacological and affinity differences at these benzodiazepine sites is that the observed differences are due to a different microenvironment.[20] Solubilization of the central type of site by Lubrol PX (see below) leads to a solubilized preparation which maintains its pharmacological specificity.[48] Kidney membranes do not yield a solubilized preparation after Lubrol PX treatment. These experiments would indicate that the microenvironment of the sites is different and the two proteins behave differently under conditions of solubilization.

Multiple Central Receptors

In addition to the distinction between peripheral and central receptors, some investigators have also examined the possibility that multiple central sites may exist based on thermostability studies.[38] These earlier studies did not consider the newly described nuclear sites. Additionally, several triazolopyridazines displace binding of [^{3}H]diazepam with properties indicating that they are displacing binding from a heterogeneous set of sites (Hill coefficient ∿0.5).[38] Such methods indicate that multiple sites may exist in brain but are not conclusive. It is not known whether these multiple sites would be genetically distinct or vary in their association with other membrane proteins such as a GABA recognition unit (see below). By this criteria of heat denaturation, two such sites are said to exist in cerebral cortex and one site in cerebellum.[25] Studies with purified receptors may clarify these issues.

MODULATION OF CENTRAL BENZODIAZEPINE BINDING SITES

Affinity Changes

The early (primarily electrophysiological) literature is strongly in favor of an interaction between the benzodiazepines and GABA.[13,42] Initial binding studies did not indicate the presence of such an interaction;[4,28] subsequently, we[17,43,44] and others[42] have obtained definitive evidence that the central benzodiazepine binding site can interact with a GABA recognition site. When GABA, muscimol and other GABAergic agonists occupy this site, the affinity of the benzodiazepine binding site for $[^{3}H]$diazepam is enhanced. This enhancement is seen in all preparations which contain clonazepam displaceable benzodiazepine binding; however, we have not seen enhancement of RO5-4864 displaceable binding in cell cultures, and our findings are in contrast to others which indicate the enhancement of $[^{3}H]$diazepam binding in these cell lines.[20] Additionally, we find no binding of $[^{3}H]$muscimol to astrocytoma or neuroblastoma cultured cells.

The magnitude of GABA-enhancement depends on the ability to remove the large amounts of endogenous GABA present in brain membrane preparations and on the region of the brain chosen for study.[22] It is not yet clear whether the regional distribution reflects altered proportions of GABA receptors and benzodiazepine sites or different amounts of residual GABA. Regionally altered proportions of high affinity GABA binding proteins and benzodiazepine sites are indicated by autoradiographic studies.[47] The contribution of nuclear binding sites to these regional distributions has not been studied, and it is not clear if multiple benzodiazepine sites may be defined upon their interaction or lack of interaction with GABA.

Although most GABA agonists enhance the affinity of central benzodiazepine sites, two compounds, isoguvacine and THIP (4,5,6,7-tetrahydroisoxazolo[5,4-c]pyridine-3-ol), behave in an anomalous fashion. Isoguvacine is a partial agonist for GABA by the criterion of enhancement of $[^{3}H]$diazepam binding and will decrease muscimol activation of binding to the isoguvacine level;[5,23] THIP, on the other hand, does not enhance binding of $[^{3}H]$diazepam, reverses muscimol activation of benzodiazepine binding (like bicuculline), and yet appears to be an agonist.[5] Neither isoguvacine nor THIP protects the benzodiazepine site from heat denaturation, a property both GABA and muscimol possess.[39] Among other explanations, it seems possible that THIP in particular may possess agonistic properties at a GABA receptor which is not coupled with a benzodiazepine site and may indicate that several different GABA receptors exist in brain. The difficulties in detecting and separating multiple GABA receptors have been discussed in great detail recently.[11,30] The antagonist bicuculline inhibits both binding to Na^+ independent GABA sites and activation of benzodiazepine binding with a similar K_i (5-10 μM).[12,43] This may indicate that Triton-X-100 treatment of the brain membranes used to detect high affinity GABA binding sites introduces a significant variable into GABA agonist binding studies rendering them less useful for studying physiological phenomena.

Lesion experiments also support the close interaction of GABA sites and benzodiazepine sites. Following kainic acid lesion of the striato-nigral GABAergic pathway an apparent increase in the number of GABA receptors in the substantia nigra was noted without changes in the affinity for the ligand.[45] Concurrent with this short-term denervation supersensitivity in nigral GABA receptors, no change in the number of benzodiazepine sites was noted under these experimental conditions. The affinity response of the benzodiazepine sites to occupancy of the GABA receptor shows a shift to the left in the GABA dose response curve (indicating a GABAergic supersensitivity).[2] Thus the lesion studies support the interdependence of GABA and the benzodiazepines.

The affinity of central sites for [^{3}H]diazepam is also enhanced by a pyrazolo(3,4-6)pyridine called SQ65,396.[1,46] Although initially thought to be via a GABAergic mechanism,[46] SQ65,396 now has been said to be a direct allosteric modifier of binding based upon studies with soluble binding sites (A. Lippa, personal communication). This compound may be a prototype for an interesting series of anxiolytic agents; it does not seem to be an effective anticonvulsant.[1]

Another agent which affects benzodiazepine binding by affinity change is pentylenetetrazole (and its analogues). They seem to block GABA enhancement of benzodiazepine binding but not basal levels. This blockade seems to be correlated to their convulsant properties.[31]

In addition to the pharmacological agents, certain anions such as chloride, iodide, nitrite and thiocyanate have been shown to enhance the affinity of central binding sites for [^{3}H]-diazepam.[9,10] This effect is separate from the GABA enhancement and is additive to it. The possibility that SQ65,396 interacts at this site has not been examined. Triton X-100 treatment of membranes resulted in a dose-dependent enhancement of the GABA effect and a progressive loss in anion effect which is completely obliterated at a concentration of 0.05%, a point where solubilization of benzodiazepine binding sites (decrease in membrane binding) occurs.[10] These Triton X-100 concentrations are used typically to unmask high affinity GABA recognition sites in brain;[12] this supports the conclusion that Triton treatment of membranes may drastically alter the nature of the GABA receptor and its physiological interactions.

Binding Site Number Changes

One of the early reports on alterations in central binding sites indicated a rapid and transient increase in the number of binding sites following either electrically or chemically induced seizures.[32] What is remarkable about this finding is the rapid increase and rapid decrease in the binding sites; most central nervous system receptors show alteration over a period of days, rather than minutes. The magnitude of this effect is approximately 15%; but it is interesting to note that only 20-30% of the benzodiazepine sites must be occupied to fully protect against seizures.[26] Thus, increases of this magnitude (or affinity changes) probably possess physiological significance.

The anticonvulsant agent, diphenylhydantoin, can also rapidly elicit a 20-30% increase in the number of benzodiazepine binding sites following pretreatment *in vivo*.[16] This increase is dose dependent and is elicited in the range of diphenylhydantoin's anticonvulsant properties. The exposure of new sites for [^{3}H]-diazepam is transient, and within a few hours, the binding returns to control levels. In addition to the increase in the number of sites, the diphenylhydantoin treatment enhances the electrophysiological properties of the benzodiazepines but does not alter the response to GABA. Accordingly, it is still possible to obtain GABA enhancement of benzodiazepine binding in membranes prepared from diphenylhydantoin treated animals. It is not known yet what chronic diphenylhydantoin will do to adult animals; however, pretreatment of pregnant rats has been shown to decrease the number of central binding sites in offspring during early postnatal life.[15] This decrease is transient and can be correlated to increased susceptibility to seizures. Diphenylhydantoin does not increase binding of [^{3}H]diazepam binding _in vitro_.

Another compound, EMD 28422 (N^6-[2-(4-chlorophenyl)-bicyclo-2.2.2.octyl-(3)]-adenosine), which is a purine derivative also elicits an increase in the number of benzodiazepine binding sites without a change in affinity. This effect was noted both _in vivo_[37] and _in vitro_[34] and has been correlated to anticonvulsant properties of this molecule.[35] In the presence or absence of GABA or chloride the magnitude of the effect was the same (about 20-30% new sites). In spite of the lack of effects of GABA upon the unmasking, the GABA antagonist, bicuculline, is capable of blocking the effects of EMD 28422, indicating a possible permissive role for the GABA receptor in the rapid modulation of the benzodiazepine binding site.

In the thermoinactivation studies of the benzodiazepine binding site,[48] it was observed that before the binding of [^{3}H]-diazepam decreased, there was a transient increase in binding. Initially, this was attributed (without data) to an increase in the apparent GABA levels or release of GABA from a cryptic heat labile site.[37] More recently, the rapid increases of the number of binding sites has prompted a re-examination of the heat denaturation studies; it is now clear that brief heating increases not the affinity but the apparent number of sites ($\sim$20%).[14] These experiments are consistent with the magnitude of the changes observed in three types of experiments described above. It is therefore curious that such a large (>100%) increase in the number of binding sites has been reported following acute diazepam injection.[36]

Decreases in [^{3}H]diazepam binding sites have been noted following physiologically stressful manipulation[24] and perhaps after chronic diazepam.[33] They have also been seen following maternal diphenylhydantoin administration in their offspring (see above). It is not yet clear how lowered number of sites may indicate altered function of the GABA-benzodiazepine system but this will be a fruitful area for further research.

PROPERTIES OF SOLUBILIZED CENTRAL BENZODIAZEPINE BINDING SITES

Because of the complex series of interactions described above, it is necessary to separate and purify as many of the components of the system as possible. Our initial studies[48] were performed with preparations solubilized with the non-ionic detergent Lubrol PX.[48] A consistent solubilization of over 50% of the central benzodiazepine sites was obtained with a single solubilization step. The solubilized material could be assayed by direct binding studies with [^{3}H]diazepam followed by precipitation of the receptor ligand complex with polyethylene-glycol and γ-globulin. In this preparation the pharmacological profile of the receptor was maintained; in particular, clonazepam was far more potent in displacing [^{3}H]diazepam from the soluble site than RO5-4864. The soluble material seems to be a protein, and its structure is disrupted by either urea or guanidine-hydrochloride. By gel filtration studies, the material runs as a single peak with a molecular weight between 200,000-250,000 daltons. This preparation does not bind to Sepharose-linked concanavalin A, in contrast to that obtained by others,[18]. Binding to concanavalin A would indicate the presence of carbohydrate associated with the protein. Thus, by this criterion, the protein preparation which we have seems devoid of α-glucosyl and α-mannosyl residues indicating a significant difference between these two preparations.

In heat denaturation studies, no initial activation of binding to the soluble preparation is seen as in the membranes and a biphasic inactivation profile is noted. Additionally, in our hands, no activation of benzodiazepine binding is obtained by either GABA or iodide. These results have been confirmed (P. Skolnick and A. Lippa, personal communication) and are similar to those obtained with Triton treatment which eliminated anion effects in membranes.[10] They are in contrast to results obtained with preparations that bind concanavalin A; such preparations have shown activation by GABA-agonists.[19] It seems likely that the "soluble" receptor obtained by these investigators is either an active aggregate of several proteins or an active membrane fragment which contains GABA and benzodiazepine binding sites.

Recently, it has been demonstrated[27] that [^{3}H]flunitrazepam covalently labels the central benzodiazepine binding site following illumination by ultraviolet light. This light-activated labeling is blocked by competitively occupying the active site with other benzodiazepines. When these radioactively labeled membranes are solubilized with Lubrol PX, solubilization of about 30-50% of the radioactivity is obtained.

Under conditions of photolabeling followed by membrane washing, the effects of flunitrazepam are entirely non-competitive. It is interesting to note that when flunitrazepam is used to photolabel the benzodiazepine binding site, between two and three sites are inactivated for each site which is labeled.

As mentioned above, the initial studies on Lubrol PX-solubilized benzodiazepine binding sites indicated a molecular weight of 200,000-250,000 daltons. When the molecular weight of the [^{3}H]flunitrazepam labeled binding site was examined by polyacrylamide gel electrophoresis in the presence of SDS, the label was associated with a protein of molecular weight approximately 50,000 daltons.[27] We have been able to confirm the 50,000 dalton molecular weight by SDS-gel electrophoresis. It is not yet known whether the normal state of the binding site is a tetramer of 200,000 daltons or whether this fraction represents an aggregated state with several other proteins associated. Preliminary evidence indicate an isoelectric point at pH 5.5 which indicates the protein containing the benzodiazepine binding site is acidic. Further purification of this site is underway. Clearly, aggregation can occur and may account for the properties of different preparations[18,27,48] under investigation.

CONCLUSIONS

A number of conclusions may be drawn from the above discussion about this rapidly moving area of research. GABA receptors and the central benzodiazepine binding closely interact in the membrane, and affinity changes may determine the ability of the system to function. Alterations in the number of benzodiazepine sites may also be of great importance in determining the magnitude of the GABA response or set point of response of the GABA system. Central benzodiazepine binding sites differ from peripheral sites and there may be several central sites. At least in the membrane central benzodiazepine binding sites may not all be normally exposed. From the covalent labeling experiments with [^{3}H]flunitrazepam and the simultaneous experiment with non-radioactive flunitrazepam, the binding sites for benzodiazepines, at least in the membrane, can probably interact with each other as well as with GABA receptors. This may indicate a complex of several benzodiazepine sites together in the membrane with a GABA recognition unit and an ion channel.

REFERENCES

1. Beer, B., Klepmer, C., Lippa, A., and Squires, R.F. (1979): Pharmacol. Biochem. Behav. 9:849.
2. Biggio, G., Corda, M., Lombetti, C., and Gessa, G. (1979): Eur. J. Pharmacol. 58:215.
3. Bosmann, H.B., Penney, D.P., Case, K.R., and Averill, K. (1980): Proc. Nat. Acad. Sci. USA, 77:1195.
4. Braestrup, C., Albechtsen, R., and Squires, R.F. (1977): Nature, 269:702.
5. Braestrup, C., Nielsen, M., Larsen, P.K., and Falch, E. (1979): Nature, 280:331.

6. Braestrup, C. and Squires, R.F. (1977): Proc. Nat. Acad. Sci. USA, 74:3805.
7. Chang, R.S.L., Tran, V.T., and Snyder, S.H. (1979): Soc. for Neursci. Abst., Abs. #1632.
8. Chang, R.S.L., Tran, V.T., and Snyder, S.H. (1980): Brain Res., in press.
9. Costa, T., Rodbard, D., and Pert, C.B. (1979): Nature, 277:315.
10. Costa, T., Rodbard, C., and Pert, C.B. (1979): In: Physical-Chemical Aspects of Cell Surface Events in Biological Regulation, edited by C. DeLisi and R. Blumenthal, pp. 37. Elsevier/North Holland, Amsterdam.
11. DeFeudis, F.V. (1978): Neurochem. Res. 3:263.
12. Enna, S. and Snyder, S.H. (1977): Mol. Pharmacol. 13:442.
13. Gallager, D.W. (1978): Eur. J. Pharmacol. 49:133.
14. Gallager, D.W., in preparation.
15. Gallager, D.W. and Mallorga, P. (1980): Science, 208:64
16. Gallager, D.W., Mallorga, P., and Tallman, J.F. (1980): Brain Res. 189:209.
17. Gallager, D.W., Thomas, J.W., and Tallman, J.F. (1978): Biochem. Pharmacol. 27:2745.
18. Garvish, M. and Snyder, S.H. (1980): Fed. Proc. 39:1098.
19. Garvish, M. and Snyder, S.H. (1980): Life Sci. 26:579.
20. Guidotti, A., Baraldi, M., and Costa, E. (1979): Pharmacology, 19:267.
21. Henn, F.A. and Henke, D.J. (1978): Neuropharmacology, 17:985.
22. Karobath, M. and Sperk, G. (1979): Proc. Nat. Acad. Sci. USA, 76:1004.
23. Krogsgaard-Larsen, P. and Johnston, G.A.R. (1978): J. Neurochem. 30:1377.
24. Lippa, A., Critchett, D., Sono, M.C., Klepner, C.A., Greenblatt, E.N., Coupet, J., and Beer, B. (1980): Pharmacol. Biochem. Behav., in press.
25. Lippa, A.L. Klepner, C.A., Benson, D.I., Critchett, D.J., Sano, M.C., and Beer, B. (1980): Biochem. Pharmacol. Behav., in press.
26. Lippa, A.S., Klepner, C.A., Younger, L., Sono, M.C., Smith, W.V., and Beer, B. (1979): Pharmacol. Biochem. Behav. 9:853.
27. Möhler, H., Battersby, M.K., and Richards, J.C. (1980): Proc. Nat. Acad. Sci. USA, 77:1666.
28. Möhler, H. and Okada, T. (1977): Science, 198:849.
29. Möhler, H. and Okada, T. (1977): Life Sci. 20:2101.
30. Nistri, A. and Constanti, A. (1979): Progress in Neurobiology, 13:117.
31. Paul, S.M., Marangos, P., and Skolnick, P. (1980): In: Proceedings of the Conference on the Psychopharmacology and Biochemistry of Neurotransmitter Receptors, edited by E. Usdin, H. Yamamura, and R. Olson. Elsevier/North Holland, Amsterdam, in press.
32. Paul, S.M. and Skolnick, P. (1978): Science, 202:892.

33. Rosenberg, H. and Chiu, T.H. (1979): Life Sci. 24:803.
34. Skolnick, P., in preparation.
35. Skolnick, P., Lock, K.L., Paugh, B., Marangos, P., Windsor, R., and Paul, S. (1980): Pharmacol. Biochem. Behav., in press.
36. Speth, R.C., Bresolin, N., and Yamamura, H.I. (1979): Eur. J. Pharmacol. 59:159.
37. Speth, R.C., Wastek, G.J., and Yamamura, H.I. (1979): Life Sci. 24:351.
38. Squires, R.F., Benson, D.I., Braestrup, C., Coupet, J., Klepner, C.A., Myers, V., and Beer, B. (1979): Pharmacol. Biochem. Behav. 10:825.
39. Squires, R.F., Klepner, C.A., and Bensen, P.I. (1980): In: Receptors for Neurotransmitters and Peptide Hormones, edited by G. Pepeu, M. Kuhar, and S. Enna. Raven Press, New York, in press.
40. Strittmatter, W.J., Hirata, F., Axelrod, J., Mallorga, P., Tallman, J.F., and Henneberry, R.C. (1979): Nature, 282:851.
41. Syapin, P.S. and Skolnick, P. (1979): J. Neurochem. 32:1047.
42. Tallman, J.F., Paul, S.M., Skolnick, W., and Gallager, D.W. (1980): Science, 207:274.
43. Tallman, J.F., Thomas, J.W., and Gallager, D.W. (1978): Nature, 274:383.
44. Tallman, J.F., Thomas, J.W., and Gallager, D.W. (1979): Life Sci. 24:873.
45. Waddington, J.L. and Cross, A.J. (1978): Nature, 276:618.
46. Williams, M. and Risley, E.A. (1979): Life Sci. 24:833.
47. Young, W.S. and Kuhar, M.J. (1980): J. Pharmacol. Exp. Ther. 212:337.
48. Yousufi, M., Thomas, J.W., and Tallman, J.F. (1979): Life Sci. 25:463.

GABA and Benzodiazepine Receptors,
edited by E. Costa et al.
Raven Press, New York © 1981.

The Regulation of Benzodiazepine Recognition Sites by Endogenous Modulators

*M. Massotti, A. Guidotti, and E. Costa

*Laboratory of Preclinical Pharmacology, National Institute of Mental Health, Saint Elizabeths Hospital, Washington, D.C. 20032; and *FDA, Bureau of Drugs, Division of Drug Biology, Washington, D.C. 20204*

A large body of experimental evidence suggests that the binding of ^{3}H-benzodiazepines to specific high affinity sites in brain is regulated by endogenous factors (1,3,4,7,10,12). It has, for example, been reported that the binding affinity of ^{3}H-diazepam or ^{3}H-flunitrazepam is increased by GABA and decreased by endogenous factors (protein factors ranging from 70,000 to 15,000 M.W., purines, nicotinamide, β-carbolin carboxylate) that can be extracted from brain homogenates.

The presence in crude synaptic membrane (CSM) preparations of endogenous factors which produce opposite effects on ^{3}H-benzodiazepine binding became a crucial element to elucidate the physiological role of the benzodiazepine receptors. That benzodiazepine recognition sites are linked with GABA receptor function is supported by the results of ^{3}H-diazepam binding experiments to CSM in the presence of GABA or bicuculline (8,13). When this blocker of GABA receptors is added to freshly prepared membranes, it decreases ^{3}H-diazepam binding, competitively. Since the opposite effect is obtained with the addition of GABA, one can infer that the two sites are functionally related. Moreover, since the action of bicuculline on CSM(s) is indistinguishable from that of the endogenous ligand of ^{3}H-diazepam, when one looks for the endogenous agonist of the benzodiazepine recognition site, one should distinguish this probable agonist from the effect of possible endogenous antagonists of GABA receptors. An essential step in this direction is the use of a purified recognition protein for ^{3}H-diazepam, because at least theoretically this preparation should be insensitive to the actions of GABA and GABA receptor antagonists. Here we will report on the use of solubilization and purification of benzodiazepine recognition sites as a tool to study the nature and characteristics of the endogenous materials which displace ^{3}H-diazepam from its specific binding site. The results suggest that an endogenous material exists in brain which is a legitimate candidate for a role as endogenous agonist(s) of benzodiazepine recognition sites.

Evidence for the Presence of an Endogenous Inhibitor of ^{3}H-diazepam binding

An indication, that an inhibitory material of ^{3}H-diazepam binding to CSM was present in CSM, was at first obtained when the K_D for ^{3}H-diazepam binding to GABA-free CSM was reduced by 50% by repeated washes (at least 3 times) with small concentrations of detergents (see Fig. 1).

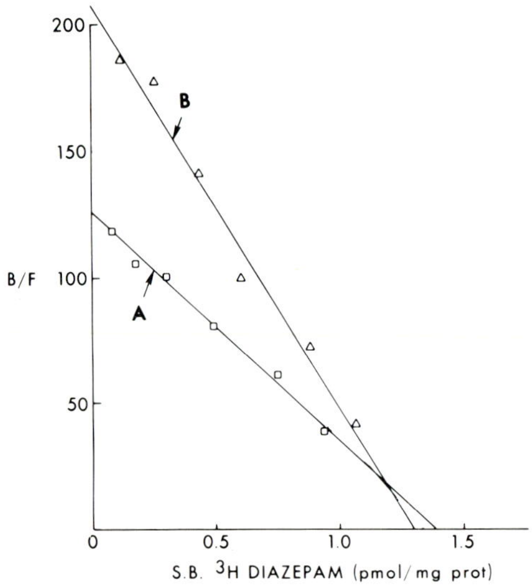

FIG. 1. Scatchard plot analysis of specific ^{3}H-diazepam binding to frozen-thawed crude synaptic membranes (A) and to frozen-thawed and three times Triton X-100 treated membrane preparations (B) from rat brain cortex. The binding characteristics were: A, K_D = 11±0.2 nM, Bmax = 1.34±0.1 pmol/mg prot; B, K_D = 6.1±0.3 nM, Bmax = 1.3±0.09 pmol/mg prot. The difference in K_D between the A and B membranes was statistically significant ($p<0.01$). Each point is the mean of at least five experiments performed in triplicate. S.E.M. was less than 10% of the mean values.

Furthermore, when Triton X-100 extract of CSM was heat-inactivated (95° x 15 min) and then added to CSM, this extract inhibited ^{3}H-diazepam binding competitively. Unlike bicuculline inhibition the inhibitory activity of this extract fails to be inhibited by the presence of GABA (Table 1).

TABLE 1. Modification of ^{3}H-diazepam binding by heat-treated (95° x 15 min) extract obtained from Triton X-100 treated synaptic membrane preparations

Inhibitory Extract			Bicuculline		
μg Prot.	^{3}H-Diaz. Binding pmoles/mg prot	% Inhib.	Dose μM	^{3}H-Diaz. Binding pmoles/mg prot	% Inhib.
0	0.30	--	0	0.30	--
12.5	0.29	13	1	0.29	13
25	0.26	22	10	0.31	--
50	0.23	31*	100	0.30	0

The assay was carried out in three times Triton X-100 treated membranes. 10 μl of endogenous inhibitor containing 50 μg of protein was added to the membranes (300-400 μg prot) 10 min before adding 6 nM ^{3}H-diazepam. S.E. of the mean was less then 10%. The reaction was terminated after 60 min by filtration. $^{*}P<0.05$.

In order to simplify the study of the endogenous inhibitor of ^{3}H-diazepam binding, we decided to use a solubilized benzodiazepine binding protein purified from CSM prepared from rat brain cortex.

Solubilization and Purification of Benzodiazepine Recognition Sites

The GABA-benzodiazepine binding complex was solubilized from frozen-thawed CSM prepared from rat brain cortex using 1% Triton X-100 according to the procedure described by Gavish and Snyder (5). The binding of ^{3}H-diazepam to this preparation was stimulated by the addition of GABA to the incubation medium. The solubilized benzodiazepine binding site, without GABA receptor, was obtained by extracting the membranes with 0.05% Triton X-100. This procedure extracted approximately 50% of membrane-bound ^{3}H-benzodiazepine binding capacity present in the starting material. Moreover this material was virtually free of GABA binding capacity. Accordingly the binding of ^{3}H-diazepam to this preparation was not stimulated by the addition of GABA. The presence of GABA or endogenous inhibitors in the solubilized extract was eliminated by rapid filtration of the 100,000 x g supernatant on a small Sephadex G-100 column using the centrifugation technique proposed by Penefsky (11). This Sephadex G-100 filtration failed to alter the Bmax of ^{3}H-diazepam binding (data not shown). However the affinity of ^{3}H-diazepam binding present in solubilized preparations was 2-3 times higher than the affinity measured in CSM preparations (Table 2).

TABLE 2. ^{3}H-Diazepam binding characteristics in different types of benzodiazepine receptor preparations

Preparation	S.B. K_D (nM)	^{3}H-Diazepam Bmax (pmol/mg prot)
Frozen-thawed Synaptic Membranes	11	1.4
Solubilized Benzodiaz.-GABA Binding Complex	3.2	3.5
Solubilized Benzodiaz. Binding Site	2.8	4.0

Frozen-thawed membranes were incubated at 37° x 30 min and washed 3 times with Tris-citrate buffer in order to remove GABA. Solubilized benzodiazepine-GABA receptor complex was prepared according to Gavish and Snyder (5). Solubilized benzodiazepine receptors were obtained from frozen-thawed membrane extracts at 37° with 0.05% Triton X-100 (6). These receptors are without GABA binding activity.

Effect of Endogenous Inhibitor on ^{3}H-diazepam Binding to Solubilized Recognition Sites

Incubation of the crude endogenous inhibitor, with isolated and purified proteins which bind ^{3}H-diazepam with high affinity, resulted in inhibition of the binding of ^{3}H-diazepam more effectively in the isolated benzodiazepine binding proteins than in the solubilized complex (see Table 3) or in crude membrane preparations

TABLE 3. Effect of endogenous inhibitor(s) on ^{3}H-diazepam binding to solubilized benzodiazepine recognition sites

Endogenous Inhibitor µg prot.	Solub. Benzodiazepine Recognition Site S.B. ^{3}H-Diaz. (pmoles/mg prot)	Solub. Benzodiazepine Recognition Site % Inhib.	Solub. Benzodiazepine-GABA Recognition Sites S.B. ^{3}H-Diaz. (pmoles/mg prot)	Solub. Benzodiazepine-GABA Recognition Sites % Inhib.
0	0.55	--	0.51	--
6	0.48	13	--	
25	0.38	30	--	
50	0.28	50	0.32	38

10 µl of crude endogenous inhibitor was added to 200-250 µg of receptor proteins 10 min before adding 0.75 nM ^{3}H-diazepam. The reaction was terminated after 60 min by filtration on G-25 column chromatography.

(compare Tables 1 and 3). Thus all subsequent efforts to characterize the endogenous inhibitor was carried out using solubilized benzodiazepine recognition sites.

Purification of the Endogenous Inhibitor of Benzodiazepine Binding

In a first group of experiments the inhibitory activity extracted from GABA-free CSM prepared from 8 rat brain cortices was heat-inactivated and then was chromatographed in a Biogel P_2 column (1 x 80 cm). GABA was removed from the CSM by incubating the CSM at 37° x 30 min and by washing three times with Tris-citrate buffer. These membranes were homogenized in H_2O (usually 1 ml/mg prot) containing 0.05% Triton X-100 and then the membranes were sonicated. The supernatant extract was heat-treated (95° x 15 min) and centrifuged at 48,000 x 10 min before lyophilization. Typically 1 mg of membrane protein yielded 12 µg of protein inhibitor. As depicted in Fig. 2 the major peak of inhibitor emerged in correspondence with the void volume.

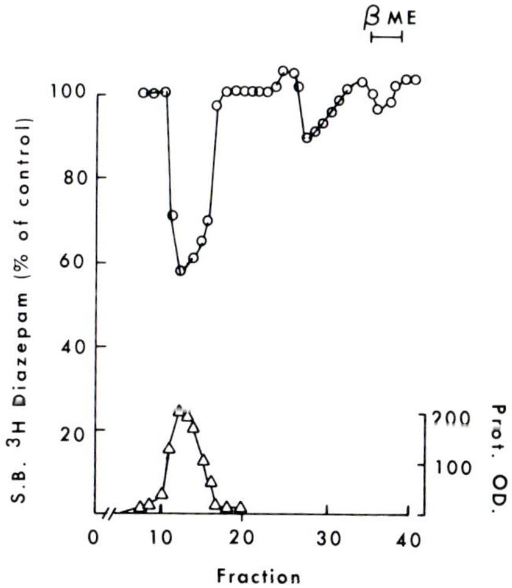

FIG. 2. Biogel P_2 (1 x 80 cm) elution profile of rat brain supernatant extracts. Synaptic membranes obtained from 8 cortices were frozen-thawed, incubated at 37° x 30 min and were used as source of the inhibitor. The extract was lyophilized, resuspended in 1 ml of Tris buffer and centrifuged at 100,000 x g x 60 min. The clear supernatant (1 ml) was applied to the column. Fractions of 0.5 ml were collected. An aliquot of these fractions (100 µl) was tested for inhibitory activity using solubilized benzodiazepine recognition sites as described in Table 3. Proteins were determined by the Bradford method (2).

Since the long time interval required to remove GABA from CSM could cause an enzymatic inactivation of the presumpt ligand for benzodiazepine receptors, it was studied whether these enzymes could be heat-inactivated without loss of ^{3}H-diazepam inhibitory activity. Thus in a second group of experiments thermo-inactivation was achieved by killing the rats with microwave and GABA was rapidly (few minutes) removed from the brain extract by repeated gel filtration of the extract 5 consecutive times on Biogel P_2. This procedure (for reference see Mazzari et al. (9)) virtually removed all the GABA present in the extract and allowed for a quantitative recovery of the material that emerged in the void volume of the P-2 column.

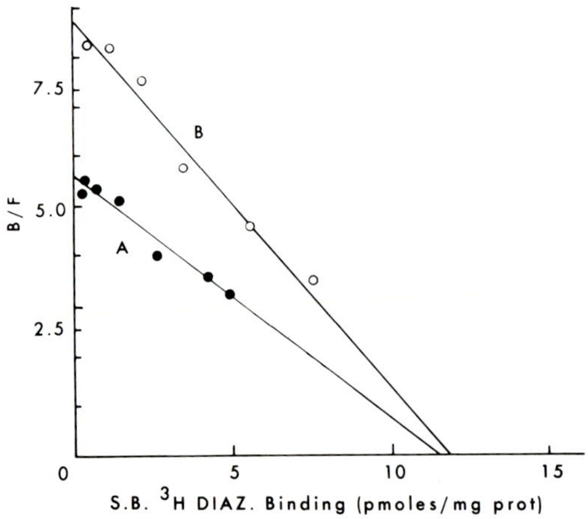

FIG. 3. Scatchard plot analysis of specific ^{3}H-diazepam binding to solubilized benzodiazepine recognition sites in the presence (A) or absence (B) of 25 μg of protein extract containing inhibitor for ^{3}H-diazepam binding.

When this procedure was applied to homogenates of rat brain, the filtrate obtained inhibited ^{3}H-diazepam binding to solubilized benzodiazepam recognition sites, competitively (Fig. 3). The inhibitory material was extracted from different brain areas; it was found that it was higher in cerebellum and cortex than in striatum and the rest of the brain. The extract obtained from 50 mg of either cerebellum or brain cortex inhibited by 50% the binding of ^{3}H-diazepam when solubilized benzodiazepine binding proteins were incubated with 1.5 nM ^{3}H-diazepam. Such an inhibitory activity is present in 200 mg of striatum or in a similar amount of the rest of the brain. Hence the inhibitory activity of cortex is four fold that of striatum. This endogenous inhibitory activity failed to be expressed when the ligand for CSM is

^{3}H-QNB, ^{3}H-dihydromorphine, ^{3}H-haloperidol.

Finally the inhibitory activity against ^{3}H-diazepam binding extracted from brain was pronase-sensitive (see Table 4).

TABLE 4. Effect of pronase on the partially purified endogenous inhibitor of ^{3}H-diazepam binding

Sample	- Pronase	+ Pronase
	S.B. ^{3}H-Diazepam (pmol/mg prot)	
Buffer	0.62	0.70
Endogenous Inhibitor (50 μg)	0.25	0.45*

Pronase (100 μg/ml) was incubated at 37° for 2 hrs.

* $P<0.05$ when pronase-treated group was compared with control group.

CONCLUSIONS

While studying the regulation of the benzodiazepine-GABA receptor complex, we found in brain extracts material which inhibits ^{3}H-diazepam binding (7,8). Attempts to characterize this material were hampered by the presence in CSM of proteases and of various inhibitory materials. The use of solubilized benzodiazepine binding proteins and of protease inhibitors appear to facilitate these studies.

Here we have reported on a simple method to solubilize benzodiazepine recognition sites from CSM and on a rapid procedure to remove from the solubilized benzodiazepine sites traces of GABA, or other interfering material of small molecular weight. The use of this solubilized and partially purified form of ^{3}H-benzodiazepine binding protein has been crucial to progress in the study and characterization of the possible endogenous inhibitor of ^{3}H-benzodiazepine binding sites. In this report, it has been possible to establish that rat brain contains a considerable inhibitory activity of ^{3}H-diazepam binding which is pronase-sensitive and has a molecular weight higher than purines, nicotinamide or -carbolin carboxylate. The activity that can be extracted from the brain is considerable. From 100 mg of rat brain cortex we can extract enough activity to displace 1 pmole of diazepam, bound to the purified binding protein. This material is thermostable (95° x 15 min), pronase-sensitive and acts like an apparent competitive inhibitor of ^{3}H-diazepam binding. We know that the molecular weight of the material responsible for the ^{3}H-diazepam binding inhibition is larger than 1,800 dalton, but its exact molecular weight and other physico-chemical characteristics have not yet been established. However, we anticipate that the utilization of the solubilized benzodiazepine receptors will facilitate our effort to isolate and characterize this endogenous material.

REFERENCES

1. Asano, T., and Spector, S. (1979): Proc. Natl. Acad. Sci. USA, 76:977-981.
2. Bradford, M. M. (1976): Anal. Biochem., 72:248-254.
3. Braestrup, C., Nilsen, M., and Olsen, C. E. (1980): Proc. Natl. Acad. Sci. USA, 77:2288-2292.
4. Colello, G. D., Hockenberg, D. M., Bosmann, H. B., Fuchs, S., and Folkers, K. (1978): Proc. Natl. Acad. Sci. USA, 75: 6319-6323.
5. Gavish, M., and Snyder, S. H. (1980): Life Sci., 26:579-582.
6. Guidotti, A., Massotti, M., and Costa, E. (1980): Psychopharmacology and Biochemistry of Neurotransmitter Receptors. Elsevier/North-Holland, New York.
7. Guidotti, A., Toffano, G., and Costa, E. (1980): Nature, 275:553-555.
8. Massotti, M., and Guidotti, A. (1980): Life Sci., in press.
9. Mazzari, S., Leon, A., Massotti, M., Guidotti, A., and Costa, E. (1980): Psychopharmacology and Biochemistry of Neurotransmitter Receptors. Elsevier/North-Holland, New York.
10. Mohler, H., Polc, P., Cumin, R., Pieri, L., and Kettler, R. (1979): Nature, 278:563-565.
11. Penefsky, H. S. (1977): J. Biol. Chem., 252:2891-2899.
12. Skolnic, P., Marangos, P. J., and Goodwin, F. K. (1979): Life Sci., 23:1473-1480.
13. Tallman, J. F., Thomas, J. W., and Gallager, D. W. (1978): Nature, 274:383-385.

GABA and Benzodiazepine Receptors,
edited by E. Costa et al.
Raven Press, New York © 1981.

Neuronal Localization of Benzodiazepine Receptors in the Murine Cerebellum

Robert C. Speth, Nereo Bresolin, Takashi Mimaki, Pushpa P. Deshmukh, and *Henry I. Yamamura

Department of Pharmacology and Psychiatry, University of Arizona Health Sciences Center, Tucson, Arizona 85724

Brain benzodiazepine receptors have been proposed to be the site at which benzodiazepines exert their psychoactive effects (10,26). We were interested in determining the neuronal localization of benzodiazepine receptors within the murine cerebellum.

Several recent studies in mutant mice strains have been directed towards this possibility (3,13,22,24) and have suggested localization on Purkinje cells.

The present study extends these observations, using two strains of mutant mice ("staggerer" and "weaver"). Three different types of chemicals (3-acetylpyridine, kainic acid and phenytoin) were also used to produce relatively selective lesions within the rat cerebellum.

MATERIALS AND METHODS

Experimental Animals

"Weaver" mice.

The "weaver" mutation is an autosomal semidominant trait characterized by a near total depletion of the cerebellar granule cell population, which occurs within the first 14 days of life. In addition, there are abnormalities in the Bergman glial fibers in the "weaver" mouse cerebellum which may be the primary defect leading to granule cell death (19).

"Weaver" mice are readily identified by their ataxic movements and tremors. Their body weight tends to be similar to their littermates, however, the weight of the "weaver" mouse cerebellum is only about 40% of the weight of that of their littermates. The "weaver" mice used in these studies were sacrificed at 54-70 days of age.

"Staggerer" mice.

The "staggerer" mutation is an autosomal recessive trait, characterized by a primary abnormality in cerebellar Purkinje cell dendrites which receive their synaptic innervation from parallel fibers arising from granule cells. The spiny branchlets

* To whom reprint request can be addressed.

or postsynaptic thickenings characteristic of post-synaptic membranes do not develop on these Purkinje cell dendrites (11). This abnormality appears to cause a "transsynaptic" degeneration of the granule cells, and subsequent degenerative changes in the mossy fibers innervating the granule cells by 26 days of age (23).

"Staggerer" mutants can be recognized by their ataxic gait and considerably decreased body weight. The weight of the "staggerer" cerebellum is only about 20% of the weight of their behaviorally normal littermates. The "staggerer" mice used in these studies were sacrificed at 25-30 days of age.

"Weaver" (B6CBA, wv/wv), "Staggerer" (C57BL, sg/sg) and their heterozygous, phenotypically normal littermates were obtained from Jackson Laboratories, (Bar Harbor, ME.).

Male, Sprague-Dawley rats were obtained from the animal colony at the University of Arizona or Hilltop Laboratory Animals (Chatsworth, CA). Rats weighed 175-200 grams at the time of lesioning with kainic acid.

Chemical Lesions

3-Acetylpyridine lesions.

3-Acetylpyridine is a nicotinamide antagonist which produces lesions in several brain regions, with the most pronounced destruction occurring in the inferior olivary nucleus in the brain stem (5). The inferior olivary nucleus gives rise to the climbing fibers which ascend into the cerebellar molecular layer where they synapse with Purkinje cell dendrites. These climbing fibers disappear following 3-acetylpyridine administration (4).

Animals treated with 3-acetylpyridine display characteristic rhythmic head movements from side to side, exhibit a splayed posture and are ataxic. There is no difference in the weight of the cerebellum after 3-acetylpyridine treatment.

To produce severe yet selective lesions, the lesioning procedure of Llinas et al. (14) was used. Rats were injected intraperitoneally (i.p.) with 75 mg/kg of 3-acetylpyridine, 90 minutes later, rats received 15 mg/kg of harmaline (i.p.) and an additional 180 minutes later, they received 300 mg/kg of nicotinamide (i.p.). Control animals received i.p. injections of saline at appropriate intervals. Rats were sacrificed 4 or 50 days after 3-acetylpyridine administration.

Kainic acid lesions.

Kainic acid is a rigid analog of glutamic acid, which when administered in high doses or directly into the brain produces a selective neurotoxicity that is thought to affect glutamatergic neurons (8,9). In the cerebellum, kainic acid is reported to destroy Purkinje cells, basket cells, stellate cells and Golgi II cells, while sparing the majority of granule cells (8,9).

Kainic acid treated rats displayed a transient hypotonia on the ipsilateral side from the lesion lasting approximately 10 days. During recovery, the animals showed convulsive symptoms with turning and rolling toward the side of the lesion.

For intracerebellar kainic acid injection, rats were anesthetized with sodium pentobarbital (35 mg/kg) and placed in a stereotaxic instrument. Kainic acid was administered unilaterally into the cerebellum in two, one microliter injections of a one microgram per microliter solution of kainic acid in saline through a fine needle at the following stereotaxic coordinates; A-P: 3.0 and 4.0 mm posterior to bregma, L: 2.5 mm, V: 3.5 mm. Control (unlesioned) animals received similar injections of the saline vehicle only. Rats were sacrificed approximately 50 days following placement of the kainic acid.

Chronic phenytoin treatment.

Male Sprague-Dawley rats (about 200 grams body weight) housed in groups of two, were treated once daily with 200 mg/kg of phenytoin (DPH) i.p. (Aldrich Chemical Co. Inc., DPH suspension in 10% (v/v) Tween 81 in saline) or 1 ml/kg of 10% (v/v) Tween 81 i.p. for 14 days or 28 days. This dose of DPH resulted in 80.0% survival rate, and the growth of DPH treated rats as compared to control was retarded about 40%. Animals were sacrificed by decapitation six hours following the last injection of drug or vehicle.

Measurement of Benzodiazepine Receptors

^{3}H-Flunitrazepam binding assay.

At the specified times, animals were sacrificed by decapitation and specified brain regions were dissected, weighed and homogenized with a Polytron ^{R} homogenizer in phosphate buffer, pH 7.4. The tissue was washed by centrifugation and resuspension of the pelleted tissue occurred in fresh buffer unless otherwise indicated. An aliquot of this homogenate was assayed for protein concentration by the method of Lowry et al. (15).

^{3}H-Flunitrazepam binding assays were performed as described previously (25). Briefly, assays contained ^{3}H-flunitrazepam in four concentrations, 0.1 nanomolar to 5.0 nanomolar, brain homogenate equivalent to 2 mg wet weight, and phosphate buffered saline solution, pH 7.4 to make a total volume of 2.0 ml. Alternate samples contained clonazepam (1.0 micromolar concentration) to assess nonspecific binding of ^{3}H-flunitrazepam.

Samples were incubated for 90 minutes at 0°C. To separate free and bound ^{3}H-flunitrazepam, samples were poured over GF/B filters in vacuo and rinsed three times with 5 ml of phosphate buffer. The filters were assayed for radioactivity by liquid scintillation spectrometry using a Triton X-100 ^{R}: toluene: Omnifluor ^{R} (1 liter: 2 liters: 16 grams) cocktail.

Determination of the dissociation constant (K_d) and receptor concentration (Bmax) for specific (clonazepam displaceable) ^{3}H-flunitrazepam binding to brain was determined by inverse Scatchard analysis of the 4 point saturation isotherms.

All values presented are the mean values ± the standard error of the mean.

Benzodiazepines. ^{3}H-Flunitrazepam (85 Ci/mmol) was obtained from New England Nuclear Corp., Boston, MA. Clonazepam was generously provided by Dr. Scott of Hoffman-LaRoche, Inc., Nutley N.J.

RESULTS

BENZODIAZEPINE RECEPTORS IN "WEAVER" MICE BRAINS

The density of benzodiazepine receptors in the "weaver" mouse cerebellum and cerebral cortex displayed a small but nonsignificant increase compared to their behaviorally normal littermates. There were also no significant differences in K_d values for ^3H-flunitrazepam binding to benzodiazepine receptors between "weaver" and control mice cerebella and cerebral cortices (Table 1).

TABLE I. ^3H-Flunitrazepam binding to the cerebellum and cerebral cortex of "weaver" and normal littermate mice.

	(n)	K_d (nM)	Bmax (pmol/g protein)
Cerebellum			
"Weaver"	4	1.16±0.19	998±61
Littermate	4	1.10±0.09	916±84
Cerebral Cortex			
"Weaver"	4	0.94±0.04	1565±84
Littermate	4	0.91±0.05	1486±79

The weight of the "weaver" mouse cerebellum was 40% of the weight of their normal littermates, so the absolute number of benzodiazepine receptors in the "weaver" mouse cerebellum was decreased 57%. The weight of the "weaver" cerebral cortex was 93% of control, and there was no change in the density of benzodiazepine receptors in the "weaver" cerebral cortex.

Benzodiazepine receptors in "staggerer" mice brains.

"Staggerer" mutant mice displayed a dramatic 45% decrease in the density of cerebellar benzodiazepine receptors. This decrease was similar in "staggerer" mice of both sexes. Benzodiazepine receptor density in the cerebral cortex of "staggerer" mice was not different from that of their normal littermates. The cerebellar benzodiazepine receptors of female "staggerer" mice displayed a significantly lower affinity (higher K_d value) for ^3H-flunitrazepam than did those of their normal female littermates or the male "staggerer" mice (Table 2).

The weight of the cerebellum of "staggerer" mice was only 18% of the cerebellum of their littermates, therefore the absolute number of benzodiazepine receptors in "staggerer" mice cerebella was decreased 90%. The weight of the cerebral cortex of "staggerer" mice was the same as that of their normal littermates, thus the absolute number of benzodiazepine receptors in the cerebral cortex was unchanged.

Benzodiazepine receptors in the brain of 3-acetylpyridine treated rats.

Administration of 3-acetylpyridine, which caused symptoms typical of inferior olivary nucleus destruction, did not significantly alter ^{3}H-flunitrazepam binding to benzodiazepine receptors in the cerebellum at either 4 or 50 days post administration, or in the cerebral cortex at 50 days post administration (Table 3).

TABLE 2. ^{3}H-Flunitrazepam binding to cerebellum and cerebral cortex of "staggerer" and normal littermate mice.

	(n)	K_d (nM)	Bmax (pmol/g protein)
Cerebellum			
Male "Staggerer"	2*	0.97±0.05	474±8 [1]
Female "Staggerer"	2*	1.28±0.04 [3]	512±56 [2]
Male Littermate	2*	0.86±0.07	884±42
Female Littermate	2*	0.86±0.07	925±35
Cerebral Cortex			
Male "Staggerer"	2*	0.80±0.04	2191±204
Female "Staggerer"	2*	1.00±0.08	2068±134
Male Littermate	2*	0.99±0.07	2220±52
Female Littermate	2*	0.93±0.02	2130±25

[1] $p<0.02$ significantly less than male littermate cerebellum
[2] $p<0.05$ significantly less than female littermate cerebellum
[3] $p<0.02$ significantly greater than female littermate cerebellum
$p<0.05$ significantly greater than male "staggerer" cerebellum
[1,2] $p<0.001$ significantly less than male and female littermate cerebella.
* Because of the small size of the cerebellum in "staggerer" mice two and three brains were pooled for each value, thus 5 to 6 mice were used for each group of mice.

TABLE 3. ^{3}H-Flunitrazepam binding to brain of 3-acetylpyridine treated and control rats.

	(n)	Cerebellum - 4 days post-injection: K_d (nM)	Bmax (pmol/g tissue)
Control	4	1.04±0.18	36.8±2.4
3-Acetylpyridine	4	1.09±0.24	38.2±5.0
		Cerebellum - 50 days post-injection: K_d (nM)	**Bmax (pmol/g tissue)**
Control	8	1.31±0.10	33.6±2.8
3-Acetylpyridine	8	1.27±0.10	31.8±2.3
		Cerebral Cortex - 50 days post-injection: K_d (nM)	**Bmax (pmol/g tissue)**
Control	4	1.01±0.03	67.9±6.7
3-Acetylpyridine	6	1.12±0.09	71.7±3.2

Benzodiazepine receptors in the brains of kainic acid treated rats.

Intracerebellar kainic acid caused a moderate decrease in the density of benzodiazepine receptors in the lesioned side of the cerebellum, compared with both the unlesioned side of the cerebellum (14% decrease) and the unlesioned cerebellum (27% decrease, Table 4). The side of the cerebellum contralateral to the injected side had a 15% lower density of benzodiazepine receptors than did the unlesioned cerebellum. This suggests that the effects of kainic acid on cerebellar benzodiazepine receptors extended throughout the cerebellum. This decrease fell short of significance however. Benzodiazepine receptors in the cerebral cortex were unaffected by intracerebellar administration of kainic acid (Table 4).

TABLE 4. ^{3}H-Flunitrazepam binding to cerebellum and cerebral cortex of rats with unilateral intracerebellar kainic acid induced lesions or saline injection only.

	(n)	K_d (nM)	Bmax (pmol/g tissue)
Cerebellum			
Lesioned Side	10	1.43±0.09[1]	724±51[2]
Unlesioned Side	10	1.31±0.09	842±54
Saline Injected	5	1.37±0.13	986±65
Cerebral Cortex			
Ipsilateral to injected side	10	1.13±0.08	1403±28
Contralateral to injected side	10	1.16±0.08	1404±33
Saline Injected	5	1.07±0.07	1420±57

[1] $p<0.02$ significantly greater than unlesioned side of cerebellum
[2] $p<0.02$ significantly less than unlesioned side of cerebellum &
[3] $p<0.01$ significantly less than saline injected cerebellum

There was a significant difference between the K_d values for ^{3}H-flunitrazepam binding to the lesioned and contralateral sides of the cerebellum, however neither side differed significantly from the K_d value in unlesioned cerebellum (Table 4).

No differences in the weight of the cerebella were observed in kainic acid treated rats compared to control rats. Thus the differences in density reflected changes in absolute numbers of receptors.

Chronic phenytoin treatment.

Table 5 shows that chronic DPH administration for 14 days or 28 days produces a significant time dependent decrease in the density of brain benzodiazepine receptors as measured by specific ^{3}H-flunitrazepam binding in both rat cerebral cortex and cerebellum. There was no significant change in the K_d value following chronic DPH administration. Preliminary experiments indicate that no changes in either K_d or Bmax values occur in the rat

TABLE 5. Effects of chronic DPH administration of ^{3}H-flunitrazepam binding[a] to rat brain benzodiazepine receptors.

Treatment	(n)	K_d (nM) Cerebral Cortex	K_d (nM) Cerebellum	Bmax (fmol/mg protein) Cerebral Cortex	Bmax (fmol/mg protein) Cerebellum
Control[b]	(8)	1.04±0.09[c]	1.39±0.10	1149.6±24.0	524.3±31.5
60 min.	(4)	1.09±0.09	1.46±0.25	1136.1±96.6	602.6±66.7
14-day	(4)	1.04±0.12	1.33±0.11	951.5±82.7[d]	392.5±28.1[d]
28-day	(4)	1.06±0.10	1.42±0.08	752.7±47.5[e]	269.6±11.2[e]

[a] ^{3}H-Flunitrazepam binding was determined in tissue that was washed 5 times with buffer.

[b] There were no significant differences in ^{3}H-flunitrazepam binding in the two control groups of 14-day and 28-day therefore the data were combined for statistical comparisons.

[c] Values are mean ± S.E.M.

[d] $p<.03$ significantly different from control (unpaired t-test)

[e] $p<.001$ significantly different from control (unpaired t-test)

cerebral cortex or cerebellum after 60 minutes or 6 hours following acute DPH (200 mg/kg) i.p. injection which suggests that the decreased benzodiazepine receptor density was caused by chronic exposure to the drug.

Since there were significant decreases in the benzodiazepine receptor density after chronic DPH administration, ultrastructural morphology of the rat cerebellum was undertaken. There were no gross morphological changes observed in the rat cerebral cortex after 14 days of DPH administration. However, the rat cerebellum at the light microscopic level showed numerous pycnotic Purkinje cells and edematous Bergmann astrocytes (Figure 1-b). Figure 1-a shows normal Purkinje cells in the control rat cerebellum. The degenerated Purkinje cells in the cerebellum at the ultrastructural level show electron dense cytoplasm and infolded nuclear envelopes (Figure 1-c). One such degenerated Purkinje cell is seen in Figure 1-c where the hyperchromacity of the cytoplasm is evident. There are also significant increases in the Golgi apparatus and the cisternae of the Golgi apparatus are pulled apart. However, the mitochondria and their cristae appear normal. More dramatic changes take place in the Bergmann astrocytes. The cytoplasm of these astrocytes in the vicinity of the Purkinje cells appears electron lucent and are filled with glycogen deposits. These changes are indicative of edema and resultant metabolic imbalance. Other neuronal elements including granule cells, the stellate and basket cells appear normal.

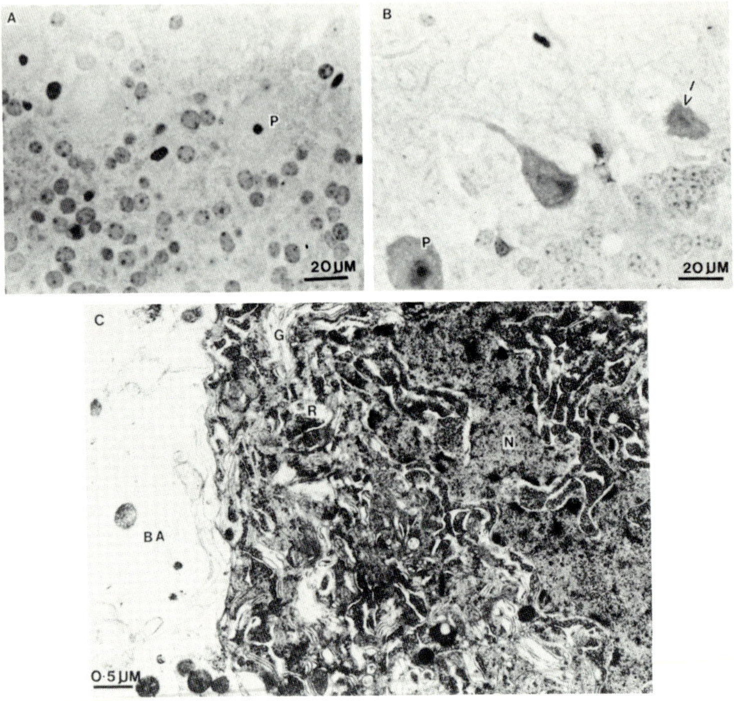

FIG. 1. (a) Control rat cerebellar cortex (X800). Purkinje neurons with round nuclei are seen at P. (b) Cerebellar cortex of DPH treated rat (14 days). Arrow indicates degenerated Purkinje cell. Edematous Bergmann astroglia seen at B. (X800). (c) Electron micrograph of degenerated Purkinje cell. Clumping of Nissl substance can be seen at R. Golgi cisternae are pulled apart at G. The nucleus (N) is irregular in outline with infolded nuclear envelope. (X56,000).

DISCUSSION

Destruction of cerebellar climbing fibers with 3-acetylpyridine (14) does not alter cerebellar benzodiazepine receptors. This suggests that climbing fibers arising into the cerebellum from the inferior olivary nucleus, do not possess benzodiazepine receptors, or if they do, their contribution to the total number of cerebellar benzodiazepine receptors is insignificant.

Intracerebellar administration of kainic acid caused significant decreases in cerebellar benzodiazepine receptors, however, histological evaluation of the lesioned cerebellum indicated that there was significant local destruction of all cerebellar tissue in the immediate vicinity of the injection site, in addition to the more widespread destruction of Purkinje cells. It is not possible to make a conclusive statement regarding the neuronal localization of benzodiazepine receptors in the cerebellum based upon the kainic acid treatments alone. The extent of the decrease in benzodiazepine receptor density seen here was substantially less than the 65% decreases reported by Braestrup et al. (2) who administered two doses of two micrograms of kainic acid into the cerebellum unilaterally. In view of the significant local destruction of all neurons in the cerebellum after administration of kainic acid seen here, interpretation of the results of kainic acid lesion studies should include a definitive analysis of the selectivity of such lesions. The decrease in ^{3}H-flunitrazepam binding affinity on the kainic acid lesioned side of the cerebellum may result from a decrease in cerebellar GABA concentrations. GABA is known to enhance benzodiazepine receptor affinity (27,30) and kainic acid has been shown to decrease endogenous GABA in the cerebellum by 50% (29).

In the "weaver" mouse cerebellum where there is extreme granule cell depletion (19) but apparently normal Purkinje cell function (20) only a small, nonsignificant increase in benzodiazepine receptor density was seen. Braestrup et al. (2) observed significant increases in benzodiazepine receptor density in "weaver" mouse cerebellum compared to control. However, the absolute number of benzodiazepine receptors (density multiplied by cerebellar weight) was decreased by 57% in the "weaver" cerebellum in their study. In the "reeler" cerebellum, where there is also a selective loss of granule cells (17) there is also an increased density of benzodiazepine receptors (24). However, when expressed as absolute numbers of receptors, "reeler" cerebella contain fewer benzodiazepine receptors than those of their behaviorally normal littermates (Speth and Yamamura, unpublished.)

In this study, "weaver" mice showed no significant differences in benzodiazepine receptor density and a decrease of 57% absolute number of benzodiazepine receptors at a density similar to or slightly less than the whole cerebellum. This conclusion contrasts with that of Braestrup et al. (2) who suggested that benzodiazepine receptors were not localized on granule cells to a great extent. However, their conclusion did not take into account the changes in absolute number of benzodiazepine receptors in the cerebellum.

Disturbances in Bergman glial fibers have been observed in the "weaver" mouse cerebellum in addition to the severe granule cell loss (19) so the possible localization of benzodiazepine receptors on normal Bergman glial fibers cannot totally be eliminated. It is also possible that granule cell input into other cerebellar neurons facilitates benzodiazepine receptor development and decreased numbers of receptors on other neurons could result from the loss of such influences.

The sizable decrease in the density of benzodiazepine receptors in the "staggerer" mouse cerebellum confirms recent preliminary observation from this laboratory (24). The primary defect in the "Staggerer" cerebellum is the absence of post-synaptic thickenings on the Purkinje cell dendrites where they synapse with parallel fibers arising from the granule cells (12). However, by 26-30 days of age, there is considerable granule cell loss as well (23). In terms of absolute numbers of benzodiazepine receptors only 10% of the normal complement of benzodiazepine receptors is present in the "staggerer" cerebellum while normal amount and density of benzodiazepine receptors is seen in the "staggerer" cerebral cortex. The decrease in the affinity of benzodiazepine receptors for ^{3}H-flunitrazepam in the female "staggerer" only is an unexpected observation, and it may indicate a sex dependent decrease in GABA concentration in the cerebellum of female "staggerer" mice.

The decreased benzodiazepine receptor density following chronic DPH administration suggests that DPH acts as a neurotoxin destroying benzodiazepine receptors on the Purkinje cells in the cerebellum. In DPH treated rats where both Purkinje cells and Bergman astroglial cells were damaged, the maximal loss of benzodiazepine receptors was 48%. This again is consistent with the hypothesis that only a portion of the cerebellar benzodiazepine receptors occur on Purkinje cells.

Since the absolute number of benzodiazepine receptors in the "staggerer" cerebellum, which is deficient in Purkinje cell dendritic spine and granule cells, is decreased 90% compared to a 57% decrease in the "weaver" cerebellum, which is deficient in granule cells only, this suggests that approximately 30 to 40% of the benzodiazepine receptors occur in cerebellar Purkinje cells, and as much as 50-60% of the cerebellar benzodiazepine receptors occur on granule cells.

"Nervous" mice are reported to undergo loss of approximately 90% of their cerebellar Purkinje cells (12). Benzodiazepine receptor density in the cerebellum of the "nervous" mouse is decreased 20 to 67% (3,13,22,24). The 67% decrease observed by Lippa et al. (13) was seen in P_2 fractions of the cerebellum and may have overlooked the contribution of other cerebellar subfractions to the total population of benzodiazepine receptors. In studies where the absolute number of cerebellar benzodiazepine receptors in "nervous" mice could be quantified, there was a 46 to 55% decrease in the absolute number of receptors (3,22). This again suggests that cerebellar Purkinje cells account for only a portion of the total number of benzodiazepine receptors in the mouse cerebellum.

This study strongly suggests that benzodiazepine receptors do not occur on glia in the cerebellum. In "staggerer" mice, where a disturbance of glial cells has not been described, benzodiazepine receptors are decreased by 90%. In the kainic acid treated rats, glial filaments accumulate in the cerebellum (9) but the benzodiazepine receptor density is decreased. Braestrup et al. (2) also concluded that benzodiazepine receptors are not located on cerebellar glial cells. However, in two of our models which showed diminished numbers of benzodiazepine receptors, there were also disturbances of Bergman astroglial cells. Henn and Henke

(7) presented evidence that brain benzodiazepine receptors were highest in brain fractions enriched in glia. Baraldi et al. (1) recently observed benzodiazepine receptors in cultures of glial cells. Thus the existence of benzodiazepine receptors on glia cannot entirely be excluded.

It is still not possible to determine whether benzodiazepine receptors play a role in synaptic transmission involving a specific neurotransmitter. The parallel fiber-Purkinje cell dendrite synapse is reported to use glutamate as its neurotransmitter (8,9,29,31). Yet neither glutamate nor its neurotoxic analog, kainic acid, interact with brain benzodiazepine receptors in the cerebellum (16,18,21). GABA also does not interact with the benzodiazepine binding site on the benzodiazepine receptor, although both GABA and benzodiazepines appear to mutually enhance each other's binding to their respective receptors (6,27,28,30). If an endogenous substance which occupies benzodiazepine receptors exists, it most likely functions in a neuromodulatory role, affecting different classes of neurons, rather than as a primary neurotransmitter.

SUMMARY

Selective genetic and chemical lesions which affect specific neuronal populations in the cerebellum were studied for changes in benzodiazepine receptors. Destruction of cerebellar climbing fibers with 3-acetylpyridine, did not affect cerebellar benzodiazepine receptors. Destruction of Purkinje, basket and stellate cells with intracerebellar kainic acid, caused moderate decreases in benzodiazepine receptor density. Destruction of Purkinje cells with chronic high doses of phenytoin also caused a significant decrease in benzodiazepine receptor density. In "weaver" mice, which have a severe loss of granule cells, benzodiazepine receptor density was unchanged, while the absolute number of benzodiazepine receptors decreased by 57%. In "staggerer" mice which have diminished Purkinje cell dendritic thickenings at their synapses with parallel fibers and subsequent granule cell loss, there was a 45% decrease in benzodiazepine receptor density and a 90% decrease in the absolute number of benzodiazepine receptors. These results suggest that benzodiazepine receptors exist on cerebellar Purkinje cells, that they probably also occur on cerebellar granule cells, and that they do not appear to be present on cerebellar glial cells or on climbing fibers.

ACKNOWLEDGEMENTS

The authors acknowledge the excellent technical assistance of Marla Bliss, Andrew Chen and Jim Davidson. N.B. is a Neuromuscular Disease Fellow of the Muscular Dystrophy Association. H.I.Y. is a receipient of a Research Scientist Development Award (MH-00095) from the NIMH. Portions of this work was supported by USPHS grants (MH-30626, MH-27257).

REFERENCES

1. Baraldi, M., Guidotti, A., Schwartz, J.P. and Costa, E., (1979): Science, 205:821-823.
2. Braestrup, C. and Squires, R.F. (1978): Europ. J. Pharmac. 48:263-270.
3. Braestrup, C., Nielsen, M., Biggio, G. and Squires, R.F. (1979): Neurosci. Lett. 13:219-224.
4. Desclin, J.C. (1974): Brain Res. 77:365-384.
5. Desclin, J.C. and Escubi, J. (1974): Brain Res. 77:349-364.
6. Guidotti, A., Toffano, G. and Costa, E. (1978): Nature (Lond) 275:553-555.
7. Henn, F.A. and Henke, D.J. (1978): Neuropharmac. 17:985-988.
8. Herndon, R.M. and Coyle, J.T. (1977): Science 198:71-72.
9. Herndon, R.M. and Coyle, J.T. (1978): Kainic acid as a tool in neurobiology. Raven Press, New York.
10. Iversen, L.L. (1977): Nature (Lond) 266:678.
11. Landis, D.M.D. and Reese, T.S. (1977): J. Comp. Neurol. 171: 247-260.
12. Landis, S.C. (1973): J. Cell Biol. 57:782-797.
13. Lippa, A.S., Sano, M.C., Coupet, J., Klepner, C.A. and Beer, B. (1978): Life Sci. 23:2213-2218.
14. Llinas, R., Walton, K., Hillman, D.E. and Sotelo, C. (1975): Science 190:1230-1231.
15. Lowry, O.H., Rosebrough, N.J., Farr, A.L. and Randall, R.J. (1951): J. Biol. Chem. 193:265-275.
16. Mackerer, C.R., Kochman, R.L., Bierschenk, B.A. and Bremner, S.S. (1978): J. Pharmac. Exp. Ther. 206:405-413.
17. Mariani, J., Crepel, F., Mikoshiba, K., Changeux, J.P. and Sotelo, C. (1977): Phil. Trans. Roy. Soc. Lond. B. 281:1-28.
18. Olson, R.W. and Mikoshiba, K. (1978): J. Neurochem. 30:1663-1636.
19. Rakic, P. (1976): Cold Spring Harb. Symp. Quant. Biol. 40: 333-346.
20. Siggins, G.R., Henriksen, S.J. and Landis, S.C. (1976): Brain Res. 114:53-69.
21. Simantov, R., Oster-Granite, M.L., Herndon, R.M. and Snyder, S.H. (1976): Brain Res. 105:365-371.
22. Skolnick, P., Syapin, P.J., Paugh, B.A. and Paul, S.M. (1979) Nature (Lond) 277:397-399.
23. Sotelo, C. and Changeux, J.-P. Brain Res. 67:519-526.
24. Speth, R.C. and Yamamura, H.I. (1979): Europ. J. Pharmac. 54: 397-399.
25. Speth, R.C., Wastek, G.J., Johnson, P.C. and Yamamura, H.I. (1978): Life Sci. 22:859-866.
26. Squires, R.F. and Braestrup, C. (1977): Nature (Lond) 266: 732-734.
27. Talman, J.F., Thomas, J.W. and Gallagher, D.W. (1978): Nature (Lond) 274:383-385.
28. Toffano, G., Guidotti, A. and Costa, E. (1978): Proc. Nat. Acad. Sci. USA 75:4024-4028.

29. Tran, V.T. and Snyder, S.H. (1979): Brain Res. 167:345-353.
30. Wastek, G.J., Speth, R.C., Reisine, T.D. and Yamamura, H.I. (1978): Europ. J. Pharmac. 59:445-447.
31. Young, A.B., Oster-Granite, M.L., Herndon, R.M. and Snyder, S.H. (1974): Brain Res. 73:1-13.

GABA and Benzodiazepine Receptors,
edited by E. Costa et al.
Raven Press, New York © 1981.

Localization of GABA and Dopamine Receptor Sites in Retinal Glial Cells Using DL-α-Aminoadipic Acid

M. Memo, F. Riccardi, M. Trabucchi, and P. F. Spano

Institutes of Pharmacology and Pharmacognosy, Universities of Cagliari and Milan, Italy

Several years ago after the discovery that glutamic acid (GLU), given to infant mice by subcutaneous administration, consistently destroyed neurons in the retina and anterior hypothalamus (AH), Olney and associates undertook a systematic evaluation of various acidic and sulfur aminoacids related structurally to GLU (21). They found that all the compounds tested could be placed in one of four groups: 1) those equipotent with L-GLU in necrosing neurons, 2) those substantially more potent than L-GLU in necrosing neurons, 3) those which affected nonneuronal components (glial ependymal, Müller cells) without appreciable effects on neurons, 4) and those with no cytotoxic effects.

Among those compounds that were found gliotoxic, but not neurotoxic, it is worth of attention DL-α-aminoadipic acid (AA) for which the gliotoxic effect was described in details by the group mentioned above.

More recently DL-α-aminoadipic acid has been used by Lund-Karlsen (18). This author found that four hours after injection of the drug into the vitreous body of adult (30 days) rats, the Müller cells could no longer be identified in the retina. This lesion was accompanied by 55% reduction in the high affinity uptake of β-alanine and 25% reduction in the uptakes of GABA and glutamate. Diamino-n-butyric acid and choline high affinity uptakes and choline acetyltransferase and glutamate decarboxylase enzyme activities were unchanged under this experimental condition.

On the bases of these findings we used DL-α-aminoadipic acid in order to investigate whether neurotransmitter receptors are located on glial cells other than on neuronal elements. The hypothesis of a glial receptor localization is suggested, indeed, either from the well established interaction between neurons and glia resulting in the regulation of transmitter turnover and metabolism or, more directly, from studies conducted in glioma cells and cellular fractionation experiments (11, 13, 14). In particular we studied in rat retina the cellular localization of the receptors for GABA and dopamine (DA) which, according to many reports, play an important role as inhibitory neurotransmitters in the retina of various animal species (2, 3, 24).

For comparison, the effect of kainic acid (KA) which, in discrete areas of the mammalian brain, has been shown to be one of the most effective dendrosomatotoxic compounds, sparing fibers of passage,axon terminals and glial cells (19) was included in our study. A report on the neurotoxic effect of kainic acid on non-mammalian retina has already appeared (19).

GLIOTOXIC ACTION OF AA

DL-α-aminoadipic acid (100 μg in 10 μl 0.9% saline) was injected through the sclera into the vitreus body with a Hamilton micro-syringe as previously described by Lund-Karlsen (18). The rats were anesthetized with ether. The other eye, utilized as control, was injected with 10 μl 0.9% saline. No difference in all parameters measured was found when the saline treated retinas were tested against retinas from untreated rats. The animals were killed at various times after the lesion by decapitation. Retinas were dissected out as floating discs and homogenates were prepared according to the biochemical assay. Glutamine synthetase (GS) (26) glutamic acid decarboxylase (GAD) (1), choline acetyl transferase (CAT) (8) and DA-stimulated adenylyl cyclase (DA-AC) (16, 17) were performed as previously described. Since with retina, in the absence of triton treatment, only very low levels of ^{3}H-GABA binding are detectable, frozen and tritonized membranes were utilized for this assay (7). However, for ^{3}H-muscimol binding it was possible to use both fresh and tritonized membranes (27). The binding of ^{3}H-bicuculline was performed as indicated by Möhler and Okada (20) in fresh membrane preparations. DA receptor binding sites were measured as indicated by Burt et al. (5) using ^{3}H-spiroperidol as radioligand. Since it is known that labelled spiroperidol binds serotonin receptors in cerebral cortex of rat brain, we used DA (10^{-4}M) to display the radioligand from its binding sites. Serotonin at the concentration of 10^{-4}M did not inhibit the binding either in lesioned or in intact retinas (data not shown). For morphological studies, retinas were prefixed in 2.5% glutaraldehyde in 0.1 phosphate buffer and, after washing with the same buffer, postfixed in 1% OsO_4 and embedded in Epon 812, according to Pedersen (22), 1 μm sections were cut with LKB ultratome and stained with toluidine blue for light microscopy.

As earlier reported by Lund-Karlsen (18) we found that four hours after injection of 100 μg AA the glial component of the retina, i.e. the Müller cells, could no longer be recognized. However, the glial toxic effect can be detected from two to eight hours after AA injection. The short-lasting effect suggests that this compound does not necessarily destroy the glial cells but it is possible that temporarily damages them. Interestingly, the retinal neuronal elements are not affected by this treatment.

ACTION OF AA ON MARKER ENZYMES FOR NEURONS AND GLIAL CELLS

Immunocytochemical studies have recently provided strong evidence that the enzyme GS is exclusively localized in the retina inside of the glial cells (i.e. the Müller cells) (23). For this reason we followed the time course of the effects of retinal AA lesions on GS activity in comparison to neuronal marker enzyme activities, such as CAT, GAD and DA-AC.

As expected from the morphological studies, reported before, biochemical changes were seen which reflect glial toxicity without neuronal losses. For example reduction of GS activity was maximal at 4 hours after AA injection (Fig. 1) consistently with the observation that the Müller cells are no longer identifiable at this stage. A tentative correlation between the number of Müller cells and the glial marker enzyme activity, measured over a period of 24 hours in AA-lesioned retinas, gave a very significant correlation coefficient (r = 0.897).

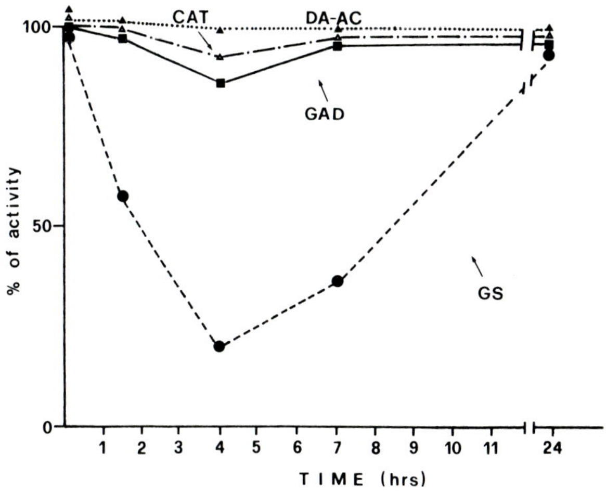

FIG. 1 - Time course of neuronal and glial marker enzyme activities following DL-α-aminoadipic acid injection (100 μg) into the vitreus body. Activities of GAD, DA-AC and GS were measured as indicated in the text. Results are expressed in terms of percent of specific activity of the enzymes in saline injected retina. Each point is the mean of five preparations; SD are less than 10% of the mean.

In contrast, the specific activities of neuronal marker enzymes, CAT, GAD and DA-AC were not reduced up to 24 hours after injection of AA into the vitreous body (Fig. 1).

ACTION OF AA ON GABA RECEPTOR BINDING

Since numerous laboratories have reported intimate functional connections between neurons and glia the concept that neurotransmitter receptors might be located on glial cells, other than on effector neurons, could not be ruled out. On the contrary cellular fractionation studies and experiments conducted with tissue cultures have indicated that some neurotransmitter receptors are present indeed on glia.

On this hypothesis we investigated the effect of AA on receptors for GABA. GABA in fact is thought to be an inhibitory neurotransmitter in the retina, with significant levels of this amino acid and its synthesizing enzyme found in the inner layer, probably associated with amacrine cell terminals (4,10). As suggested by different groups, retinal GABAergic system appears involved in the transmission of visual information (9). The experiments were set up measuring GABA receptor binding in fresh or frozen membrane preparations, as indicated above from AA- or saline-injected retinas. Three different radioligands, described to suitably label GABA receptors, were used, namely ^{3}H-GABA, ^{3}H-muscimol and ^{3}H-bicuculline.

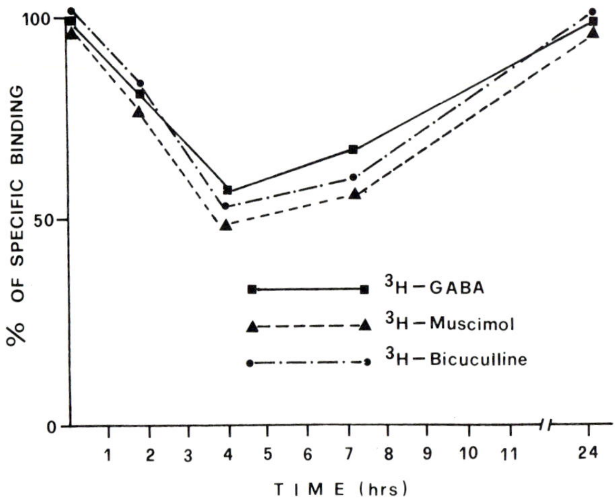

FIG. 2 - The time course of ^{3}H-GABA, ^{3}H-muscimol and ^{3}H-bicuculline specific bindings in rat retinal membrane preparations after DL-α-aminoadipic acid injection (100 μg) into the vitreus body. Specific bindings for radioligands were performed as described in the method section. Results are expressed in terms of percent of specific binding in saline injected retina. Values are the mean of four determinations with samples in triplicate; SD are less than 10% of the mean.

The time course of the action of AA on GABA receptor specific binding, over 24 hours, is illustrated in Figure 2. As is it evident AA injection elicited a quite significant reduction of retinal specific binding for all the three radioligands used. The magnitude of the reduction, when the data are normalized as percent of maximal specific binding, was practically the same for ^{3}H-GABA, ^{3}H-muscimol and ^{3}H-bicuculline, with time courses virtually superimposible.

It is noteworthy that the peak effect of AA on GABA receptor binding was observed at 4 hours postinjection, a stage at which the Müller cells are no longer morphologically identifiable and the activity of the glial marker enzyme (GS) was maximally reduced (-80%). It is also relevant that the time course of the reduction of GABA receptor binding also roughly parallels that observed either in morphological studies or in marker enzyme activity measurement.

Scatchard analysis of binding data, obtained in preparations of retinas from rats killed 4 hours after AA injection, revealed that the reduction of GABA receptor binding is due to a marked decrease in the number of binding sites rather than to a change in the affinity constant (Fig. 3 and Table 1). It is conceivable that this fact reflects a degradation or at least a denaturation of retinal glial membrane proteins following AA treatment.

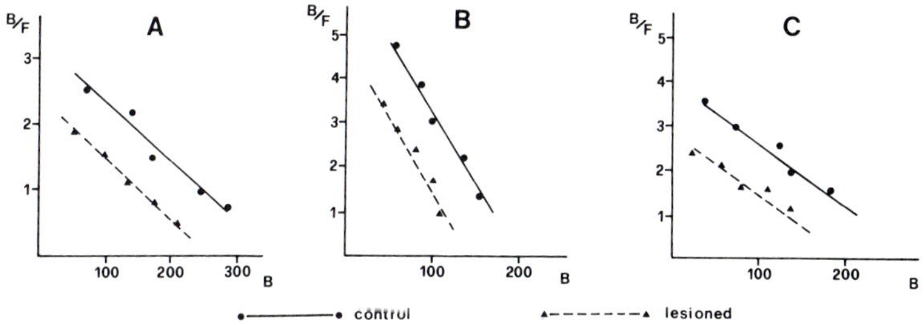

FIG. 3 - Scatchard analysis of ^{3}H-GABA (A), ^{3}H-muscimol (B) and ^{3}H-bicuculline (C) specific bindings 4 hours after DL-α-aminoadipic acid injection (100 μg) into the vitreus body. Numbers are from a representative experiment and are the means of triplicate determinations which varied less than 10%. For K_D and B_{max} values see Table 1.

ACTION OF AA ON DOPAMINE RECEPTOR BINDING

Chemical and histochemical studies have shown that DA is the predominant monoamine in terms of amount present (6, 12) in the neural retina of various animal species. The DA neurons in the retina appear to be part of amacrine cell population located in the inner nuclear layer and interconnected with many other cell types. Electrophysiological experiments indicate that DA may function as inhibitory transmitter, which is released as a consequence of light stimulation (15). In addition a wealth of data has clearly established that retina contains an adenylyl cyclase preferentially stimulated by DA and sensitive to pharmacological and physiological influences (28). Moreover, significant binding of ^{3}H-spiroperidol can be demonstrated in rat retinal homogenates (29). This binding appears to be associated with DA receptors.

TABLE 1. Kinetic parameters of ^{3}H-GABA, ^{3}H-muscimol and ^{3}H-bicuculline specific bindings in rat retinal membrane preparations after DL-α-aminoadipic acid injection (100 µg) into the vitreus body

	K_D		B_{max}	
	Intact	Lesioned	Intact	Lesioned
^{3}H-GABA	112	120	394	264$^+$
^{3}H-muscimol	28	31	203	110$^+$
^{3}H-bicuculline	75	71	320	190$^+$

$^+p < 0.01$ in respect to B_{max} value of intact retina

Previous studies by Henn et al. (13) - utilizing cellular fractionation techniques - have indicated on the other hand, that DA receptors are located other than on neural membranes also on glial membranes of bovine neostriatum.

On the bases of these findings and of our results, previously described, we were prompted to examine the effect of AA on retinal DA receptors as labeled by ^{3}H-spiroperidol.

We found that a significant portion of retinal ^{3}H-spiroperidol specific binding was reduced following intravitreal injection of AA. The time course of the action of AA on DA receptor binding is illustrated in Figure 4. As earlier found for GABA receptor binding the maximal reduction of ^{3}H-spiroperidol binding, elicited by the gliotoxic agent, was observed at 4 hours, a stage as stressed above, at which GS activity and number of Müller cells are maximally reduced.

Also in the assay of DA receptor binding Scatchard analysis revealed that AA lesions result in a marked decrease of the number of binding sites with no effect on the equilibrium dissociation constant. It is pertinent to recall that the activity of retinal DA-AC is unmodified by AA injection all over the period of the time course studied.

ACTION OF KAINIC ACID ON GABA AND DA RECEPTOR BINDING

In the last years kainic acid has been utilized by different groups for receptor localization studies because of its specific neurotoxic effect. In particular, the injection of kainic acid

(100 nmoles) into the vitreus body induces a lesion involving the entire retina from optic disc to the ora serrata retinae with a marked decrease in thickness due to a severe loss of the cells in the inner layer. Changes were not restricted in the inner regions of the retina, since there was a disruption and swelling of the elements of the outer nuclear layer. The effects can be observed starting 2 hours after the treatment. Müller cells and the optic fibers layer appear unaffected by kainic acid injection. The morphological observations may be correlated with the enzymatic activity measurements reported in Fig. 5. Biochemical markers of neuronal integrity, such as GAD, DA-AC and CAT appear strongly affected by the lesion. The maximal reduction can be observed 48 hours after the treatment. In contrast, the specific activity of GS does not change over 4 days after KA injection.

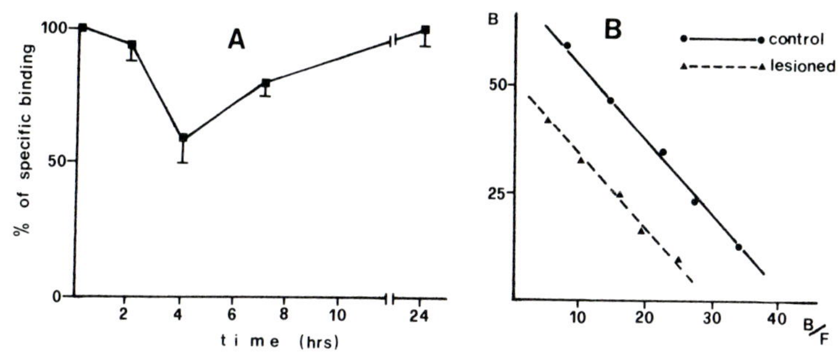

FIG. 4 - Time course (A) and Scatchard analysis (B) of ^{3}H-spiroperidol specific binding in rat retinal membrane preparations after DL-α-aminoadipic acid injection (100 μg) into the vitreus body. A: results, obtained at various times after treatment, are expressed in terms of percent of specific binding in saline-injected retina. B: kinetic studies of retinal ^{3}H-spiroperidol specific binding were performed 4 hours after DL-α-aminoadipic acid injection. The apparent K_D are 1.86 nM and 1.76 nM for control and lesioned retina, respectively. Maximum specific binding (B_{max}) is 78 fmol/mg prot for control and 51 fmol/mg prot for lesioned retina. Numbers are from a representative experiment and are the means of triplicate determinations which varied less than 10%.

Interestingly, as shown in Table 2, GABA receptor binding sites decreased in KA-lesioned retinas by about 45% in respect to control, after 24 hours. The modification could be detected using ^{3}H-GABA as radioligand or labelled compounds which do not bind high affinity uptake sites for GABA, such as ^{3}H-muscimol and ^{3}H-bicuculline. Retinal DA receptor function seems to be altered by kainic acid injection. In fact ^{3}H-spiroperidol specific binding was decreased (-33%) in KA-treated retina in respect to control.

In the same experimental conditions DA-AC is virtually abolished. These results support the hypothesis of an exclusive neuronal localization of those DA receptors linked to adenylyl cyclase activity (D1).

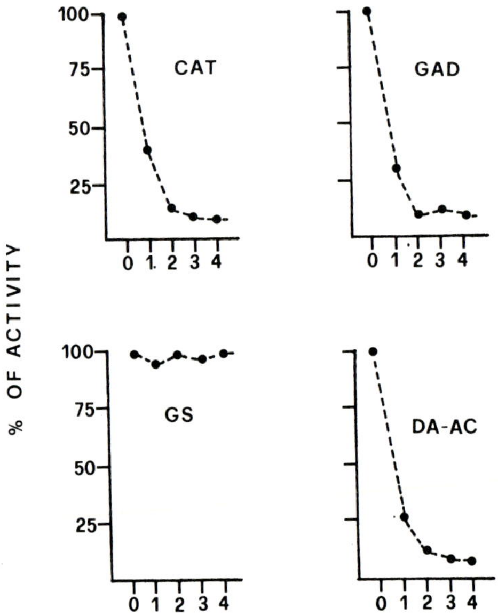

FIG. 5 - Time course of neuronal and glial marker enzyme activities following kainic acid injection (100 nmoles) into the vitreus body. Activities of CAT, GAD, GS and DA-AC were measured at various days after treatment as indicated in the text. Results are expressed in terms of percent of the specific activity of the enzyme in saline injected retina. Each point is the mean of five preparations, SD is less than 10% of the mean.

SUMMARY AND CONCLUSIONS

An earlier report by Olney et al., had clearly shown that DL-α-aminoadipic acid exerts a specific gliotoxic action at the level of neural retina. This effect observed after systemic administration in infant mice has been fully confirmed by Lund-Karlsen and by us after intravitreal injection in adult rats. In our study we have further provided evidence that the specific activity of GS - an enzyme exclusively located in glial Müller cells - follows after AA injection a similar pattern of reduction as the number of Müller cells themselves. No effect of AA was observed on neuronal marker enzymes such as CAT, GAD and DA-AC. In these experimental conditions a marked reduction of specific GABA and DA receptor binding was observed with time courses paralleling the gliotoxic effects of AA on the morphology and on the marker enzyme activity of retinal glial cells. The kinetic analysis of the data indicate a decrease in the number of binding sites for GABA and DA with no changes in the affinity. These results are in agreement with the interpretation that the action of AA ultimately elicits a denaturation of GABA and DA receptor protein present on the membrane of retinal glial cells. In view of the recent evidence on the existence of multiple receptors for DA our results further suggest that a substantial portion of DA receptors in the retina are not functionally linked to adenylyl cyclase activity (D2 type).

TABLE 2. Effect of kainic acid injection (100 nmoles) into the vitreus body on rat retinal GABA and DA receptor binding using different radioligands.

	^{3}H-GABA (20 nM)	^{3}H-Muscimol (10 nM)	^{3}H-Bicuculline (5 nM)	^{3}H-Spiroperidol (0.8 nM)
Intact	188 ± 8	204 ± 8	259 ± 19	80 ± 6
Lesioned	103 ± 10$^+$	139 ± 5$^+$	148 ± 8$^+$	54 ± 5$^+$

$^+$P < 0.01 in respect to intact values.

Values are expressed as fmol/mg prot. Number are the mean ± SD of three experiments run in triplicate. Animals were killed 24 hours after kainic acid injection.

It is of great interest at this time to study the specific gliotoxic effect of AA on the neuroglia surrounding GABAergic or DAergic synapses in selected brain regions. Experiments in this direction are in progress in our laboratory. In this regard, it is also important to note that no loss of glia have been reported after kainic acid injection in discrete areas of the brain. However, it is possible that glial cells, which contain receptor sites and are in intimate contact with neurons, disappear and are replaced with other glial cell types lacking the receptors. In this case, receptors associated with glial cells could be depleted by kainic acid treatment.

In addition it is pertinent to recall that the mechanism of the gliotoxic action of AA is presently unknown and therefore investigation to clarify this point are urged.

Therefore, on the ground of these considerations and of our results, AA may represent a new useful and powerful tool both for the progress of biochemical anatomy and to get a better insight on the interaction between neurons and glial cells, which seem to play an important role in the normal, and probably also abnormal, function of the central nervous system.

REFERENCES

1. Albers,R.W. and Brady,R.D.(1959): J.Biol.Chem., 234: 926-928

2. Ames,A., and Pollen,A. (1969): J.Neurophysiol. 32: 424-429

3. Bonaventure,V., Wioland V. and Mandel,P. (1974): Brain Research 80: 281-289

4. Brandon,C., Lam,D.M.K. and Jang-Yen Wu (1979): Proc.Natl.Acad. Sci. USA, 26: 3557-3561

5. Burt,D.R., Creese,I. and Snyder S.H. (1976): Science, 192: 481-483

6. Ehinger,B. and Falck,B. (1969): Albrecht von Graefes Arch. Klin.Ophthalmol. 178: 295-301

7. Enna,S.J. and Snyder S.H. (1976): Brain Res. 115: 174-179

8. Fonnum,F. (1975): J.Neurochem. 24: 407-409

9. Graham,L.T.Jr., Baxter,C.F. and Lolley,R.N. (1970): Brain Res. 20: 379-388

10. Graham,L.T.Jr., and Aprison,M.H. (1969): J.Neurochem. 16:559-566

11. Guidotti,A., Baraldi,M. and Costa,E. (1979): Pharmacology, 19: 267-277

12. Haggendal,J. and Helmfors,T. (1965): Acta Physiol.Scand. 64: 58-65

13. Henn,F.A., Anderson,D.J., and Sellström,Å. (1977): Nature, 266: 637-638

14. Hertz,L. (1979): Progress in Neurobiology, 13: 277-323

15. Iuvone,P.M., Galli,C.L. and Neff,N.H. (1978): Med.Pharmacol. 14: 1222-1219

16. Kebabian,J.W., Petzold,G.L. and Greengard,P. (1972) Proc.Natl. Acad.Sci.USA, 69: 2145-2149

17. Kuo,J. and Greengard,P.(1972): Adv.Cyclic Nucleotide Res. edited by P.Greengard, R.Paoletti and G.A.Robinson 2:41-50, Raven Press, N.Y.

18. Lund-Karlsen,R. (1978): J.Neurochem. 31: 1055-1061

19. McGeer,G., Olney,J.W. and McGeer,P.eds. (1978): Kainic Acid as

a Tool in Neurobiology, Raven Press, New York

20.Mohler,H. and Okada,T. (1977):Nature, 267: 65-67

21.Olney,J.W., Ho,L.I. and Rhee,V. (1971):Exp.Brain Res. 14: 61-76

22.Pedersen,O.Ø. (1973): Acta Ophthal. 51: 878-888

23.Riepe,E.R. and Horenburg,M.D. (1977): Nature, 268: 654-655

24.Scholes,V. and Roberts,E. (1964): Biochem.Pharmacol., 13: 1319 1329

25.Schubert,D., Tarikas,H. and La Corbiere,M. (1976): Science, 192: 471-472

26.Sellinger,O.Z. and de Balbian Verster,F. (1962): J.Biol.Chem., 237: 2836-2844

27.Snodgrass,S.R. (1978): Nature, 273: 392-394

28.Spano,P.F., Govoni,S., Hofmann,M., Kumakura,K. and Trabucchi,M. (1977): in: Advances in Biochemical Psychopharmacology,edited by E.Costa, and G.L.Gessa, pp. 307-310, Raven Press, New York

29.Spano,P.F., Memo,M., Riccardi,F., and Trabucchi,M. submitted for publication.

GABA and Benzodiazepine Receptors,
edited by E. Costa et al.
Raven Press, New York © 1981.

Radiohistochemical Studies of Benzodiazepine and GABA Receptors and Their Interactions

Jose M. Palacios, James R. Unnerstall, W. Scott Young, III, and Michael J. Kuhar

Departments of Pharmacology and Experimental Therapeutics, and Psychiatry and the Behavioral Sciences, The Johns Hopkins University School of Medicine, Baltimore, Maryland 21205

INTRODUCTION

Recently, investigators have been studying the interactions and relationships between GABA and benzodiazepines in the brain. For example, GABA stimulates benzodiazepine receptor binding by increasing the receptors' affinity for the drugs (4,14,17,27,30). Conversely, the benzodiazepines have been reported to increase the affinity of the GABA receptor for GABA by displacing an endogenous inhibitor (11,12,28). Behavioral and electrophysiological studies also indicate an interaction between GABA and the benzodiazepines (1,7,9,10,18,22,23,24, 29,31) and at low iontophoretic doses, the benzodiazepines augment GABA mediated synaptic inhibition in spinal cord cell cultures (6,16). Recent studies have examined this interaction in more detail. Some receptor binding methods suggest that a unique GABA receptor or a subpopulation of GABA receptors may be responsible for stimulating benzodiazepine receptor binding (13). Similarly, high and low affinity GABA sites have different regional distributions (11). Also, the ontogeny of benzodiazepine and of GABA receptors are different in the rat brain as the benzodiazepine receptors are found at 50% of adult levels at birth while GABA receptors are barely detectable (3,5,8,20). Our laboratory has investigated the anatomical localization of the benzodiazepine and GABA receptors by a light microscopic radiohistochemical method (19,21,33,34). The distribution of the high affinity GABA receptor (a low affinity receptor would not be detectable by our methods) was not simply and directly related to the distribution of the benzodiazepine receptor in a one to one fashion. In addition, the regional stimulation of benzodiazepine receptor binding by GABA does not correspond simply and in a one to one way to the distribution of the high affinity GABA receptors.

METHODS

The *in vitro* labeling light microscopic autoradiographic studies follow a generally applicable procedure which involves receptor binding on slide-mounted tissue sections and the generation of autoradiograms by the apposition of emulsion-coated coverslips. The details of this procedure have been presented (32). We have also determined the optimal conditions for localizing the benzodiazepine receptor and the high affinity GABA receptor (19,21,33,34).

Preliminary biochemical studies revealed that the benzodiazepine and high affinity GABA receptor binding in our slide-mounted sections had all of the characteristics previously demonstrated in biochemical in vitro binding studies with tissue homogenates (26). The binding was of a high affinity, saturable, showed the appropriate regional distribution, and had the expected pharmacological properties.

The conditions selected for producing autoradiograms are as follows. Four or six micron sections were incubated with 1.0nM ^{3}H-flunitrazepam in 0.17 M Tris-HCl, pH 7.6, at ice-water temperatures for 40 min. The incubations were followed by a 2min wash in the same buffer. Blanks were generated by incubating adjacent sections in ^{3}H-flunitrazepam and 1uM clonazepam to displace specific binding. GABA receptors were labeled following a 20-min preincubation in 0.31 M Tris-citrate buffer, pH 7.1, at ice-bath temperatures. The preincubation was necessary to produce a substantial level of specific binding. High affinity GABA receptors were labeled in an incubation with 5nM ^{3}H-muscimol for 40 min followed by a 1-min wash in the same buffer. Nonspecific binding was examined by utilizing 0.2mM GABA in parallel incubations.

RESULTS

Both benzodiazepine and GABA receptors had heterogenous distributions throughout the rat central nervous system which were different from each other and different from other receptor distributions (19,21,33,34). Nonspecific binding was as low as that seen in white matter areas and all of the areas showing elevated levels of binding were displaced in the blank slides.

The radiohistochemical localization of the benzodiazepine receptor varied dramatically in the rat forebrain. In the olfactory bulb, the molecular layer as well as the mitral cell layer of the accessory olfactory bulb revealed very high levels of receptor. Dense levels were observed in the insulae Calleja and nucleus olfactorius, although relatively few receptors were present in the olfactory lobe. In the limbic lobe, the greatest densities were seen in the rostral medial forebrain bundle. High densities were also seen in the hippocampus, dentate gyrus, pyriform cortex, nucleus septi medialis and nuclei amygdaloideus centralis, medialis and lateralis. The rest of the telencephalon contained only low to moderate densities of benzodiazepine receptor with a few exceptions. The frontal cortex at the level of the forceps minor as well as lamina IV at most levels had elevated levels of receptor. Laminae I and VI were occasionally elevated. Of the basal ganglia structures, only the nucleus entopeduncularis had a high level of receptor. The diencephalon exhibited several areas of dense benzodiazepine receptor concentrations. These areas were mostly in the hypothalamus and in the nucleus subthalamicus and zona incerta. The hindbrain had generally lower levels of benzodiazepine receptor with several exceptions. A very high density was found in the nucleus ventralis rostralis lemnisci lateralis. The inferior and superior colliculi also had high levels. In the rest of the rat brain, the molecular layer of the cerebellum had a very high level of receptor. Dense amounts were seen in the nucleus dentatus of the cerebellum, parts of the floor of the fourth ventricle, the substantiae gelatinosae of the spinal cord and trigeminal nucleus as well as laminae III, IV and X of the spinal cord. The inner plexiform layer of the retina was also labeled.

High affinity GABA receptors also showed a striking variation in their distribution in the brain. In the cerebellum, for example, the granule cell layer had a very high density. In the olfactory bulb, the external plexiform layer had a very high level. The glomeruli showed lower levels. In the cerebral cortex, the distribution and density varied with the area; but generally, it appeared that the more superficial layers (layers I through IV) had higher densities than the deeper layers. In the thalamus, a number of nuclei showed strikingly high levels. These included the ventral nucleus; the lateral nuclei; the ventral nuclei, pars dorsomedialis and magnocellularis; the medial nuclei, pars lateralis and medialis, and the medial dorsal and ventral anterior nuclei. The dorsal lateral geniculate also had high levels. In the hippocampal formation, the molecular layer of the dentate gyrus and the substantia nigra, zona reticulata, had a high level of receptor. In the retina we observed a labeling of receptor in the inner plexiform layer. The substantia gelatinosa of the spinal cord also had elevated levels of GABA receptors.

Thus, although some areas showed high levels of both benzodiazepine and high affinity GABA receptors, many areas showed elevations in only one receptor. For example, in the cerebellum, high levels of GABA receptors were in the granule cell layer while the benzodiazepine receptors were highest in the molecular layer. In the diencephalon, benzodiazepine receptors were higher in the hypothalamus than in the thalamus, in general, while GABA receptors showed the opposite distribution.

Since there was not a fixed ratio between the quantity of benzodiazepine and GABA receptors in all areas, it suggested that there was not a simple constant relationship between the two receptors. Accordingly, we carried out some experiments where we stimulated benzodiazepine binding with 0.2mM GABA. We examined the sections autoradiographically to carefully quantitate the changes in benzodiazepine receptor following the GABA stimulation.

In the olfactory bulb, approximately equal increases in benzodiazepine binding were produced in the glomerular and external plexiform layers even though the highest GABA receptor concentration was in the external plexiform layer. The largest increase was in the granule cell layer, an area containing lower levels of benzodiazepine receptor than the external plexiform layer (Table I and Fig. 1). Similarly, in the cerebellum, benzodiazepine receptor binding was increased slighty more in the molecular layer than in the granule cell layer even though the GABA receptor density was highest in the granule cell layer (Table I). Thus, we found that the stimulation of benzodiazepine receptor binding due to the presence of 0.2uM GABA varied from 40% to nearly 230%. This regional variation in the ability of GABA to effect benzodiazepine receptors was also observed by Karobath and Sperk (14).

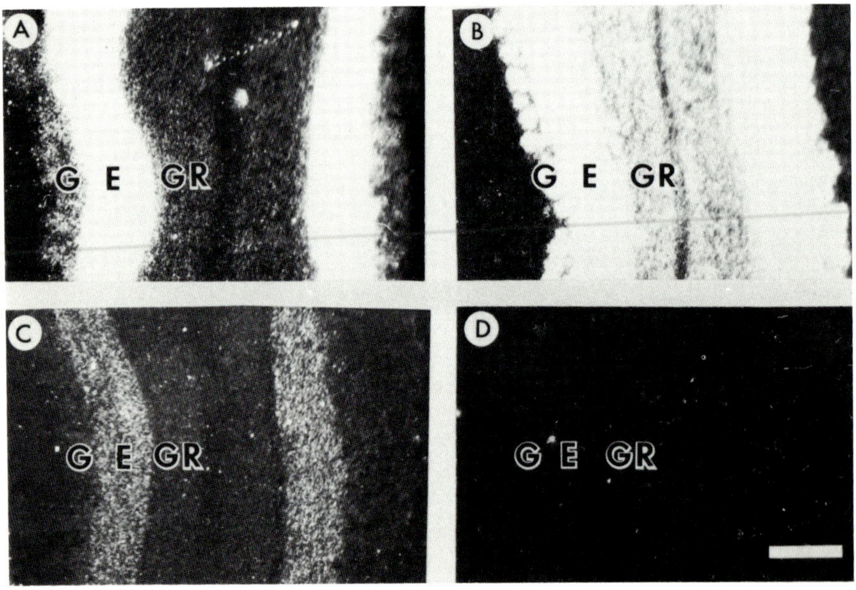

Figure 1. Darkfield photomicrographs of high affinity benzodiazepine and GABA receptors in adjacent sections of rat olfactory bulb. Autoradiograms were produced as described in the text. A and C show that the binding of ^{3}H-flunitrazepam and ^{3}H-GABA, respectively, are highest in the external plexiform layer (E) and lower in the glomeruli (G). Very low levels are present in the granule cell layer (GR). In B, 0.2mM GABA stimulates ^{3}H-flunitrazepam binding (see Table 1 for values). Notice that the granule cell layer is particularly affected. D is a blank generated with 1nM ^{3}H-flunitrazepam and 1uM clonazepam. Bar = 250u.

TABLE I - The effect of GABA on ^{3}H-FLU binding in discrete regions of rat brain

Region	Specific Binding (fmoles/mg tissue wet weight)[a] ^{3}H-FLU[b]	^{3}H-FLU + GABA[b]	Increase (%)
Olfactory Bulb			
Glomeruli	56.9	85.0	49
Ext. plexiform layer	204.9	342.5	67
Granule cell layer	26.8	54.0	101
Cerebellum			
Molecular layer	27.9	91.7	229
Granule cell layer	7.4	18.6	151

[a]Autoradiograms were produced along with standards containing known amounts of radioactivity. This allowed conversion from grains/1000u^2 to fmoles/mg tissue wet weight. Specific binding was calculated by subtracting counts of nonspecific from total binding in autoradiograms.
[b]Six micron sections were incubated in 1 nM ^{3}H-FLU with or without 0.2mM GABA as described in the text. Nonspecific binding was produced by including 1uM clonazepam in parallel incubations. This experiment was repeated once more.

DISCUSSION

Our autoradiographic studies have localized with a high degree of anatomical resolution and sensitivity high affinity benzodiazepine and GABA receptors. We find that they have strikingly different regional distributions in brain. This observation, along with the fact that GABA potentiates benzodiazepine receptor binding differently in various brain regions led us to suggest that there is not a simple fixed ratio relationship between high affinity GABA receptors and benzodiazepine receptors (33). Karobath and Sperk (14) showed that muscimol stimulates benzodiazepine receptor binding to a small extent in the cerebellum, medulla, and spinal cord while the stimulation in the olfactory bulb and cerebral cortex was greater. Interestingly, those quantitative results are different from ours in that we find large changes in the cerebellum. A likely explanation for these discrepancies is that we have measured changes in smaller areas that are missed when larger parts of the brain are examined in homogenate studies.

It is not surprising that we do not observe a fixed ratio between high affinity GABA and benzodiazepine receptors. For example, Karobath et al. (13) have reported that the pharmacology of the GABA-benzodiazepine link is different from that observed for the high affinity GABA site. Thus, only a fraction of the benzodiazepine receptors may be connected to GABA receptors and, similarly, only a fraction of GABA receptors may be connected to BZ receptors. Another GABA receptor with a unique pharmacology has been found, possibly localized to presynaptic nerve terminals (2). Also, it has been suggested, using heat inactivation experiments and various pharmacological studies that there are multiple types of benzodiazepine receptors (15,25). Previous ontogenetic studies are in agreement with this in that the GABA stimulation of benzodiazepine receptor binding develops at a different rate than the high affinity GABA binding (3,5,8,20).

A potential difficulty with both our autoradiographic and other biochemical studies is that there may be endogenous compounds such as GABA, GABAmodulins or other materials whose concentrations differ in different parts of the brain which could distort the regional pattern of GABA and benzodiazepine binding. Our studies to date do not suggest that this has caused serious problems in our regional localization studies. For example, preincubation of our sections for removing endogenous compounds did increase high affinity GABA receptor binding, but it did not vary the regional distributions (21). Obviously, further effort is needed to investigate the possible existence of multiple receptors and endogenous ligands and their interactions.

REFERENCES

1. Banna, N.R., Jabbur, S.J. and Saade, N.E. (1974): Br. J. Pharmacol., 51:101-103.

2. Bowery, N.G., Hill, D.R., Hudson, A.L., Doble, A., Middlemiss, D.M., Shaw, J. and Turnbull, M. (1980): Nature, 283:92-94.

3. Braestrup, C. and Nielsen, M. (1978): Brain Res., 147:170-173.

4. Briley, M.S. and Langer, S.Z. (1978): Europ. J. Pharmacol., 52: 129-132.

5. Candy, J.M. and Martin, I.L. (1979): J. Neurochem., 32:655-658.

6. Choi, D.W., Farb, D.H. and Fischbach, G.D. (1977): Nature, 269:342-344.

7. Costa, E., Guidotti, A. and Mao, C.C. (1975): Adv. Biochem. Psychopharmacol., 14:113-130.

8. Coyle, J.T., and Enna, S.J. (1976): Brain Res., 111:119-133.

9. Gallager, D.W. (1978): Europ. J. Pharmacol., 49:133-143.

10. Geller, H.M., Taylor, D.A. and Hoffer, B.J. (1978): Naunyn-Schmiedeberg's Arch. Pharmacol., 304:81-88.

11. Guidotti, A., Gale, K., Suria, A. and Toffano, G. (1979): Brain Res., 172:566-571.

12. Guidotti, A., Toffano, G. and Costa, E. (1978): Nature, 275:553-555.

13. Karobath, M., Placheta, P., Lippitsch, M. and Larsen, P.K. (1979): Nature, 278:748-749.

14. Karobath, M and Sperk, G. (1979): Proc. Natl. Acad. Sci. (U.S.A.), 76:1004-1006.

15. Klepner, C.A., Lippa A.S. Benson, D.I., Sano, M.C., and Beer, B. (1980): Pharmacol. Biochem. Behav., 11:457-462.

16. Macdonald, R. and Barker, J.L. (1978): Nature, 271:563-564.

17. Martin, I.L. and Candy, J.M. (1978): Neuropharmacol. 17:993-998.

18. Montarolo, P.G., Raschi, F. and Strata, P.G. (1979): Brain Res., 162:358-362.

19. Palacios, J.M. and Kuhar, M.J. (1980): Brain Res. Bul., 5:in press.

20. Palacios, J.M., Niehoff, D.L., and Kuhar, M.J. (1979): Brain Res., 179:390-395.

21. Palacios, J.M., Young, W.S., III and Kuhar, M.J. (1980): Proc. Natl. Acad. Sci. (U.S.A.), 77:670-674.

22. Polc, P. and Haefely, W. (1976): Naunyn-Schmiedeberg's Arch. Pharmacol., 294:121-131.

23. Polc, P., Mohler, H., Haefely, W. (1974): Naunyn-Schmiedeberg's Arch. Pharmacol., 284:319-337.

24. Raabe, W. and Gummit, R.J. (1979): Epilepsia, 18:117-121.

25. Squires, R.F., Benson, D.I., Braestrup, C., Coupet, J., Klepner, C.A., Myers, V. and Beer, B. (1979): Pharmacol. Biochem. Behav., 10:825-830.

26. Tallman, J.F., Paul, S.M., Skolnick, P. and Gallager, D.W. (1980): Science, 207:274-281.

27. Tallman, J.F., Thomas, J.W. and Gallager, D.W. (1978): Nature, 274:383-385.

28. Toffano, G., Guidotti, A. and Costa, E. (1978): Proc. Natl. Acad. Sci. (U.S.A.), 75:4024-4028.

29. Waddington, J.L. (1978): Europ. J. Pharmacol., 51:417-422.

30. Wastek, G.J., Speth, R.C., Reisine, T.D. and Yamamura, H.I. (1978): Europ. J. Pharmacol., 50:445-447.

31. Wolf, P. and Haas, H. (1977): Naunyn-Schmiedeberg's Arch. Pharmacol., 299:211-218.

32. Young, W.S., III and Kuhar, M.J. (1979): Brain Res., 179:255-270.

33. Young, W.S., III and Kuhar, M.J. (1979): Nature, 280:393-395.

34. Young, W.S., III and Kuhar, M.J. (1980): J. Pharmacol. Exp. Ther., 212:337-346.

GABA and Benzodiazepine Receptors, edited by E. Costa et al.
Raven Press, New York © 1981.

GABA and Benzodiazepine Receptors. Studies on Their Localization in the Hippocampus and Their Interaction with Central Dopamine Neurons in the Rat Brain

K. Fuxe, [1]C. Köhler, [2]L. F. Agnati, K. Andersson, [1]S.-O. Ögren, [3]P. Eneroth, [4]M. Pérez de la Mora, [5]M. Karobath, and [6]P. Krogsgaard-Larsen

Department of Histology, Karolinska Institutet, [3]Hormone Laboratory, Department of Obstetrics and Gynaecology, Karolinska Hospital, S-104 01 Stockholm; [1]Astra Läkemedel AB, S-151 85 Södertälje, Sweden; [2]Department of Human Physiology, University of Modena, Bologna, Italy; [4]Centro de Investigaciones en Fisiologia Celular, Universidad Nacional Autónoma de México, Apartado Postal 70-600, México 20, D.F.; [5]Department of Experimental Psychiatry, Psykiatrische Universitätskilinik Universität Wien, Wien A1090, Austria; and [6]Department of Chemistry BC, Royal Danish School of Pharmacy, DK-2100 Copenhagen, Ø, Denmark

During recent years, biochemical and immunohistochemical studies have demonstrated a wide-spread distribution of GABA and glutamate systems in the brain (5, 10). Pharmacological investigations have indicated that central GABA neurons participate in a wide range of brain functions (16). Recently, high affinity binding of ^{3}H-GABA has been demonstrated in several brain regions shown by immunohistochemistry to be rich in GABA nerve terminals. The observation that benzodiazepines can stimulate high affinity GABA binding in the brain suggest a close interrelationship between the receptors for benzodiazepines and GABA (14). The exact neuronal localization of the GABA and the benzodiazepine binding sites remain largely unknown at the present. An understanding of this relationship would be of importance for the elucidation of both the role of GABA receptors in the brain and the pharmacological action of the benzodiazepines. In the present study, we have analyzed the binding of ^{3}H-GABA, ^{3}H-muscimol and ^{3}H-flunitrazepam in the hippocampus of the rat after lesions of intrinsic cell bodies and transections of various cholinergic and glutamergic afferents to the hippocampus.

GABA nerve terminals have been localized both within the area of the dopamine (DA) rich cell bodies of the ventral midbrain and in the DA terminal rich areas of the striatum, nucleus accumbens and the limbic regions (8, 21). Previous experiments have demonstrated that GABA-mimetic drugs can exert both inhibitory and excitatory influences on the various dopamine nerve terminals in the neostriatum and the limbic forebrain (6, 7, 8, 9). In the present paper we have extended the analysis of GABA-monoamine interactions in studies of the effects of the GABA transaminase inhibitor, gabaculine (20), the GABA agonist THIP (15) and a new GABA-mimetic drug, GA 30-905 on monoamine turnover. GA 30-905 (4β-hydroxy-8-methoxy-10β-methyl-3β-(N-piperidine)-methylene-2,9-dioxa,tricyclo-(4,3,1,$0^{3,7}$)-decane hydrogen tartrate) has no affinity for GABA, muscimol or benzodiazepine binding sites but demonstrates GABA-mimetic activity in several animal models (Gähwiler 1977, Sandoz report). We have also analyzed the effects of SQ 20009 (1-ethyl-4-(isopropylidene-hydrazino)-1H-pyrazolo(3,4,5)pyridine-5carboxylic acid, ethylester HCl) alone and in combination with flunitrazepam of gabaculine on monoamine turnover. SQ 20009 have been shown to be an allosteric modulator of the GABA-benzodiazepine receptor complex (19, 29).

Finally, we present evidence that glutamatergic pathways may control turnover of the central dopamine pathways by measuring the dopamine turnover in the lateral septal region following ibotenic acid lesions of hippocampal pyramidal cells which are known to give rise to the glutamate innervation of the lateral septum (28).

LOCALIZATION OF ^{3}H-GABA, ^{3}H-MUSCIMOL AND ^{3}H-FLUNITRAZEPAM BINDING SITES IN THE HIPPOCAMPAL FORMATION FOLLOWING IBOTENIC ACID LESIONS OF INTRINSIC NEURONS AND TRANSECTIONS OF AFFERENT SYSTEMS

In Triton treated membranes high affinity and low affinity classes or specific sodium independent GABA binding sites have been detected (4, 19). ^{3}H-muscimol binding in rat brain is associated with synaptic GABA receptors and the behavioural effects of this compound are probably therefore related to activation of GABA receptors (see 1). By using radioligands, such as diazepam, the existence of specific high affinity binding sites for benzodiazepines have been shown and characterized within the brain (26). There is evidence that benzodiazepines enhance GABA neurotransmission in the brain and furthermore, stimulation of benzodiazepine receptor binding by GABA have been demonstrated (14). The observation that GABA stimulate benzodiazepine binding suggest that GABA and benzodiazepine binding sites may be anatomical and functionally linked together. In order, to better understand the interrelationships between the benzodiazepine and GABA binding sites we analyzed their localization in the hippocampal formation of the rat after various types of lesions. The same membrane fractions were used for ^{3}H-flunitrazepam, ^{3}H-GABA and ^{3}H-muscimol binding (19). After two injections of ibotenic acid (5 μg in 0.5 μl) into the dorsal hippocampus, a degeneration of all hippocampal nerve cell bodies were found whereas the afferents to the hippocampus remained intact (see 17, 24). In other experiments the perforant pathway to the hippocampal formation and the cholinergic pathway running in the fornix-fimbria were cut by means of a dura knife. All lesions are confirmed histologically and by determination of GAD and CAT activity.

Ibotenate injections into the dorsal hippocampus reduced the ^{3}H-flunitrazepam binding approximately by 30 % at 5 and 75 days after injections (Fig. 1). Five days after the injections there was also a reduced K_D value of ^{3}H-flunitrazepam binding. In the normal hippocampus the B_{max} for ^{3}H-flunitrazepam was 50.5 pmol/g wet weight with a K_D value of around 1.0 nM. The ibotenic acid lesions caused a gradual loss of low affinity (40-45 %) but not of the high affinity ^{3}H-muscimol binding sites (Figs. 2 - 3). These results indicate that the high and the low affinity component of ^{3}H-muscimol binding can be differentially located. The K_D values for the high and low affinity ^{3}H-muscimol binding sites were both reduced by 40 %, indicating an increased affinity for these sites. The results obtained with ^{3}H-GABA binding have shown that in contrast to the ^{3}H-muscimol binding a loss of both the high and low affinity GABA sites were found after ibotenic acid lesions. This reduction was in the order of 30 % and (Fig. 4) similar to the reduction of ^{3}H-flunitrazepam and of the low affinity component of ^{3}H-muscimol binding. Also the K_D values for both high and low affinity components of ^{3}H-GABA binding were reduced. Taken together, these results may indicate the following;

1. The high and low affinity ^{3}H-GABA binding sites and the ^{3}H-flunitrazepam binding sites show a similar reduction in density after ibotenic acid lesions, suggesting that these two receptors may be localized on the same cellular constituents. The high affinity ^{3}H-muscimol binding sites may not label the GABA-benzodiazepine receptor complex located on intrinsic hippocampal neurons, since this binding is not reduced by ibotenic acid lesions. These results indicates the possibility that ^{3}H-muscimol may not label all the high affinity ^{3}H-GABA binding sites in the brain, at least not within the hippocampal formation. Furthermore, since the numbers of high affinity ^{3}H-muscimol binding sites are somewhat higher than the numbers of high affinity binding sites for GABA, it may also be that ^{3}H-muscimol can bind to high affinity sites which are not associated with GABA receptors.
2. The increased affinity of ^{3}H-GABA and ^{3}H-flunitrazepam binding sites may be related to a dennervation supersensitivity of the remaining GABA receptors after removal of intrinsic hippocampal GABAergic interneurons.
3. The results indicate that a large number of ^{3}H-GABA, ^{3}H-muscimol and ^{3}H-flunitrazepam binding sites may be located on the axon terminals innervating the hippocampal formation.

After bilateral transections of the perforant path which innervates the dorsal hippocampus from the entorhinal cortex, the number and the affinity of ^{3}H-flunitrazepam binding sites remained

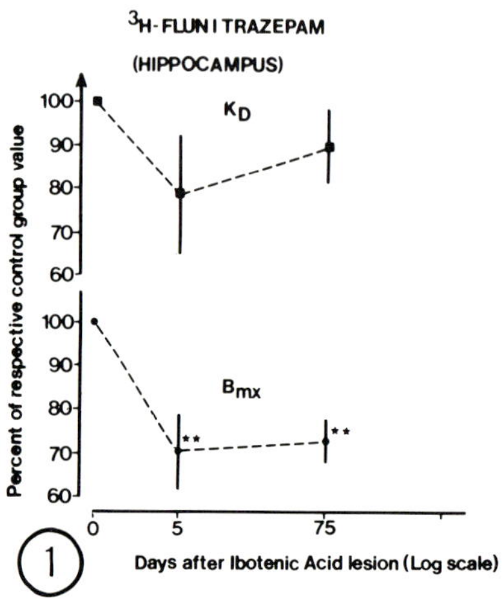

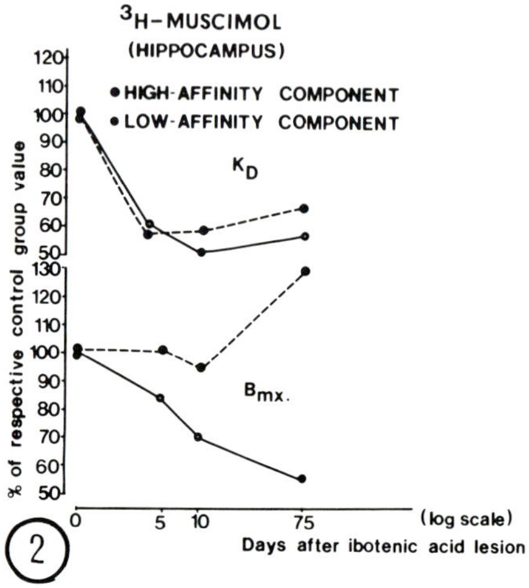

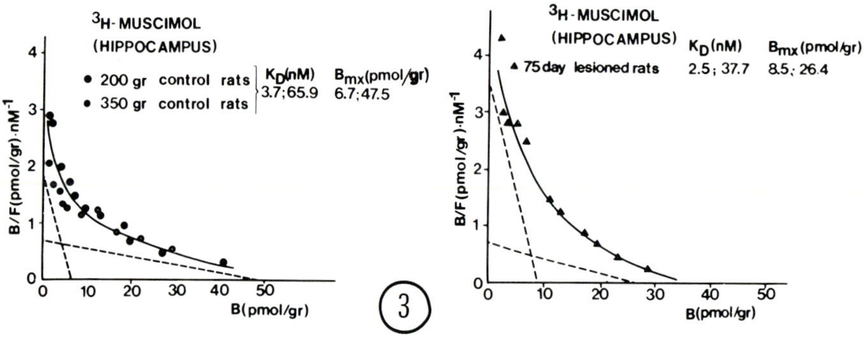

FIG. 1. The results obtained in the experiments on ^{3}H-flunitrazepam binding in ibotenate lesioned hippocampus are summarized. Specific binding was defined as the binding in the presence of 1 μM flunitrazepam. The binding of ^{3}H-flunitrazepam was made in concentrations from 0.03 to 5 nM. The statistical analysis has been carried out by means of standard parametrical procedures (25). The 95 % confidence intervals are shown. The best fit line in the Scatchard plot has been obtained by means of the least square method. **= $p<0.01$. FIG. 2. The effects of ibotenate lesions of the hippocampal formation on ^{3}H-muscimol binding. FIG. 3. Scatchard plot of ^{3}H-muscimol binding to membranes not treated with Triton X-100 from the normal and ibotenate lesioned hippocampus. The concentrations of ^{3}H-muscimol ranged from 0.5 to 100 nM, three replicates per concentration. Unspecific binding was defined as the binding in the presence of 10^{-5} M of muscimol. A curved Scatchard plot was obtained and the two ^{3}H-muscimol binding sites have been separated using a modification of Hart's procedure (10). From the two binding lines the theoretical curve has been calculated according to Rosenthal's procedure (22). The theoretical curve is shown and give an appreciable improvement of the goodness of fit.

unchanged. Thus, the number of binding sites (B_{max}) was 46 (conf. int; 44-48) pmol/g versus 43 (39-47) pmol/g in the hippocampus with perforant path transections. Similarly no differences in the K_D values in the ^{3}H-flunitrazepam binding were observed when comparing experimental and control animals. The K_D value of the control group was 1.08 (1.01-1.15) nM versus 1.07 (0.91-1.23) nM in the experimental group. In contrast, a 20 % decrease in the low affinity ^{3}H-muscimol binding sites (B_{max}, 36 pmol/g) and a 50 % reduction in the high affinity ^{3}H-muscimol binding sites (B_{max}, 3.0 pmol/g) were seen after perforant path transections. The K_D value of the low affinity binding site in the experimental group was 100 nM, whereas it was 48 nM in the control group, suggesting a possible reduction of affinity in the remaining low affinity ^{3}H-muscimol binding sites. The corresponding K_D value for high affinity binding was 3.1 and 3.7 nM in the experimental and control groups respectively. Control experiments demonstrated a 40 % reduction of glutamate uptake in this type of experiment. Thus, as evaluated 5 days following the lesion ^{3}H-flunitrazepam binding sites are probably not located on glutamate containing perforant path fibres terminating within the hippocampal formation. Furthermore, glutamate released from perforant path fibres may be controlled by GABA receptors. These results suggest a partial dissociation between flunitrazepam and muscimol binding sites. It is of substantial interest that these GABA receptors may not be coupled to benzodiazepine binding sites. Our findings suggest that the GABA and benzodiazepine binding sites are differentially located and regulated. Lesions of the cholinergic afferents to the hippocampus were found to reduce both low and high affinity ^{3}H-GABA binding in the hippocampus by 35 and 20 % respectively. A reduction of the K_D values of both binding sites from 81 to 44 nM and from 3.8 to 2.0 nM respectively were observed. Thus, GABA receptors may also be located on cholinergic afferents to the hippocampus, possibly regulating the release of acetylcholine. In conclusion, a measurable number of GABA receptors appear to have a presynaptic localization on cholinergic and glutamatergic nerve terminals in the hippocampus. Their role may be the regulation of the release of the respective transmitters.

GABAERGIC CONTROL OF DOPAMINE PATHWAYS

As pointed out in a large number of articles (16) GABA neurons can control dopamine systems at many levels, directly or indirectly. It has been shown that inhibitory influences of GABA-mimetic drugs were most pronounced following activation of dopamine systems by means of neuroleptic drugs, and that some GABAergic drugs may preferentially reduce dopamine turnover within the limbic dopamine system. Low doses of the GABA agonist muscimol have been shown to increase dopamine turnover within the nuc. caudatus, nuc. accumbens and the median eminence (8). One explanation that has been offered for this effect is that unlike the GABA transaminase inhibitors, muscimol preferentially activated those GABA

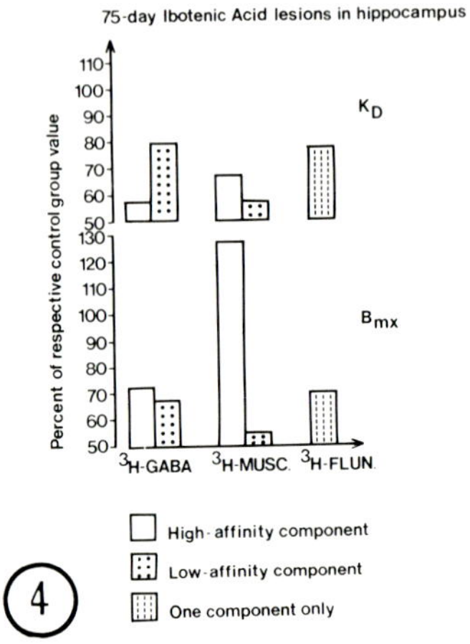

FIG. 4. Summary of the results obtained on ^{3}H-muscimol, ^{3}H-GABA and ^{3}H-flunitrazepam binding in the hippocampal formation of 75 day ibotenate lesioned rats. The percentage changes in binding parameters are shown following the lesion. For further details, see text to previous figures and (4, 19). The concentrations of ^{3}H-GABA ranged from 0.5 to 300 nM. Unspecific binding was defined as the binding in the presence of 10^{-3} M of GABA. A curved Scatchard plot was obtained and the two ^{3}H-GABA binding sites have been separated using a modification of Hart's procedure (10). From the two binding lines the theoretical curve has been calculated according to Rosenthal's procedure (22).

receptors which were not directly located on the dopamine cell bodies, dendrites and terminals. Thus, muscimol may increase dopamine activity via an indirect neuronal mechanism.

It has been suggested that many GABA receptors may be located on GABA containing cell bodies and dendrites within the zona reticulata of substantia nigra which projects to the ventromedial thalamus (3, 23). In view of these findings it became of interest to analyze also the actions of the GABA receptor agonist THIP on the dopamine activity in the brain. THIP (4,5,6,7-tetrahydrosiooxazolo(5,4-c)pyridin-3-ol) is a semirigid analogue of muscimol and like muscimol, THIP produces inhibition of locomotion and stereotypies, enhances the cataleptic actions of neuroleptics and produces hypothermia in rats (see 15, 16). As can be seen in Table 1, THIP selectively reduced dopamine turnover in the nuc. caudatus but had no effect on dopamine turnover in the nuc. accumbens. Thus, THIP may preferentially activate in vivo those GABA receptors which produce inhibitory effects on dopamine turnover in the nuc. caudatus. Alternatively, THIP may exert blocking actions at those GABA receptors which have an excitatory influence on the

TABLE 1. Effects of various doses of THIP on the $H^{44}/68$ induced DA fluorescence disappearance in the forebrain of the normal male rat

Treatment	Dose mg/kg	CAUD. marg.	CAUD. med.	CAUD. cent.	ACC. dif.	ACC. dot.	TUB. dot.	TUB. dif.
NaCl + $H^{44}/68$ 2 h		100 ± 5	100 ± 3	100 ± 3	100 ± 2	100 ± 4	100 ± 2	100 ± 3
THIP + $H^{44}/68$ 2 h	1	113 ± 5	98 ± 2	104 ± 2	114 ± 4	100 ± 2	90 ± 3	90 ± 4
THIP + $H^{44}/68$ 2 h	3	105 ± 2	114 ± 2	107 ± 3	116 ± 3	105 ± 3	93 ± 3	87 ± 3
THIP + $H^{44}/68$ 2 h	10	108 ± 4	126 ± 5 **	119 ± 6 *	104 ± 6	116 ± 5	98 ± 3	103 ± 3

THIP was administered in various doses i.p. together with $H^{44}/68$ (250 mg/kg, i.p., 2 h before killing). Means$\pm$s.e.m. are shown out of 5 rats. The fluorescence values are given in per cent of the respective $H^{44}/68$ alone group mean value. The fluorescence was expressed relatively to a dopamine standard present in the section (relative fluorescence units, see Löfström et al., 1976). The statistical analysis involved the use of the Wilcoxon test, one-way classification: treatment versus controls. *= $p<0.05$; **: $p<0.01$. Abbreviations used. CAUD. marg.= marginal zone of the caudate nucleus; CAUD. med.= medial part of the caudate nucleus; CAUD. cent.= central part of the caudate nucleus; ACC. dif.= diffuse type of DA fluorescence in the anterior nucleus accumbens; ACC. dot.= dotted type of DA fluorescence in the posterior nucleus accumbens; TUB. dot.= dotted type of DA fluorescence in the medial posterior tuberculum olfactorium; TUB. dif.= diffuse type of DA fluorescence in the lateral posterior tuberculum olfactorium. Fort details on anatomical localization, see Fuxe et al., 1979 (9).

caudate dopamine nerve terminals. This speculation is supported by the partial GABA agonist properties of THIP on benzodiazepine receptor binding in the brain (13). In agreement with this hypothesis it has been shown (Ögren et al., unpublished observation) that THIP in contrast to muscimol antagonizes the anticonvulsant action of diazepam on bicuculine induced convulsions (Fig. 5). These studies demonstrate that also in vivo conditions, THIP may be a GABA receptor antagonist at GABA receptors controlling benzodiazepine binding. The studies with GA 30-905 further suggest that GABAergic drugs may preferentially reduce dopamine turnover in limbic areas (Table 2). Thus, in doses from 3 mg/kg of GA 30-905, which produces mild sedation with increased periods of sleep and reduced motility (Gähwiler 1977, Sandoz report) caused a selective reduction of dopamine turnover within the nuc. accumbens-tuberculum olfactorium area (Table 2). A dose of 3 mg/kg of GA 30-905 caused a significant increase of dopamine turnover in the nuc. caudatus. Furthermore, high doses (30-100 mg/kg) increased noradrenaline turnover in the antero-medial frontal cortex and in the nuc. accumbens-tuberculum olfactorium area.

In two different experiments we have also studied whether SQ 20009 can modulate the actions of flunitrazepam and gabaculine on dopamine turnover in various parts of the forebrain, in the substantia nigra as well as the area surrounding the nuc. interpeduncularis (DA cell groups A9 and A10 respectively). As can be seen in Fig. 6, flunitrazepam in a dose of 1 mg/kg significantly and selectively reduce dopamine turnover in the medial part of the nuc. caudatus, whereas no effect was observed in the limbic areas. SQ 20009 counteracted the flunitrazepam induced reduction of dopamine turnover in the nuc. caudatus. Combined treatments, however, increased dopamine turnover in the dotted type of DA terminals of the nuc. accumbnes (9) which have been shown to be cholecystokinin (CCK) positive by Hökfelt et al. (12). The DA turnover in A9 and A10 was not changed by any type of treatment (data not shown). These results suggest the possibility that SQ 20009 can preferentially enhance the effects of flunitrazepam at GABA receptors in the forebrain excitatory to some neostriatal and accumbens DA nerve terminals. The experiments with SQ 20009 and gabaculine are shown in Fig. 7. It can be seen that gabaculine reduce DA turnover in the central part of the nuc. caudatus as well as in the medial part of the nuc. caudatus and in its marginal zone (data not shown). However, the limbic dopamine terminal systems and the dopamine cell body groups (A10) show no changes of DA turnover after gabaculine (data not shown). SQ 20009 was found to antagonize the actions of gabaculine on dopamine turnover in the nuc. caudatus. In contrast, in the limbic areas combined treatment with SQ 20009 and gabaculine (10-30 mg/kg) was found to result in a reduction of dopamine turnover exclusively within the diffuse type of dopamine terminals in the tuberculum olfactorium and in the nuc. accumbens both of which are not cholecystokinin immunoreactive (12).

These results indicate that increases of GABA levels can re-

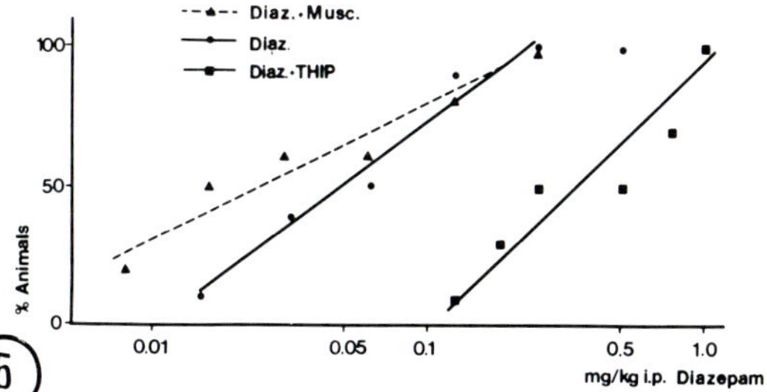

5

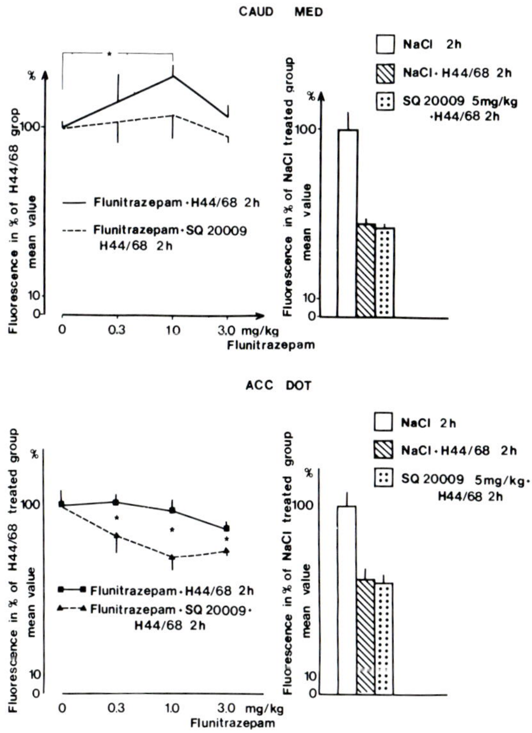

6

FIG. 5. Diazepam was injected i.p. 30 min before bicuculine (0.35 mg/kg i.v.). THIP (0.25 mg/kg) and muscimol (0.06 mg/kg) were injected i.p. 15 min before bicuculine. The number of animals with clonic-tonic convulsions were scored in groups of 10 animals for a period of 10 min after the injection of bicuculine. FIG. 6. The effects of flunitrazepam on the H44/68 induced DA fluorescence disappearance with or without simultaneous treatment with SQ 20009. Means±s.e.m. are shown (4-6 rats). To the right of the Fig. the DA fluorescence values are given in per cent of the untreated group mean value. The statistical analysis used was Wilcoxon test, one-way classification: treatment versus controls and multiple comparisons. *= $p<0.05$; **= $p<0.01$; ***= $p<0.001$.

TABLE 2. The effects of GA 30-905 on the $H^{44}/68$ induced DA and NA depletion in nuc. caudatus, the nuc. accumbens-tuberculum olfactorium area and the antero-medial frontal cortex

Treatment	Dose mg/kg	Caudatus DA	Caudatus NA	Tuberculum olfactorium -nuc. accumbens area DA	Tuberculum olfactorium -nuc. accumbens area NA	Antero-medial frontal cortex DA	Antero-medial frontal cortex NA
$H^{44}/68$		4058±104	123±9	588±59	2253±67	15±1.7	190±16.2
GA 30-905 + $H^{44}/68$	1	3314±188	125±19	714±69	2382±192	17±2	213±14
GA 30-905 + $H^{44}/68$	3	3001±206*	143±29	894±105	2216±245	17±1.7	192±10.9
GA 30-905 + $H^{44}/68$	10	4058±104	151±18	1011±174	1645±137	14±0.7	* 185±11.2
GA 30-905 + $H^{44}/68$	30	3435±309	117±12	1094±158	1448±141**	16±1.5	181±11.5
GA 30-905 + $H^{44}/68$	100	3266±265	108±11	1216±228*	1574±129*	12±2.2	138±7.9

GA 30-905 was given i.p. at the same time as the $H^{44}/68$ injection (250 mg/kg, i.p., 2 h before killing). Means±s.e.m. are shown out of 6 rats. The results are expressed as ng/g tissue. Wilcoxon's test was used in the statistical analysis (one-way classification, comparing experimental groups with a control group or comparing all possible pairs of treatment (NA, anterior medial frontal cortex)). *= $p<0.05$; **= $p<0.01$.

duce dopamine turnover in the nuc. caudatus (8) effects which are mimicked by receptor agonists such as flunitrazepam and THIP. In limbic areas SQ 20009 can preferentially enhance the action of GABA at those receptors which inhibit the activity in a subgroup of mesolimbic dopamine systems which are cholecystokinin negative. The opposite effects were observed in the neostriatal dopamine pathways, where SQ 20009 antagonized the action of gabaculine and it may thus, preferentially enhance the effects of GABA at those GABA receptors which stimulate dopamine turnover in nuc. caudatus. However, within the limbic system, different results were obtained in the SQ 20009-gabaculine versus the SQ 20009-flunitrazepam experiments. Thus, flunitrazepam tends to increase dopamine turnover in the CCK positive dopamine terminals of the nuc. accumbens while gabaculine reduces the dopamine turnover in the diffuse type of dopamine terminals in the limbic forebrain (those which are CCK negative), when given together with SQ 20009. In summary, the present findings suggest that SQ 20009 can differentially modulate the actions of gabaculine and of flunitrazepam at various types of forebrain dopamine nerve terminals.

INHIBITION OF PROLACTIN SECRETION BY GABAERGIC DRUGS AND ITS MODULATION BY SQ 20009

Prolactin gland cells have GABA receptors which may be involved in regulation of prolactin secretion (see 16). We have therefore analyzed whether SQ 20009 can modulate the effects of benzodiazepines and gabaculine on prolactin secretion. Gabaculine has been shown to lower prolactin secretion probably thorugh a mechanism involving an increased release of GABA from the median eminence. In Fig. 8, it can be seen that SQ 20009 enhances the inhibitory actions of gabaculine on the secretion of prolactin and other findings (not shown) indicate that SQ 20009 slightly reduces the inhibitory actions of flunitrazepam on the hypersecretion of prolactin induced by tyrosine hydroxylase inhibition. These results are of considerable interest since it may be suggested on the basis of these findings that at least with regard to pituitary GABA receptors, SQ 20009 via its action on the chloride conductance mechanism, may favor the coupling of the GABA binding sites to the opening of the chloride channel. The negative results with flunitrazepam may suggest that the effects of SQ 20009 are mediated over the benzodiazepine binding sites of pituitary GABA receptors, since no additional effects are seen following flunitrazepam plus SQ 20009.

POSSIBLE GLUTAMERGIC CONTROL OF SEPTAL DOPAMINE TERMINALS

As seen in Table 3, lesions of the dorsal hippocampus by ibotenic acid produce a 40 % bilateral depletion of dopamine levels within the septal region and a 20 % bilateral depletion of the noradrenaline levels in the same region. A change in dopamine turnover was also demonstrated since the degeree of dopamine

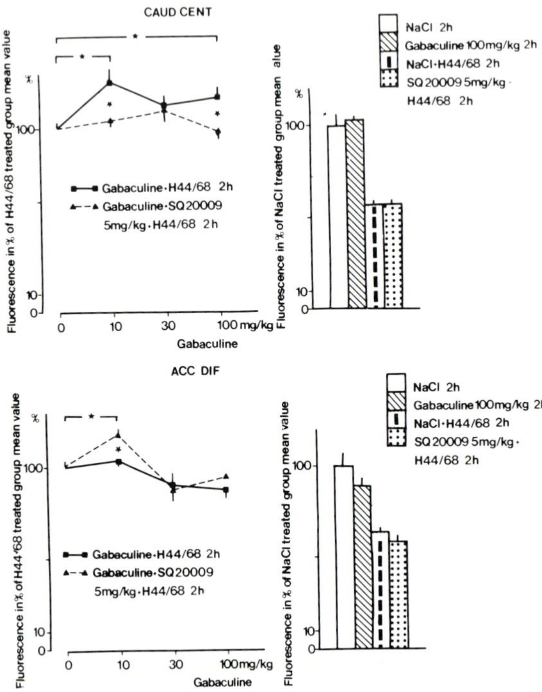

7

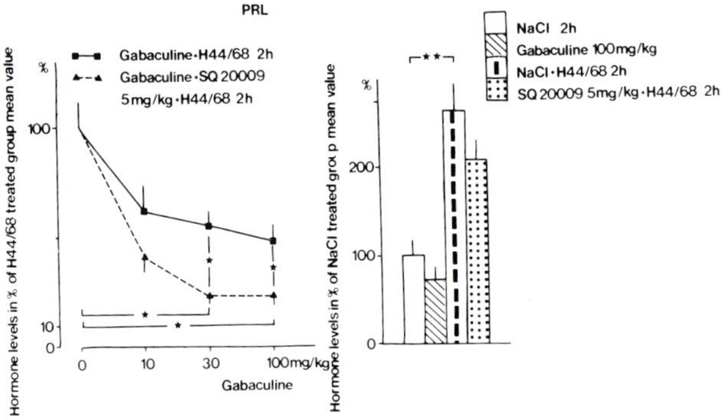

8

FIG. 7. The effects of gabaculine on the $H^{44}/68$ induced DA fluorescence disappearance. Means$\pm$s.e.m. are shown (4-6 rats). See text to Fig. 8. FIG. 8. The effects of gabaculine on the $H^{44}/68$ induced increase of prolactin secretion in the normal male rat in the absence or presence of SQ 20009. $H^{44}/68$ (250 mg/kg, i.p., 2 h before killing. Gabaculine and $H^{44}/68$ was administered at the same time as $H^{44}/68$ with or without SQ 20009 (5 mg/kg, i.p.). Means $\pm$s.e.m. are shown out of 4-6 rats. To the right in the Fig. the prolactin levels are given in per cent of the untreated group mean value. The statistical analysis was performed by means of Wilcoxon test, one-way classification: treatment versus controls and multiple comparisons. *= $p<0.05$; **= $p<0.01$; ***= $p<0.001$.

TABLE 3. Effects of unilateral ibotenic acid induced hippocampal lesions on CA levels and turnover in the ipsilateral and contralateral septum 8 days following the lesion

	CA LEVELS		CA LEVELS AFTER $H^{44}/68$	
	NA	DA	NA	DA
	%	%	%	%
Control normal side	100 ± 8	100 ± 17	78 ± 6	28 ± 3
Control sham op. side	100 ± 5*	100 ± 12*	79 ± 6	26 ± 3**
Ibotenic acid unlesioned side	80 ± 8*	63 ± 7*	100 ± 10	45 ± 3*
Ibotenic acid lesioned side	86 ± 3	69 ± 9	86 ± 9	41 ± 4

Ibotenic acid (5 µg/1 µl) was injected into the dorsal hippocampus (see 17, 24). Means $\pm$ s.e.m. (6-7 rats) are shown. The noradrenaline levels of the control side were 727 ± 37 ng/g and the dopamine levels 646 ± 41 ng/g. The catecholamine levels are given in per cent of the control mean value, and the catecholamine depletion induced by $H^{44}/68$ is indicated by showing the remaining amounts of catecholamines in per cent of the respective untreated group mean value. Student's paired t-test was used in the statistical analysis. * = $p<0.05$; ** = $p<0.01$.

but not of noradrenaline depletion by H44/68 was reduced bilaterally in the septum of lesioned rats. These findings of a bilateral depletion of dopamine in the septum and a bilateral reduction of septal dopamine turnover is in full accordance with the interpretation that there may exist a glutamate dopamine interaction within the septum, since the projection is bilateral. Thus, an important role of hippocampal glutamate fibres to the lateral septum may be their regulation of dopamine release in this area. It remains to be established if this glutamate dopamine interaction is a general phenomenon in the brain. However, preliminary experiments indicate that in the piriform cortex, no such interactions exist since transections of the lateral olfactory tract did not affect piriform dopamine turnover as evaluated 5 days after the operation.

ACKNOWLEDGEMENTS

This work has been supported by a grant, 04X-715, from the Swedish Medical Research Council, by a grant, MH 25504, from the National Institute of Health and by a grant from Magnus Bergwall's Stiftelse, Stockholm, Sweden.

REFERENCES

1. Beaumonte, K., Chilton, W.S., Yamamura, H.I. and Enna, S.J. (1978): Brain Res., 148:153-162.

2. Beer, B., Chasin, M., Clodi, D.E., Vogel, J.R. and Horovitz, Z.P. (1972): Science, 176:428-430.

3. Di Chiara, G., Porceddu, M.L., Morelli, M., Mulas, M.L. and Gessa, G.L. (1979): In: GABA-Neurotransmitters, edited by P. Krogsgaard-Larsen, J. Scheel-Krüger, and H. Kofod, pp. 465-481. Munksgaard, Copenhagen.

4. Enna, S.J. and Snyder, S.H. (1975): Brain Res., 100:81-97.

5. Filer, L.J.Jr., Garattini, S., Kare, M.R., Reynolds, W.A. and Wurtman, R.J., editors (1979): Glutamic Acid: Advances in Biochemistry and Physilogy, Raven Press, New York.

6. Fuxe, K., Hökfelt, T., Ljungdahl, A., Agnati, L.F., Johansson, O. and Pérez de la Mora, M. (1975): Medical Biology, 53:177-183.

7. Fuxe, K., Pérez de la Mora, M., Hökfelt, T., Agnati, L.F., Ljungdahl, A. and Johansson, O. (1977): In: Psychopathology and Brain Dysfunction, edited by C. Shagass, S. Gershon, and A.J. Friedhoff, pp. 97-111. Raven Press, New York.

8. Fuxe, K., Andersson, K., Ögren, S.-O., Pérez de la Mora, M., Schwarcz, R., Hökfelt, T., Eneroth, P., Gustafsson, J.-Å. and Skett, P. (1979): In: GABA-Neurotransmitters, edited by P. Krogsgaard-Larsen, J. Scheel-Krüger, and H. Kofod, pp. 74-94. Mungsgaard, Copenhagen.

9. Fuxe, K., Andersson, K., Schwarcz, R., Agnati, L.F., Pérez de la Mora, M., Hökfelt, T., Goldstein, M., Ferland, L., Possani, L. and Tapia, R. (1979): In: Advances in Neurology 24, edited by L.J. Poirer, T.L. Sourkes, and P.J. Bédard, pp. 199-215. Raven Press, New York.

10. Hart, H.E. (1965): Bull. Math. Biophysics., 27:87-98.

11. Harvey, J.A., Scholfield, C.N., Graham, L.T.Jr. and Aprison, M.H. (1975): J. Neurochemistry, 24:445-449.

12. Hökfelt, T., Skirboll, L., Rehfeld, J.F., Goldstein, M., Markey, K. and Dann, O. (1980): Nature, in press.

13. Karobath, M. and Lippitsch, M. (1979): Eur. J. Pharmacol., 58:485-488.

14. Karobath, M. and Sperk, G. (1979): Proc. Natl. Acad. Sci. USA, 76(2):1004-1006.

15. Krogsgaard-Larsen, P., Honoré, T. and Thyssen, K. (1979): In: GABA-Neurotransmitters, edited by P. Krogsgaard-Larsen, J. Scheel-Krüger, and H. Kofod, pp. 201-216. Munksgaard, Copenhagen.

16. Krogsgaard-Larsen, P., Scheel-Krüger, J. and Kofod, H., editors (1979): GABA-Neurotransmitters: Pharmacochemical, Biochemical and Pharmacological Aspects, Munksgaard, Copenhagen.

17. Köhler, C., Schwarcz, R. and Fuxe, K. (1979): Brain Res., 175: 366-371.

18. Löfström, A., Jonsson, G., Wiesel, F.-A. and Fuxe, K. (1976): J. Histochem. Cytochem., 24:430-442.

19. Placheta, P. and Karobath, M. (1980): Eur. J. Pharmacol. 62: 225-228.

20. Rando, R.R. (1979): In: GABA-Neurotransmitters, edited by P. Krogsgaard-Larsen, J. Scheel-Krüger, and H. Kofod, pp. 228-235. Munksgaard, Copenhagen.

21. Roberts, E. (1979): In: GABA-Neurotransmitters, edited by P. Krogsgaard-Larsen, J. Scheel-Krüger, and H. Kofod, pp. 28-45. Munksgaard, Copenhagen.

22. Rosenthal, H.E. (1967): Anal. Biochem., 20:525-532.

23. Scheel-Krüger, J., Arnt, J., Braestrup, C., Christensen, A.V. and Magelund, G. (1979): In: GABA-Neurotransmitters, edited by P. Krogsgaard-Larsen, J. Scheel-Krüger, and H. Kofod, pp. 447-464. Munksgaard, Copenhagen.

24. Schwarcz, R., Hökfelt, T., Fuxe, K., Jonsson, G., Goldstein, M. and Terenius, L. (1979): Exp. Brain Res., 37:199-216.

25. Sokal, R.R. and Rohlf, F.M. (1969): Biometry, W.H. Freeman, San Fransisco.

26. Squires, R.F. and Braestrup, C. (1977): Nature (London), 271: 732-734.

27. Storm-Mathisen, J. (1977): Brain Res., 120:379-386.

28. Storm-Mathisen, J. (1977): Prog. Neurobiol., 8:119-181.

29. Supavilai, P. and Karobath, M. (1979): Eur. J. Pharmacol., 60:111-113.

GABA and Benzodiazepine Receptors,
edited by E. Costa et al.
Raven Press, New York © 1981.

Electrophysiological Analysis of Gabaergic Local Circuit Neurons in the Central Nervous System

B. E. Alger, C. E. Jahr, and R. A. Nicoll

Departments of Pharmacology and Physiology, University of California, San Francisco, California 94143

A great deal has recently been written on the importance of local circuit neurons in neuronal integration (28,31,32,34). Many, probably a majority, of local circuit neurons (LCNs) are GABAergic and have an inhibitory function. The pioneering work of Eccles and his collaborators on inhibitory pathways in the CNS (10-12) clearly established the central role of inhibition in neuronal integration. However, in vivo experiments have limitations for precise analysis of interneuronal circuitry. The recent development of in vitro preparations offers a number of advantages, including mechanical stability for intracellular recording, control of the extracellular environment and the ability to analyze various parts of a neuron.

Using in vitro preparations we have focused on the role of dendritic inhibitory inputs, which are provided by local circuit neurons, in controlling principal cell excitability in hippocampus and olfactory bulb. Principal cells in these two cortical structures provide an interesting comparison due to the differing functions served by their respective dendritic trees. In the case of the hippocampus there is good reason to believe the dendrites are active elements, possessing the capability for post-synaptic amplification of excitatory inputs via intrinsic action potential, and "burst" firing, properties. Such intrinsic dendritic amplification is seen as exerting a substantial excitatory influence on the pyramidal cell somata, and hence on cell outputs. Therefore, inhibitory control over the pyramidal cell dendrites is emerging as an important control function, but one which, in the hippocampus, is at present little understood.

In contrast, mitral cell dendrites have long been thought to participate in local circuits as presynaptic, as well as post-synaptic elements. Inhibitory control over the mitral cells is provided largely via the reciprocal dendrodendritic synapse made between mitral and granule cell dendrites. This reciprocal connection can presumably act to impart a rhythmicity to mitral cell outputs. Unlike pyramidal cells, mitral cells can act synaptically to control their own excitability.

In each case, while it is clear that dendritic inhibitory processes must be important in neuronal integration, precise electrophysiological characterization of these processes is lacking. We have been analyzing the pathways involved in dendritic inhibitory control of hippocampal pyramidal cells and olfactory bulb mitral cells.

HIPPOCAMPUS

Shortly after the detailed description of inhibitory postsynaptic potentials (IPSPs) in hippocampal pyramidal cells by Kandel and Spencer (16), Andersen, et al. (3) proposed that these IPSPs are mediated by a recurrent collateral activation of basket cells, which synapse on the somata of pyramidal cells. Although this hypothesis has withstood the test of time, there is growing evidence that dendritic inhibition may also exist in these cells. Purpura et al. (27) have found that large IPSPs can be recorded in pyramidal cells in new born cats even though at this stage of development few somatic synapses exist. Fugita (13) has reported that the late phase of the orthodromic IPSP is more difficult to reverse than the early component and proposes that the late phase originates in the dendrites. Biochemical and histochemical studies also suggest that GABAergic pathways may exist in the dendritic region of pyramidal cells (35).

We have used the hippocampal slice preparation (2) to examine the possibility that pyramidal cell dendrites are under inhibitory synaptic control. Because GABA is probably the major hippocampal inhibitory transmitter (35), we first compared the sensitivity of the dendrites and soma to GABA applied from two independently positioned iontophoretic pipettes. Iontophoresis at the soma produces either a hyperpolarizing-depolarizing sequence (Fig. 1A.) or a pure hyperpolarization. Biphasic neuronal responses to GABA have also been seen in other types of neurons (7,26). Dendritic application indicated that the dendrites are also sensitive to GABA, but invariably, pure depolarizing responses are observed (Fig. $1A_2$; cf., 5,17,36). Both somatic and dendritic GABA responses are blocked by GABA antagonists. To ensure that the responses resulted from activation of GABA receptors on the pyramidal cells themselves and not from indirect effects, we have demonstrated that the depolarizing action of GABA persists after synaptic transmission has been eliminated by changing to a low Ca^{++}/high Mg^{++} saline. Both hyperpolarizing and depolarizing responses exert an inhibitory influence on the pyramidal cell, as measured by their ability to block action potentials caused either by intrasomatic depolarizing current pulses or by EPSPs (Fig. 1A). The inhibitory effectiveness of the depolarization is not surprising in view of the very large conductance increase accompanying it. This conductance increase is large enough to be easily measurable in the soma of the neuron and readily shunts the action potentials.

Our next question was whether these depolarizing dendritic receptors might be activated by synaptically released GABA. In normal conditions we have been unable to find any evidence for a depolarizing component to the IPSP. However, we considered the possibility that a relatively weak dendritic depolarizing IPSP might be masked by the large hyperpolarizing somatic IPSP. In an attempt to unmask depolarizing IPSPs, we added pentobarbital

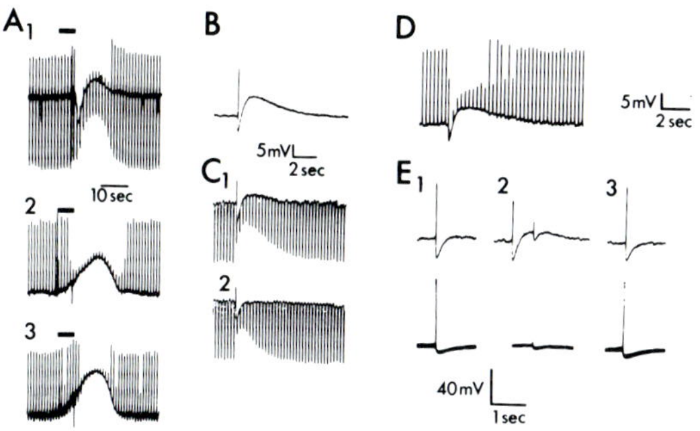

Fig. 1 Biphasic inhibitory responses in hippocampal pyramidal cells. A. Effects of iontophoretic GABA (1 M) (horizontal bar) in normal medium without pentobarbital. A_1. Application through a pipette in s. pyramidale. Downward deflections are membrane responses to 100 ms current pulses given at 1 Hz. Resting potential (RP) -55mV. A_2,A_3. GABA iontophoresed in s. radiatum region of another cell. During the depolarization, both directly and synaptically activated action potentials are blocked (A_2 and A_3, respectively). RP -61mV. Iontophoretic pipettes were lowered independently 200 µm into the slice before impaling a cell. Ejection currents were 500 nA for 5 s. B. Orthodromic stimulation (s. radiatum) elicits a hyperpolarization followed by a prolonged depolarization. RP -57mV. C. Orthodromic and antidromic stimulation compared in a single cell. Downward deflections produced by hyperpolarizing 100 ms current pulses (2 Hz) through a bridge circuit. Reduced membrane resistance accompanies both responses; however, no depolarization is seen with antidromic stimulation. RP -59mV. D. A train (2 Hz) of depolarizing current pulses initiated full-sized somatic action potentials (amplitudes not accurately reproduced by the pen recorder) which were blocked during most of the stimulation evoked response. E. Inhibition of spikes elicited by just suprathreshold EPSP during a depolarizing IPSP (E_2). Unconditioned control responses are shown before and after inhibition (E_1 and E_3). Same cell as in B.

(10^{-4} M) to the perfusate, since this drug markedly augments GABA-mediated events (25). If, as we suppose, the somatic hyperpolarization is nearly maximal normally, then augmentation of GABA effects by pentobarbital might cause a relatively greater increase of a weak dendritic response than of the strong somatic response. In pentobarbital the IPSP is prolonged and the hyperpolarization elicited by orthodromic stimulation in s. radiatum is usually followed by a depolarization (Fig. 1B). Ayala and Thalman have independently made similar observations (6). The depolarization is more reliably elicited with strong (suprathreshold), rather than weak, stimuli. Passage of a series of 100 ms current pulses across the membrane shows that the entire sequence is accompanied by a drop in membrane resistance (Fig. 1C), as was the case with the biphasic, iontophoretic GABA responses.

The involvement of GABA in the synaptically evoked depolarizing phase is further suggested by the observations that: 1) pentobarbital, a specific potentiator of GABA effects, must be present in order to elicit it electrically, and 2) GABA antagonists, picrotoxin (10^{-5} M) or bicuculline (10^{-5} M), which block both aspects of the biphasic iontophoretic GABA response, also block both phases of the synaptic response (n = 4; data not shown). These results strongly implicate GABA as the neurotransmitter for the biphasic action. Again, as was true of iontophoretically applied GABA, both phases of the orthodromically activated responses are inhibitory and can block action potentials caused either by intrasomatic depolarizing current pulses (Fig. 1D) or by EPSPs (Fig. 1E).

Since the classical studies of Andersen, et al. (3) had indicated that the recurrent (antidromic) IPSP was focused primarily on the cell soma, rather than the dendrites, we wondered if the dendritic IPSPs revealed with pentobarbital resulted from activation of the same recurrent collateral system. To test this we have recorded over 40 cells from slices in which two stimulating electrodes had been placed so that both orthodromically and antidromically evoked IPSPs could be compared in the same cell. In over 90% of the cases a biphasic response resulted from orthodromic (s. radiatum) stimulation, while antidromic stimulation evoked a pure hyperpolarizing IPSP (Fig. 1C). In all cases the duration of the underlying conductance increase measured with brief constant current pulses is much longer with the orthodromic, than the antidromic, response, even when the hyperpolarization of the antidromic IPSP is greater than that of the orthodromic IPSP. Hence the orthodromic response is due to a more prolonged activation of inhibitory transmitter channels and is not a peculiarity of cell electrotonic geometry. (It should also be noted that these responses in pentobarbital are extremely long, on the order of seconds, whereas the membrane time constant is on the order of tens of milliseconds, so the duration of these potentials cannot be attributed to passive membrane properties.) Furthermore, even with weak, near threshold stimuli, when no overt depolarization is seen even in response to orthodromic stimulation, an occult depolarizing phase of the orthodromic response can be revealed by hyperpolarizing the membrane. Such relative depolarizations are only rarely produced by antidromic stimulation. In the few cases in which slight depolarizations were seen in response to "antidromic" stimuli, high intensity stimulation was used and it was likely that the current activated nearby orthodromic fibers in s. oriens and thus contaminated the antidromic response (2). This distinction between orthodromically and antidromically evoked IPSPs is especially significant because it indicates the orthodromic depolarization is not an artifact of pentobarbital. The antidromically evoked IPSP is also thought to be GABAergic (35). Taken together, all of these findings suggest that orthodromic stimulation, in addition to activating the well-documented recurrent inhibitory pathway (3), also activates another set of inhibitory neurons. The results of direct application of GABA to the dendrites in the absence of pentobarbital (i.e., depolarization), suggests the synaptically produced depolarization seen in pentobarbital is due to activation of dendritic GABA receptors by this non-recurrent inhibitory system. To obtain direct evidence for or against this hypothesis, we injected TTX (10^{-5} M) through a broken pipette, into the CA1 apical dendritic region to block neuronal activity locally. In several cells in which a large hyperpolarizing-depolarizing response was present, a small (approx. 0.5 nl) bolus of TTX on the dendrites selectively blocked the depolarizing phase and its underlying conductance increase, but had little effect on the hyperpolarizing IPSP (which closely resembled the response to antidromic stimulation), or the action potential produced by somatic current injection (Fig. 2A). Neither resting potential nor input impedence changed and the TTX effect was reversible. The somatic action potential, which is TTX-sensitive, serves as a marker for the localization of the TTX. Since, at the time when the depolarization is initially blocked, the somatic action potential is unaffected, we can conclude that the TTX had its initial effects in the dendritic region away from the soma, and that production of the depolarization requires neuronal activation in this dendritic region. In the converse experiment, TTX injection through a pipette carefully positioned near the soma resulted in a complete block of somatic action potentials and a substantial reduction in stimulation-evoked hyperpolarization, without major effect on the depolarization (n = 4; Fig. 2B). Large TTX injections in the somatic region could occasionally result in the simultaneous reduction of both phases of the orthodromic response, which may indicate the cells whose synapses produce the depolarization exist in or near s. pyramidale. We have recently obtained results very similar to those with TTX using localized iontophoresis of bicuculline methiodide in the somatic and dendritic regions. With dendritic application, the depolarization was abolished while the antidromic hyperpolarizing IPSP was still unaffected. Somatic application of bicuculline blocked the antidromic IPSP and the hyperpolarizing phase of the orthodromic response, without affecting the depolarization. The results with TTX injections and bicuculline iontophoresis imply that orthodromic stimulation in s. radiatum activates dendritic synapses which mediate IPSPs having a depolarizing component. The mechanism by which pentobarbital brings out the depolarizing component to orthodromic stimulation is not clear. One possibility is that pentobarbital merely enhances a depolarizing response which is normally present but is too small to detect by an intrasomatic microelectrode. The depolarizing action of applied GABA iontophoretically to the dendrites in the absence of pentobarbital supports this explanation. Alternatively, pentobarbital may convert a normally hyperpolarizing dendritic response into a depolarizing response. Regardless of the mechanism underlying the action of pentobarbital, this drug has been useful in uncovering a dendritic, feedforward inhibitory pathway.

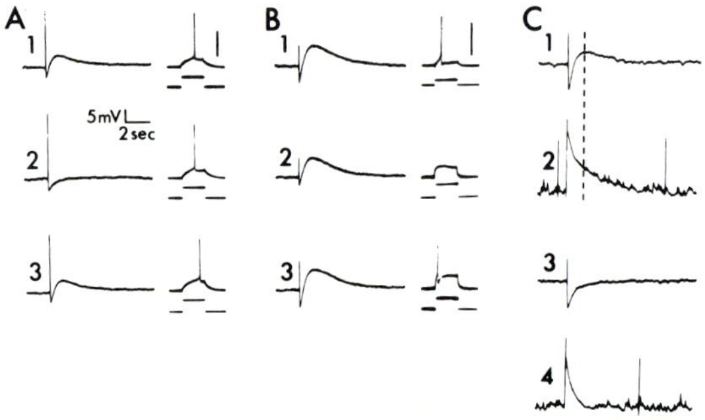

Fig. 2 Effects of TTX and chloride injections on biphasic responses. A. TTX (10^{-5}M) pressure injected in the dendritic region abolishes the depolarization with no effect on the hyperpolarization. Action potentials produced by current pulses were unaffected immediately after TTX injection (A_2) although the depolarization was eliminated. The spike was subsequently blocked but recovered (B_3). RP -63mV. B. TTX injection in the somatic region greatly attenuates the hyperpolarization and blocks direct action potentials with little effect on the depolarization (B_2). Both the hyperpolarization and the action potential recovered substantially (B_3). RP -56mV. All records were obtained in the presence of 10^{-4} M pentobarbital. Calibration for pen traces is 5 mV and 2 s. Calibration for oscilloscope traces is 40 mV and 1.0 nA. Current pulse duration is 100 ms in A, 30 ms in B. C. Two cells from the same slice in pentobarbital. C_1, recorded with a 2 M potassium methylsulphate-filled pipette. C_2, with a 3 M KCl pipette. Note large amplitude and prolonged time course of depolarizing response in C_2 after Cl^- leakage into the cell. Small reversed IPSPs visible on the baseline of the KCl-filled cell are capable of triggering action potentials. Antidromic responses from the same cells are shown for comparison (C_3, C_4). RP -59 mV (C_1, C_3); RP -56 mV (C_2, C_4).

The ionic mechanisms of the biphasic IPSP are also not yet clear. However, elevation of intracellular chloride (Cl^-) by leakage of Cl^- from a 3 M KCl-filled electrode reverses the hyperpolarization to a pronounced depolarization, as noted previously by others. This finding is usually taken to indicate a major contribution of Cl^- to the hyperpolarization. Interestingly, intracellular Cl^- injection also appears to increase the amplitude of the depolarizing phase (Fig. 2C). Even more dramatic effects on the depolarization are seen when a slice is perfused with a low Cl^- saline (70% substitution of sodium isethionate for sodium chloride; data not shown). These results, in addition to the large conductance increase, suggest that Cl^- is at least partially involved in both phases. Indeed, it is relatively easy to reverse the depolarization with current through the micropipette, with typical apparent reversal potentials occurring at -50 to -55 mV resting potential. If Cl^- is involved in both phases, then, to account for the depolarizing sign of the dendritic IPSP, it must be assumed either that the Cl^- equilibrium potential is positive relative to the dendritic membrane potential, or, more likely, that the conductance increase also involves other ions such as sodium or calcium. These cations alone could not be responsible for the depolarization because: 1) excitatory, perhaps regenerative, activity would be expected to occur with a large increase in their conductances, and 2) it would be much more difficult to reverse the depolarization. Chloride plus either sodium or calcium currents could easily produce slight net depolarizations. (Experiments such as that seen in Fig. 1E imply the depolarization cannot be due simply to a depolarizing shift in the local IPSP equilibrium potential, since in that case the superimposed test IPSP (Fig. $1E_2$) would not continue to be hyperpolarizing.) It may be significant in this regard that Dudel (9) has recently reported a current relaxation analysis in which the inhibitory postsynaptic currents in crayfish muscle were found to have a fast chloride conductance phase followed by a slower conductance phase in which cations may be involved.

Despite this unresolved problem of the actual ionic mechanism of the biphasic IPSP, our data have confirmed the presence of GABA-mediated dendritic IPSPs. We suggest that these are part of a feedforward inhibitory system which is distinct from the classical recurrent somatic feedback pathway. Furthermore there is a depolarizing aspect to the orthodromically activated IPSP in pentobarbital which can be localized to the dendritic region. Several circumstances, including differences in experimental conditions, as well as its relatively hyperpolarized reversal potential and requirement for high stimulus intensities, may all contribute to the fact that previous investigations <u>in vivo</u> did not report the depolarizing component.

From the recent discoveries of an intrinsic "burst" generating mechanism present in pyramidal cell dendritic membranes (37) it seems clear that control over dendritic excitability is a requirement for normal functioning of these cells, since bursting properties are only expressed when IPSPs are blocked. Selective orthodromic activation of a dendritic IPSP, such as demonstrated here, would provide optimal control over local dendritic events. However, the functional significance of the depolarizing phase of the dendritic IPSP is unknown. Certainly the pronounced conductance increase accompanying this depolarization can predominate in inhibiting action potential generation. It remains possible, however, that the depolarization could act to reduce the inhibitory effectiveness of the conductance increase.

We have not identified the inhibitory neurons involved in the dendritic IPSP pathway. Doing so definitively will require immunohistochemical staining procedures. There are, however, likely candidate neurons for this role including the non-pyramidal cells which have somata near s. pyramidale and vertically oriented axons branching in s. radiatum (4,18,33).

OLFACTORY BULB

The hypothesis of dendrodendritic inhibition is particularly interesting since it involves dendrites, not only as recipients of inhibitory input, but also as presynaptic elements whose activity evokes their own inhibition. Such a form of inhibition is thought, on the basis of anatomical evidence, to occur in many sensory pathways in the CNS (28,31,32,34). However, a definitive physiological verification of this hypothesis has been lacking, and the specific properties of dendrodendritic inhibition are not understood. In the olfactory bulb the physiological evidence is founded largely on the analysis of the extracellular field potentials with some supporting intracellular data (22,23,28). These data suggest that depolarization of mitral cells (M) (Fig. 3A), and their dendrites, activates excitatory synapses which depolarize granule cell dendrites (G). Granule cell depolarization in turn would activate inhibitory synapses made by granule cells that release GABA back onto the same, and neighboring, mitral cells. It has also been proposed that this pathway can be activated by graded electrotonic depolarization.

Testing the hypothesis of dendrodendritic inhibition in the olfactory bulb requires detailed intracellular recordings which are technically extremely difficult to obtain in the intact animal. Therefore, we have used an in vitro preparation of the turtle olfactory bulb in carrying out the following experiments. The concept of reciprocal dendrodendritic inhibition has been clearly stated and from it a number of predictions can be made: 1) In mitral cells the IPSP observed when an antidromic action potential is allowed to invade the soma-dendritic (SD) membrane should be much larger than that seen when invasion is limited to the axon initial segment (IS). Antidromic activation as far as the initial segment will evoke recurrent collateral inhibition. If, indeed, there is a dendrodendritic component to the IPSP, this inhibition should be seen only when antidromic action potentials trigger SD spikes. This prediction can be tested by controlling the degree of invasion of the mitral cell with hyperpolarizing current passed into the cell through the recording microelectrode. It has been shown in other systems (10), that antidromic action potentials can be fractionated into discrete components by injecting hyperpolarizing currents directly into the soma. These steps correlate with the sequential invasion of the initial segment and the SD membrane; 2) when propagated action potentials are blocked with tetrodotoxin (TTX), direct depolarization of a mitral cell should still be followed by an IPSP if the major inhibitory pathway includes the SD membrane but not the axon. That is, it may be expected that depolarization at the soma will spread, either actively (via TTX-resistent potentials, see below) or passively to at least nearby dendritic loci and activate the reciprocal synapse. Indeed, this

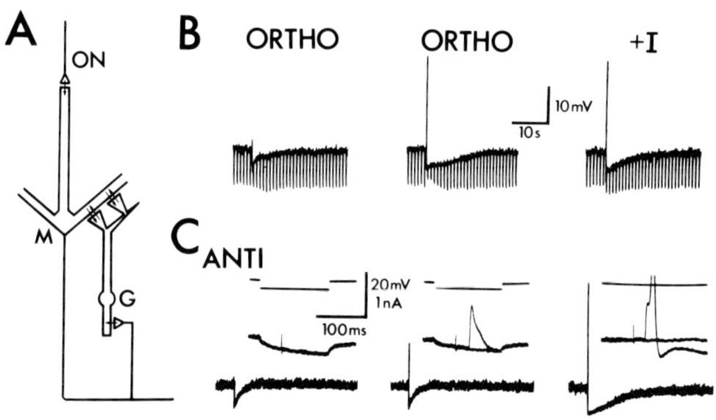

Fig. 3 IPSPs recorded in turtle olfactory bulb mitral cells with potassium methylsulfate-filled electrodes. A. Schematic diagram of neuronal circuit. ON, olfactory nerve; M, mitral cell; G, granule cell. Arrows indicate synaptic polarity. B. Chart records of IPSPs evoked by orthodromic and direct stimulation. The first trace is the IPSP resulting from ON stimulation slightly below threshold for the cell. The second trace is the result of a just suprathreshold ON stimulus. The third trace is the IPSP resulting from an action potential produced by a depolarizing current pulse injected through the recording electrode. C. IPSPs resulting from antidromic stimulation. Invasion of the soma (the presumed site of impalement) and the initial segment were blocked in the first trace by injecting a hyperpolarizing current pulse through the recording electrode. In the second trace a smaller current pulse allowed activation of the initial segment. The third trace illustrates full soma-dendritic invasion. Calibration in B applies to all chart records in B and C. Calibration in the inset of C applies to all insets. The resting potentials of the cells in B and C were -58 and -55mV, respectively.

test would indicate whether or not sodium-dependent action potentials are necessary for the release of transmitter or whether graded depolarizations can elicit a graded release of transmitter. Axonal processes will not be extensively invaded by passive current and axonal action potentials are TTX-sensitive; 3) if mitral cell SD membranes are presynaptic structures, they should possess well-developed calcium channels. Voltage dependent calcium currents are ubiquitous phenomena found in conjunction with transmitter release processes of many kinds. A recording electrode in a mitral cell should be capable of detecting evidence for such presynaptic processes according to the hypothesis of dendrodendritic inhibition. Therefore, in the presence of TTX one might expect to observe calcium-dependent spikes or at least an apparent anomalous rectification of the membrane due to activation of voltage-dependent calcium channels during membrane depolarization (14).

Stimulation both of the olfactory nerve and the mitral cell axons evoked action potentials in mitral cells that were followed by a prolonged hyperpolarization. With potassium methylsulfate-filled electrodes the response remained hyperpolarizing for the duration of the impalement (recording periods of several hours were frequently possible) and was associated with a marked increase in membrane conductance (Fig. 3B). Since many neurons possess calcium-dependent potassium responses (19,21) which could be confused with true inhibitory postsynaptic potentials (IPSPs), we usually used KCl-filled electrodes to invert the IPSPs to depolarizing potentials. As chloride diffuses out of these electrodes into the cells, the chloride gradient, (normally from outside to inside) becomes inverted. Because IPSPs in the CNS are chloride-dependent, this procedure will alter the IPSP, but will leave potassium potentials unaffected (3,10,16). Immediately following impalement with a KCl-filled electrode, the responses were slightly hyperpolarizing (Fig. 4A, first trace) but with time became depolarizing (Fig. 4A, second trace) In addition, shifting the mitral cell membrane to a more hyperpolarized level resulted in a much larger depolarizing response (Fig. 4A, third trace). These properties indicate that following orthodromic and antidromic stimulation there is a prolonged IPSP in mitral cells. IPSPs could be generated by orthodromic and antidromic stimuli that were below threshold for action potentials in the impaled mitral cells, but a large increase in the size of the IPSP generally occurred when the cell responded with an action potential (Fig. 3B). This suggests that the IPSP is linked, in part, to the firing of the cell under observation. Indeed, single spikes occurring either spontaneously, or in response to depolarizing current pulses, were capable of eliciting IPSPs (Fig. 3B and 4C). Increasing the intensity of the depolarizing current pulses increased the size of the IPSP (Fig. 4B). These findings imply that mitral cells are self-inhibited and suggest that recurrent axon collateral pathways are not necessary for inhibition since in neurons which receive only collateral inhibition, IPSPs do not follow spikes evoked by intracellularly applied depolarizing

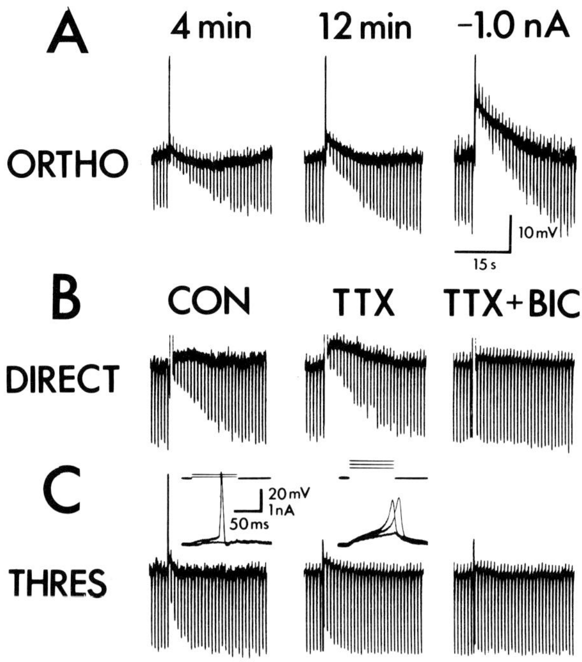

Fig. 4 IPSPs recorded in turtle olfactory bulb mitral cells with a potassium chloride-filled electrode. A. Chart records of responses to orthodromic stimulation at 4 minutes after impalement, at 12 minutes, and during passage of 1 nA DC hyperpolarizing current through the recording electrode. Downward deflections are hyperpolarizing responses to constant current pulses through the recording electrode. The increase of resting membrane resistance between the 4 minute record and the following records is due to improvement of the impalement. B. Responses to large depolarizing current pulses through the recording electrode (6 nA x 800 ms) in control Ringer (CON), in 10^{-6} M TTX for 15 minutes and in 10^{-6} M TTX with 10^{-4} M bicuculline methiodide added for 23 minutes (TTX + BIC). C. Responses to threshold depolarizing current pulses in the same conditions as in B. The first inset shows the directly produced action potential in control Ringer. The second inset shows the calcium spikes to direct stimulation in TTX. Note the great increase in threshold for the calcium responses. The calibration in A applies to all chart records. The resting potential of this cell was -55 mV.

---

pulses. To verify the linkage between activity in mitral cell SD membranes and self-inhibition, we compared the size of the IPSP generated in the absence and presence of SD impulses. By injecting hyperpolarizing current into the soma through the recording electrode, invasion of the soma and initial segment can be blocked sequentially (Fig. 3C). The size of the IPSP is unaffected by the presence or absence of an impulse in the IS membrane. However, a large increase in the size of the IPSP is observed when the impulse is permitted to invade the SD membrane. It can be concluded, then, that the observed increment in the IPSP is due to a synaptic pathway involving the soma-dendritic membrane.

In a second approach we added tetrodotoxin (TTX) to the Ringer to block impulse propagation out the mitral cell axon. This should localize the effects of depolarizing current injected through the recording electrode to the cell body and proximal dendrites. TTX (10^{-6} M) blocked propagated action potentials in the olfactory nerve and mitral cell axons and thus both orthodromic transmission and antidromic invasion. The fast action potentials elicited by the intracellular stimulation of mitral cells were also blocked. However, increasing the strength of the depolarizing current pulses evoked smaller and broader action potentials (Fig. 4C, insets) which were entirely blocked by the calcium antagonist, cobalt (5mM). These TTX-resistant action potentials, therefore, appear to be calcium spikes. The presence of these calcium spikes indicates that mitral cell SD membranes do possess calcium channels as expected from the prediction of a presynaptic role for these membranes. In addition, calcium spikes were capable of activating the reciprocal synapse (Fig. 4C, second trace) which indicates that granule, as well as mitral cell dendrites can release transmitter in the absence of propagated sodium spikes. The reciprocal synapse could not be activated by graded depolarizations below threshold for calcium spike initiation. The fact that the IPSP is produced in TTX demonstrates quite clearly that the inhibitory pathway can be activated by the mitral cell body body and dendrites and does not require axonal pathways, since mitral cell axons are inexcitable in TTX. Finally, we have found that iontophoretically applied GABA produces inhibitory hyperpolarizations in mitral cells (data not shown) and that the GABA antagonist bicuculline blocks the evoked IPSP (Fig. 4B and 4C). These findings support and extend previous suggestions that GABA is released from granule cells (20,24,30).

The present results provide strong physiological support for the concept of dendrodendritic inhibition in the olfactory bulb. They demonstrate that a major component of the mitral cell IPSP is strictly dependent on action potential production in the mitral cell SD membrane, that the granule cell inhibitory transmitter release can be evoked by activity intrinsic to the mitral cell, and that mitral cell SD membranes have properties expected of presynaptic elements. The results suggest the entire local circuit involving reciprocal synapses can be mediated dendritically, since the pathway remains intact when all sodium-dependent propagated action potentials are blocked by TTX. Such a pathway provides for an all-or-none self-inhibition of mitral cells. These cells are also subjected to lateral inhibition, as is apparent from observations that orthodromic and antidromic stimuli which are below threshold for action potential generation in the impaled cell, nevertheless evoke small IPSPs.

CONCLUSION

In conclusion, we can compare and contrast our results on hippocampal pyramidal cells and olfactory bulb mitral cells as follows: Through what appear to be local circuit effects, both of these cortical cell types receive a synaptically mediated dendritic inhibitory input in addition to somatic inhibitory inputs. Because the dendritic inhibition can be mimicked by iontophoretically applied GABA and blocked by GABA antagonists, we conclude the inhibition is GABAergic in both structures. The output of most neurons occurs exclusively via the axon. As has been stressed repeatedly (10-12), the somatic synaptic inhibition is strategically positioned for control of this output, since spike initiation occurs at the initial segment. It has been found that the dendrites of many cortical neurons have active properties and that there is a somatopetal tendency for spike conduction, i.e., dendritic impulses travel towards the soma. Thus, the observation that dendrites spike, indicates that there are two levels of integration in nerve cells. In general, dendritic inhibition would control transmission of dendritic spikes to the cell body, while somatic inhibition would control the firing of the cell's axon.

In the hippocampus, synaptic activation of cells during blockade of inhibition leads to immediate and pronounced bursts of action potentials, which are also generated in the dendrites. These bursts are capable of triggering somatic bursts, and therefore, presumably, excitatory output of the cell. Therefore, in the hippocampus, the function of dendritic inhibition is exclusively to exert control over these excitatory effects, which culminate in firing the axons.

On the other hand, the output of mitral cells occurs via both the axon and the dendrites. The secondary dendrites of mitral cells (the ones on which the reciprocal granule cell synapses are primarily made) probably do not receive excitatory input. The dendrites are, instead, activated by a somatofugal depolarization. This depolarization spreads out the secondary dendrites from the primary dendrites and soma, triggering excitatory transmitter release, and subsequently the reciprocal inhibitory synapse on the same and neighboring mitral cells. This pathway, therefore, provides for a lateral inhibition as well as a self-inhibition. Thus, in mitral cells, somatic inhibition would block both axonal and dendritic outputs, while dendritic inhibition would selectively block somatofugal dendritic excitation and, thereby, the lateral inhibition generated by this pathway.

Hence, these differences in dendritic inhibiton imply that GABA will have a variety of functions in different parts of the CNS, each peculiar to the specific architecture of the local circuits present.

REFERENCES

1. Alger, B.E. and Nicoll, R.A. (1979): Nature, 281:315-317.
2. Alger, B.E. and Teyler, T.J. (1977): Brain Res. Bull., 2:355-365.
3. Andersen, P., Eccles, J.C. and Loyning, Y. (1974): J. Neurophysiol., 27:592-607.
4. Andersen, P., Gross, G.N., Lomo, T. and Sveen, O. (1969): In: The Interneuron, edited by M.A.B. Brazier, pp. 415-467. UCLA Forum Med. Sci. No. 11, University of California Press.
5. Andersen, P., Bie, B., Ganes, T. and Mosfeldt-Laursen, A. (1978): In: Iontophoresis and Transmitter Mechanisms in the Mammalian Central Nervous System, edited by R. Ryall and J. Kelly, pp. 179-181. Elsevier, Holland.
6. Ayala, G.F. and Thalmann, R.A. (1979): Neurosci. Abst., 5:736.
7. Barker, J.L. and Ransom, B.R. (1978): J. Physiol.(Lond.), 280:331-354.
8. Barrett, E.F. and Barrett, J.N. (1976): J. Physiol.(Lond.), 255:737-774.
9. Dudel, J. (1978): Pflugers Arch. ges. Physiol., 376:151-157.
10. Eccles, J.C. (1957): The Physiology of Nerve Cells. Johns Hopkins, Baltimore.
11. Eccles, J.C. (1966): Inhibitory Pathways in the Central Nervous System. (Liverpool University Press, London).
12. Eccles, J.C., Ito, M. and Szentagothai, J. (1967): The Cerebellum as a Neuronal Machine. Springer-Verlag, New York.
13. Fujita, Y. (1979): Brain Res., 175:59-69.
14. Hotson, J.R. Prince, D.A., and Schwartzkroin, P.A. (1979): J. Neurophysiol., 42:225-242.
15. Jahr, C.E. and Nicoll, R.A. (1980): Science, 207:1473-1475.
16. Kandel, E., Spencer, W.A., and Brinley, F.J. (1961): J. Neurophysiol. 24:225-242.
17. Langmoen, I.A., Andersen, P., Gjerstad, L., Mosfeldt-Laursen, A. and Ganes, T. (1978): Acta physiol. scand., 102:C27.
18. Lorente de No, R. (1934): J. Psychol. u. Neurol., 46:113-177.
19. MacAfee, D.A. and Yarowsky, P.J. (1979): J. Physiol.(Lond.), 290:507-523.
20. McLennan, H. (1971): Brain Res., 29:177-184.
21. Meech, R.W. and Standen, N.B. (1975): J. Physiol.(Lond.), 249: 211-239.
22. Mori, K. and Takagi, S.F. (1978): J. Physiol.(Lond.), 279:569-588.
23. Nicoll, R.A. (1969): Brain Res., 14:157-172.
24. Nicoll, R.A. (1971): Brain Res., 35:137-149.
25. Nicoll, R.A., Eccles, J.C., Oshima, K. and Rubia, F.J. (1975): Nature, 258:625-627.
26. Nicoll, R.A., Padjen, A. and Barker, J.L. (1976): Neuropharmacology, 15:45-63.

27. Purpura, D.P., Prelevic, S. and Santini, M. (1968): Expl. Neurol., 22:408-422.
28. Rakic, P. (1975): Neurosci. Res. Prog. Bull., 13:289-446.
29. Rall, W. and Shepherd, G.M. (1968): J. Neurophysiol., 31: 884-915.
30. Ribak, C.E., Vaughn, J.E., Saito, K., Barber, R. and Roberts, E. (1977): Brain Res., 126:1-18.
31. Schmitt, F.O., Dev, P. and Smith, B.H. (1976): Science, 193:114-120.
32. Schmitt, F.O. and Worden, F.G. (1979): The Neurosciences-Fourth Study Program, (MIT Press, Cambridge, MA).
33. Schwartzkroin, P.A. and Mathers, L.H. (1978): Brain Res., 157:1-10.
34. Shepherd, G.M. (1978): Sci. Am., 238:92-103.
35. Storm-Mathisen, J. (1977): Progr. Neurobiol., 8:119-181.
36. Thalmann, R.H., Peck, E.J. and Ayala, G.F. (1979): Neurosci. Abst., 5:747.
37. Wong, R.K.S. and Prince, D.A. (1979): Science, 204:1228-1231.

GABA and Benzodiazepine Receptors,
edited by E. Costa et al.
Raven Press, New York © 1981.

Convulsant and Anticonvulsant Drug Binding Sites Related to GABA-Regulated Chloride Ion Channels

Richard W. Olsen and Frederick Leeb-Lundberg

Division of Biomedical Sciences and Department of Biochemistry, University of California, Riverside, California 92521

Picrotoxin is a central nervous system stimulatory drug (10) which is believed to cause convulsions via a noncompetitive block of inhibitory synaptic transmission mediated by gamma-aminobutyric acid (GABA) (17). Picrotoxin inhibits the postsynaptic response to GABA (the opening of chloride ion channels [11]) without affecting the binding of GABA to its receptor site (18). This GABA receptor-regulated chloride channel appears to be a likely site of action for several types of convulsant drugs (30) and also for numerous depressant drugs, such as barbiturates (16) and benzodiazepines (8, 28), which appear to act at least in part by enhancing GABAergic synaptic transmission (9, 31). We present here a summary of radioactive drug binding studies on mammalian brain in vitro which suggest that two classes of drug receptor sites, one for picrotoxin-like convulsants and barbiturates, and one for benzodiazepines, are related to many of the pharmacological actions of these drugs and that these receptors are coupled to the postsynaptic membrane GABA receptor-chloride ion channel complex.

[^{3}H]α-DIHYDROPICROTOXININ BINDS TO CONVULSANT-ANTICONVULSANT RECEPTOR SITES

A biologically active analogue of picrotoxin, α-dihydropicrotoxinin (DHP), was made radioactive and found (20) to bind specifically to synaptic membrane fragments from crayfish muscle (a tissue containing GABA synapses blocked by picrotoxin [17]) and mammalian brain, but not to nonneuronal tissues (34). The binding dissociation constant was 1-2 μM, and the number of binding sites in brain was 5-10 pmol/mg protein, about two-three times the level of GABA binding sites having receptor properties (19). DHP binding sites appear to be distinct from GABA receptor sites by various criteria (35), while showing a similar brain regional and subcellular distribution (19, 35).

DHP binding is inhibited by biologically active chemical analogues of picrotoxin, but not inactive analogues (21, 34). Table 1 lists the IC_{50} values for selected drugs which inhibit DHP binding. Notable other convulsants which are active include the cage compounds such as bicyclophosphates, and tetramethylene disulfotetramine (21, 37) which inhibit GABA synapses [4]). Other convulsants which inhibit DHP binding

TABLE 1. Selected Inhibitors of DHP Binding[a]

Excitatory drug	IC_{50} (μM)	Depressant drug	IC_{50}
α-Dihydropicrotoxinin	2	Hexobarbital	2
Picrotoxinin	0.5	Pentobarbital	50
Tutin	0.4	Phenobarbital	400
Picrotin	70	Diphenylhydantoin	100
t-Butyl Bicyclophosphate	2	Diazepam	1
TETS	4	Clonazepam	4
Decamethrin	0.1	Chlordiazepoxide	4
DMBB	0.1	RO 11-6896 (+)	1
CHEB	0.7	RO 11-6893 (-)	> 100
MPPB	0.9	RO 5-4864	> 100
RO 5-3663	0.1	SQ 20009	8

[a] [^{3}H] DHP binding was measured by centrifugation (34, 36), using fresh rat cortex membranes fraction $P_2 + P_3$, washed once with assay buffer (0.2 M NaCl, 5 mM $NaPO_4$, pH 7.0). Quadruplicate samples were incubated for 15 min at 0° with 50 nM [^{3}H] DHP (15 Ci/mmol, Amersham) and varying concentrations of displacing drug; background was determined with 0.1 mM nonradioactive DHP. Each IC_{50} value is the mean of at least two determinations. TETS = tetramethylenedisulfotetramine; DMBB = dimethyl butyl barbiturate; CHEB = cyclohexylidene-ethyl barbiturate; MPPB = N-methyl, phenyl, propyl barbiturate. The structures of RO 5-3663 and SQ 20009 are given in Figure 1; RO 11-6896 (+) and RO 11-6893 (-) are stereoisomeric benzodiazepines (courtesy of Dr. H. Mohler, Hoffmann-La Roche). RO 5-3663 was the gift of Dr. W. Schlosser, Hoffmann-LaRoche, and SQ 20009 was the gift of Dr. B. Meiners, ICI America.

are the pyrethroid insecticides, excitatory barbiturates (such as DMBB, CHEB, and MPPB [21, 36]), and an excitatory benzodiazepine (RO5-3663 [12, 23]). These compounds inhibit DHP binding in the micromolar and submicromolar range, suggesting that the DHP site is indeed a convulsant drug receptor site, and also raising the question of what might be the naturally occurring ligand in the brain which uses this receptor site (see below).

DHP binding was also inhibited by numerous CNS depressant drugs including hypnotic barbiturates (at 1-100 μM [36]), anticonvulsant barbiturates (1-500 μM), diphenylhydantoin (100 μM [21, 34]), and benzodiazepines (0.1-50 μM [12, 23]). The effective concentrations of these drugs, although high, are consistent with pharmacological potencies of these compounds. The barbiturates inhibit DHP in concentrations similar to those which enhance GABA synaptic responses involving chloride conductance increases (2) and to concentrations which reverse the effects of GABA synaptic antagonists such as bicuculline and picrotoxin (25). These in vitro effects of barbiturates occur at concentrations lower than those required (millimolar) for "nonspecific" membrane and protein perturbations (27). The relative potency of various barbiturates for inhibiting DHP binding (e.g. hexobarbital > pentobarbital > phenobarbital) agreed roughly with drug potency (5, 7), suggesting that the DHP binding site might reasonably be involved in at least some of the actions of depressant barbiturates. Anticonvulsant activity was more difficult to correlate with this drug receptor site, but the action of convulsant barbiturates seems likely to involve the DHP binding site.

With respect to benzodiazepine inhibition of DHP binding, whereas chemical and stereospecificity was observed for a series of compounds (some examples are given in Table 1) (12, 23), the effective concentrations were not only much higher than those active (14, 29) on the high affinity brain benzodiazepine binding site (both measured at 0°) but no correlation was found between relative potencies at the two types of site. Since the high affinity benzodiazepine binding sites appear to correlate well with the anxiolytic, anticonvulsant, muscle relaxant, and hypnotic activities of these drugs (14, 29), the low affinity benzodiazepine binding sites (DHP sites) apparently do not. The possibility remains that the DHP binding sites (or a subpopulation thereof) may correspond to the site of action for part of the

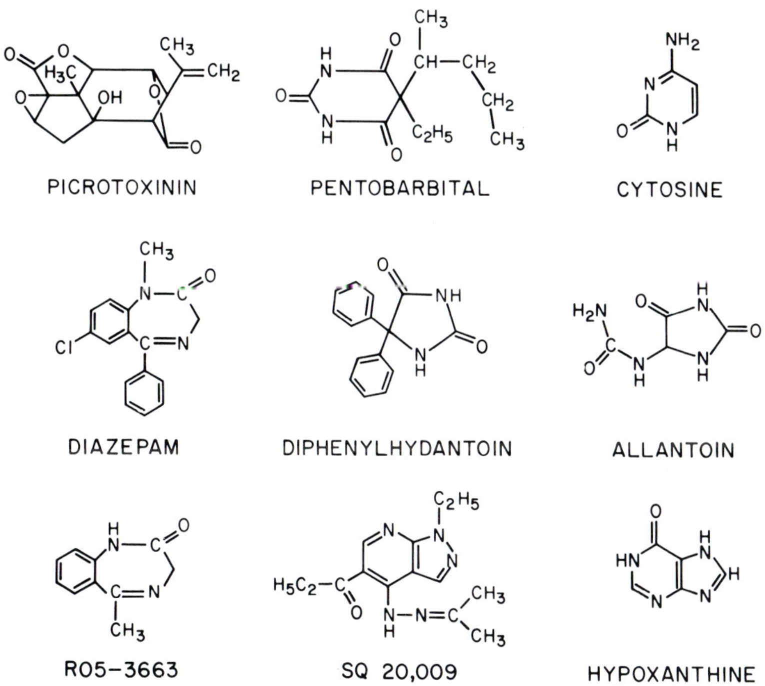

FIG. 1. Structures of drugs active on DHP binding sites.

pharmacological profile of benzodiazepines. However, the two types of drug receptor site appear distinct. Interestingly, the excitatory benzodiazepine RO5-3663 binds competitively to the DHP sites (12, 23) with a higher affinity than for the high affinity benzodiazepine sites, suggesting that its convulsant and GABA blocking action (26) probably involves the DHP sites.

AN ENDOGENOUS PICROTOXININ/BARBITURATE-LIKE SUBSTANCE IN BRAIN?

Might there be a natural substance in brain which utilizes the DHP receptor site in vivo? The supernatant fraction of crude brain homogenates was found to inhibit competitively the binding of DHP, giving half-maximal inhibition at 40-50 μg of soluble protein with $[^3H]$ DHP at 50 nM and 10 nM membrane binding sites. This crude inhibitor was found to be stable to boiling, dialyzeable, and effective at 0° without preincubation (22, 23).

The endogenous inhibitor(s) of DHP binding has not yet been identified, but some other naturally occurring inhibitors of DHP binding have been found, namely, purines and pyrimidines. DHP binding was inhibited competitively by adenine at 0.12 mM (but not adenosine) and by hypoxanthine, inosine, cytosine, uric acid, and allantoin (22, 23), at about 0.1-0.3 mM. These observations are of interest for two reasons.

First, the therapeutic exogenous substances, the barbiturates, are chemically classified as pyrimidines (like cytosine) and are similar in structure to purines (like adenine and hypoxanthine); also, diphenylhydantoin is an analogue of the purine metabolite allantoin. Some of these natural analogues of the depressant drugs also have CNS depressant neuropharmacological effects (24). All of these substances (Figure 1) weakly inhibit DHP binding, suggesting that one of the purines, pyrimidines, hydantoins, or some related natural substance might function as an endogenous depressant or excitatory substance at brain DHP sites, thus modulating GABAergic inhibitory synaptic transmission.

Second, some of the same natural substances such as the purines (hypoxanthine, inosine) have also been observed to inhibit at millimolar concentrations the high affinity benzodiazepine binding sites (1, 24), and so does diphenylhydantoin at 10μM (38). Although the DHP and high affinity benzodiazepine binding sites do not seem to be the same (as discussed above), the sensitivity of both types of sites to certain purines and hydantoins may not be coincidental, since both appear to be part of the postsynaptic membrane GABA receptor-ionophore complex. Allosteric coupling between GABA receptor binding sites and benzodiazepine binding sites has been observed in vitro (33), and we have recently found allosteric perturbations of benzodiazepine binding by drugs binding at the DHP sites (12), as described below.

COUPLING BETWEEN SOME PICROTOXIN-BARBITURATE RECEPTOR SITES AND SOME BENZODIAZEPINE RECEPTOR SITES

Whereas drugs binding to GABA receptor sites can allosterically perturb benzodiazepine binding, (either by increasing the binding affinity, or by inhibiting this enhancement by those GABA analogues

TABLE 2. Interaction with benzodiazepine receptors by SQ 20009 occurs at the picrotoxinin binding site.[a]

Additions	Percent of control specific binding [³H] Diazepam	[³H] DHP
SQ 20009 (μM)	100	100
0.3	105	89
1	120	83
10	135	50
20	105	35
SQ 20009 (10 μM) + picrotoxinin (μM)		
0.01	135	
0.1	124	
1	121	
10	113	
100	109	

[a] DHP binding was measured as described in Table 1, with quadruplicate assays done twice. Rat cortex membranes (fraction $P_2 + P_3$) were prepared by freezing and thawing and five washes (32) to remove endogenous GABA (15). Diazepam binding was measured by filtration following 30 min incubations at 0° with 0.5 nM [^{3}H] diazepam (85 Ci/mmol, NEN) in 5 mM $NaPO_4$, 0.2 M NaCl, pH 7.0, using 10 μM nonradioactive diazepam to determine nondisplaceable background.

which do enhance benzodiazepine binding [6]), some other anxiolytic drugs of the triazolopyridazine variety (purine analogues) either inhibit benzodiazepine binding with a shallow displacement curve (3), and those of the pyrazolopyridine variety (Hill number < 1) enhance benzodiazepine binding (3, 40). This enhancement does not involve GABA receptor sites and might theoretically require another drug receptor site of action, although all drugs affecting benzodiazepine binding in any manner could have in common some relationship to GABA-regulated chloride ion channels.

The enhancement of benzodiazepine binding by one of these purine analogue anxiolytics, SQ 20009, has been reported to be chloride-dependent and sensitive to picrotoxin (32). We have reproduced these findings and also extended them to show that SQ 20009 very likely acts via the picrotoxinin binding site. Table 2 describes how SQ 20009 inhibits [^{3}H] DHP binding (IC_{50} = 8 μM) at concentrations similar to those enhancing benzodiazepine binding (EC_{50} = 2 μM), and picrotoxinin reverses the enhancement by SQ 20009 with an IC_{50} (3 μM) similar to its IC_{50} for the DHP site (0.5μ M) (Leeb-Lundberg, Snowman, and Olsen, submitted). This observation provides an important link between DHP binding sites and GABA receptor sites, since both have now been shown to interact with benzodiazepine binding sites. SQ 20009 has also been found to allosterically perturb GABA receptor binding in a chloride-dependent manner (25).

This interaction of some DHP sites with some benzodiazepine sites is supported by studies on other drugs which bind to the DHP site, which show that all of these drugs perturb benzodiazepine binding, either enhancing it (like SQ 20009), or blocking the effect of SQ 20009 (like picrotoxinin). Thus convulsants like bicyclophosphates and benzodiazepine RO5-3663 reverse the SQ 20009 enhancement, whereas barbiturates enhance benzodiazepine binding. The enhancement of benzodiazepine binding by barbiturates, like that by SQ 20009 (3, 40), involves a change in K_D rather than any alteration in the number of binding sites (13, Leeb-Lundberg, Snowman, and Olsen, submitted).

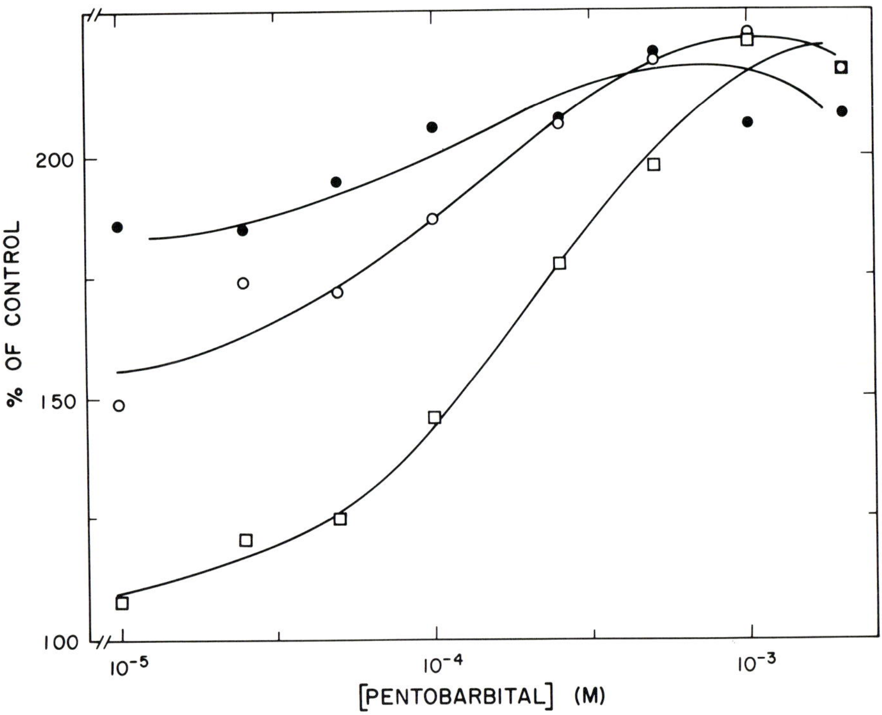

FIG. 2. Enhancement of benzodiazepine binding by varying concentrations of pentobarbital in the absence and presence of SQ 20009. Diazepam binding was measured by filtration (Whatman GF/c), following equilibration for 30 min at 0° with 0.5 nM [^{3}H] diazepam (85 Ci/mmol, NEN), using 10 μM nonradioactive diazepam to determine nondisplaceable background. Fresh rat cortex membranes (fraction P_2 + P_3) were subjected to osmotic shock (disruption by tissuemizer Ultra-turrax in 20 vol H_2O) and two buffer washes with 10 mM $NaPO_4$, 0.2 M NaCl, pH 7.0. Pentobarbital alone (□); varying pentobarbital plus constant SQ 20009 (O, 1 μM, ●, 10 μM). Each plot is the average of three experiments in triplicate, with variation ± 10%.

Figure 2 shows a concentration-dependent enhancement by pentobarbital of benzodiazepine binding. The EC_{50} of pentobarbital is about 100 μM, with a maximal effect of about 100% enhancement. Addition of SQ 20009 to such assays shows that the effect of just-maximal concentrations of the two drugs are not additive, consistent with action on the same site, the DHP site. Furthermore, effects of both drugs are completely dependent on chloride ions (not shown). By contrast, enhancement of benzodiazepine binding by GABA is completely additive with that of SQ 20009 or barbiturates, consistent with action on two different sites, and the effect of GABA is not chloride dependent (Leeb-Lundberg, Snowman, and Olsen, submitted).

Figure 3 shows that picrotoxinin reverses the pentobarbital enhancement of benzodiazepine binding with an IC_{50} ($\simeq$5 μM) roughly equal to the affinity of picrotoxinin for the DHP site, especially considering that DHP must displace pentobarbital from a half-saturated receptor under these conditions. A series of barbiturates shows a relative activity for this effect (secobarbital > pentobarbital>>phenobarbital ≥ barbital) which correlates better than any heretofore described in vitro action of barbiturates with the

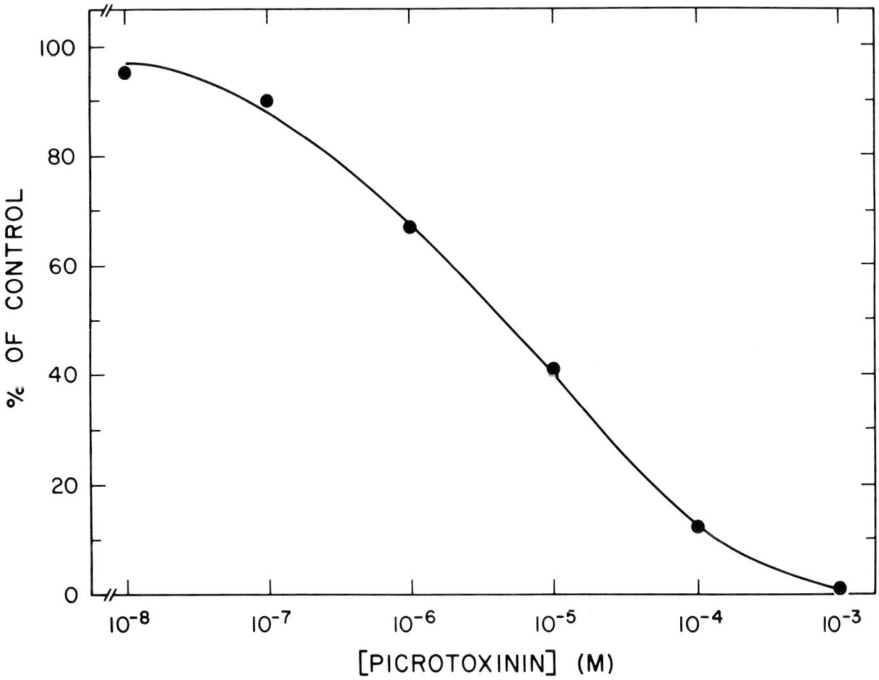

FIG. 3. Inhibition by picrotoxinin of pentobarbital enhancement of benzodiazepine binding. Membranes were prepared and assayed for [^{3}H] diazepam binding as described in FIG. 2 and TABLE 2.

pharmacological action of these drugs (sedative-hynotic activity [7] or reversal of GABA synaptic antagonists [5]). Furthermore the enhancement of benzodiazepine binding by barbiturates is stereospecific, since a greater effect was seen with the active hypnotic (+) hexobarbital than with the less active (-) isomer (39). Thus at least some of the picrotoxin-sensitive barbiturate receptor sites seem related both to pharmacological activity and to the GABA receptor-ionophore complex (by virtue of the interaction with benzodiazepine binding).

Figure 4 shows a hypothetical model of this complex, incorporating the three drug receptors: GABA, picrotoxin-barbiturates, and benzodiazepines, and the functional portion of the system, the chloride ion channel. This model extends our previously described model (21, 36) for picrotoxin-barbiturate action (see also related models of Simmonds

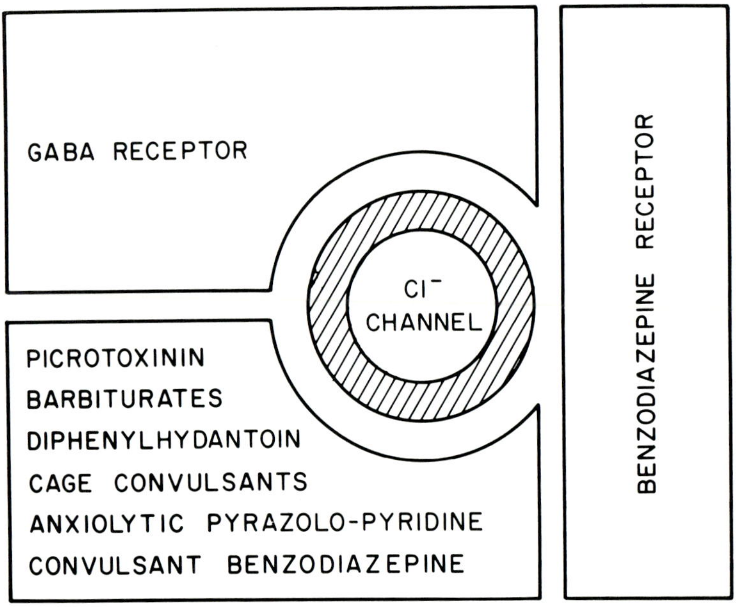

FIG. 4. Theoretical model of the GABA receptor-ionophore complex, including receptors for convulsant and anticonvulsant drugs. The complex contains three drug binding sites, the GABA receptor, the picrotoxinin-barbiturate receptor, and the benzodiazepine receptor, as well as the chloride ion channel. This ion channel may be a separate component or part of one of the drug-binding proteins. We propose that GABA function (opening of the chloride channel) can be modulated by drugs binding to the other two receptor sites, either endogenous ligands or exogenous substances. These drugs can be either positive (depressants) or negative (excitants) modulators of GABA chloride ionophores. Whereas electrophysiological studies (2, 5, 9, 31) are consistent with such a model, and the coupling of these components is suggested by allosteric interactions in vitro, it is possible that 100% of each component in the CNS is not coupled to all the other components.

[28] and Karobath, this volume). We propose that excitatory and depressant drugs act on one of these three drug receptors to either enhance (depressants) or block (excitants) GABA regulated chloride ion channels. It seems reasonable that this system and its associated endogenous ligands are intimately involved in nervous system structures related to excitability control and seizure disorders, and possibly also to sleep and anxiety.

ACKNOWLEDGEMENTS

We thank Drs. C. Napias and M.K. Ticku for assistance with early stages of this work and A. Snowman for expert technical assistance. Supported by NSF Grant BNS 77-24414, the Wills Foundation, and NIH Grants # RR 09077, # NS 12422, and RCDA # NS 00224.

REFERENCES

1. Asano, T. and Spector, S. (1979): Proc. Nat. Acad. Sci. 76: 977-981.
2. Barker, J.L. and McBurney, R.N. (1979): Proc. Roy. Soc. Lond. B, 206: 319-327.
3. Beer, B., Klepner, C.A. Lippa, A.S. and Squires, R.F. (1978): Pharmacol. Biochem. Behav. 9: 849-851.
4. Bowery, N.G., Collins, J.F. and Hill, R.G. (1976): Nature 261: 601-603.
5. Bowery, N.G. and Dray, A. (1978): Br. J. Pharmac. 63: 197-215.
6. Braestrup, C., Nielsen, M., Krogsgaard-Larsen, P., and Falch, E. (1979): Nature 280: 331-333.
7. Butler, T.C. (1942): J. Pharmac. 74: 118-128.
8. Costa, E. and Guidotti, A. (1979) Ann. Rev. Pharmacol. Toxicol. 19: 531-545.
9. Haefely, W., Polc, P., Schaffner, R., Keller, H.H., Pieri, L. and Mohler, H. (1979): In: GABA-Neurotransmitters, edited by P. Krogsgaard-Larsen, J. Scheel-Kruger, and H. Kofod, pp. 357-375. Munksgaard, Copenhagen.
10. Jarboe, C.H. Porter, L.A. and Buckler, R.T. (1968): J. Med. Chem. 11: 729-731.
11. Kelly, J.S., and Krnjevic, K., Morris, M.E. and Yim, G.K.W. (1969): Exptl. Brain Res. 7: 11-31.
12. Leeb-Lundberg, F. and Olsen, R.W. (1980): In: Psychopharmacology and Biochemistry of Neurotransmitter Receptors, edited by H.I. Yamamura, R.W. Olsen, and E. Usdin, Elsevier, New York, in press.
13. Leeb-Lundberg, F., Snowman, A. and Olsen, R.W. (1980): Soc. Neurosci. Abstr. 6: in press.
14. Mohler, H. and Okada, T. (1977): Science 198: 849-851.
15. Napias, C., Bergman, M.O, Van Ness, P.C., Greenlee, D.V. and Olsen, R.W. (1980): Life Sci. 26: in press.
16. Nicoll, R.A., Eccles, J.C., Oshima, T.C. and Rubia, F. (1975): Nature 258: 625-627.
17. Nistri, A. and Constanti, A. (1979): Prog. Neurobiol. 13: 117-235.
18. Olsen. R.W., Ticku, M.K., Van Ness, P.C. and Greenlee, D.V. (1978): Brain Res. 139: 277-294.

19. Olsen, R.W. Greenlee, D., Van Ness, P. and Ticku, M.K. (1978): In: Amino Acids as Chemical Transmitters, edited by F. Fonnum, pp. 467-486. Plenum Press, New York.
20. Olsen, R.W., Ticku, M.K. and Miller, T. (1978): Mol. Pharmacol. 14: 381-390.
21. Olsen, R.W. Ticku, M.K., Greenlee, D. and Van Ness, P. (1979): In: GABA-Neurotransmitters, edited by P. Krogsgaard-Larsen, J. Scheel-Kruger, and H. Kofod, pp. 165-178. Munksgaard, Copenhagen.
22. Olsen, R.W. and Leeb-Lundberg, F. (1980): Eur. J. Pharmac. in press.
23. Olsen, R.W. Leeb-Lundberg, F. and Napias, C. (1980): In: GABA-Neurotransmission, edited by H. Lal, Brain Res. Bull. in press.
24. Paul, S.M., Marangos, P. and Skolnick, P. (1980): In: Phychopharmacology and Biochemistry of Neurotransmitter Receptors, edited by H.I. Yamamura, R.W. Olsen, and E. Usdin, Elsevier, New York, in press.
25. Placheta, P. and Karobath, M. (1980): Eur. J. Pharm. 62: 225-228.
26. Schlosser, W. and Franco, S. (1979): J. Pharm. Exptl. Ther. 211: 290-295.
27. Seeman, P. (1972): Pharmac. Rev. 24: 583-655.
28. Simmonds, M.A. (1980): Nature 284: 558-560.
29. Squires, R.F. and Braestrup, C. (1977): Nature 266: 732-734.
30. Straughan, D.W. (1974): Neuropharmacology 13: 495-508.
31. Straughan, D.W. (1978): Adv. Pharmacol. Therap. 2: Neurotransmitters, edited by P. Simon, pp. 19-27, Peragmon, Oxford.
32. Supavilai, P and Karobath, M. (1979): Eur. J. Pharm. 60: 111-113.
33. Tallman, J.F., Paul, S.M., Skolnick, P. and Gallager, D.W. (1980): Science 207: 274-281.
34. Ticku, M.K., Ban, M. and Olsen, R.W. (1978): Mol. Pharmacol. 14: 391-402.
35. Ticku, M.K., Van Ness, P.C., Haycock, J.W., Levy, W.B. and Olsen, R.W. (1978): Brain Res. 150: 642-647.
36. Ticku, M.K. and Olsen, R.W. (1978): Life Sci. 22: 1643-1652.
37. Ticku, M.K. and Olsen, R.W. (1979): Neuropharmacology 18: 315-318.
38. Tunnicliff, G., Smith, J.A. and Ngo, T.T. (1979): Biochem. Biophys. Res. Comm. 91: 1018-1024.
39. Wahlstrom, G., Buch, H. and Buzello, W. (1970): Acta Pharmacol. Toxicol. 28: 493-498.
40. Williams, M. and Risley, E.A. (1979): Life Sci. 24: 833-842.

GABA and Benzodiazepine Receptors,
edited by E. Costa et al.
Raven Press, New York © 1981.

Demonstration and Characterization of an Endogenous Inhibitor of GABA-Enhanced [^{3}H]-Diazepam Binding from Bovine Cerebral Cortex

*S. Paul, *P. Marangos, **M. Brownstein, and †P. Skolnick

**Clinical Psychobiology Branch, **Laboratory of Clinical Science, NIMH, and †Laboratory of Bioorganic Chemistry, NIAMDD, National Institute of Health, Bethesda, Maryland 20205*

Introduction

The demonstration of high affinity, saturable, and stereospecific binding sites for benzodiazepines in the mammalian CNS has dramatically altered current thinking on both the mechanism(s) of action of this class of psychotropic agents and the neurochemical bases of anxiety, seizures, and muscle relaxation (17). The excellent correlation(s) obtained between the in vitro affinities of a series of benzodiazepines for these binding sites and their relative clinical and behavioral potencies in vivo (9, 16) strongly suggest(s) that these sites are pharmacologic receptors. Furthermore, recent work from our laboratory and others (6, 13) has provided direct evidence that occupation of benzodiazepine receptors is highly correlated with both the anticonvulsant and anticonflict (anxiolytic) effects of parenterally administered diazepam. Although these data strongly support a role for benzodiazepine receptors in the therapeutic actions of these agents, little is known about the physiological (or pathophysiologic) role(s) of these receptors.

Since benzodiazepine receptors possess pharmacological and biochemical characteristics reminiscent of the "classical" neurotransmitter receptor system, it has been suggested that, like these systems, endogenous compound(s) which function as physiologic receptor ligands (or modulators) may exist. Shortly after the identification of the benzodiazepine receptor, several substances were isolated from brain and identified as putative endogenous ligands of the receptor. Low molecular weight (less than 10^4 daltons) compounds which have been identified as competitive inhibitors of [^{3}H] benzodiazepine binding include the purines inosine and hypoxanthine, and the vitamin, nicotinamide (1, 10, 14). These compounds have also been shown to possess some benzodiazepine-like activity in several neuropharmacologic and electrophysiologic tests (7, 10, 15). Other low molecular weight factors isolated and characterized by our laboratory (8) and others (3) remain unidentified. In addition, relatively higher molecular weight factors (greater than 10^4 daltons) which competitively inhibit [^{3}H] benzodiazepine binding have also been described (2, 5, 18). One of these factors, "GABA-modulin" (M.W. ∿15,000 daltons) may affect both the GABA and benzodiazepine receptors.

GABA does not bind to the recognition site for benzodiazepines, but will alter the affinity of the receptor for benzodiazepines (and presumably other compounds which bind to this recognition site). Hence GABA may be considered an endogenous modulator of the benzodiazepine receptor. Recently, both the convulsant benzodiazepine Ro-5-3663 (11) and pentylenetetrazole (Paul and Skolnick, in preparation) have been demonstrated to antagonize GABA enhanced increases in [^{3}H] benzodiazepine binding at concentrations below those needed to displace [^{3}H] benzodiazepines from their recognition sites. These observations, taken together with the high (4) concentrations of GABA (mM) present in the CNS, suggests that the modulation of the GABA-benzodiazepine "coupling" mechanism may be important for both the pharmacologic and physiologic regulation of the benzodiazepine receptor. We now report the presence in bovine brain of a low molecular weight substance(s) which is 10-20 fold more potent in antagonizing the GABA-enhanced binding of [^{3}H] diazepam than in antagonizing basal (non-GABA enhanced) binding of [^{3}H] diazepam to receptor sites.

Methods

Tissue Preparation.

Fresh bovine brain was obtained from a local slaughterhouse within 20 min after sacrifice and placed on ice. The cerebral cortex (frontal, temporal, parietal, and occipital lobes) was dissected (all procedures were carried out at 0-4°) and approximately 100 g of tissue was homogenized in 10 vol 0.32 M sucrose (Fig. 1). A crude synaptosomal membrane preparation was prepared by differential centrifugation (12). The P_2 fraction was then osmotically shocked by resuspension in hypotonic buffer (5 mM Tris-HCl, pH 7.4), shaken on ice for 60 min, and frozen for at least 12 hours at -20°. The membranes were thawed and stirred gently prior to centrifugation at 100,000 x g for 1 hr. The supernatant was filtered through an Amicon PM-10 membrane and the ultrafiltrate lyophilized to yield the "crude extract".

Chromatography

The lyophilized crude extract was resuspended in a small volume of 10 mM acetic acid and chromatographed on a Biogel P-6 column (2.5 x 90 cm). The column was eluted with 10 mM acetic acid at a flow rate of 21 ml/hr. The column fractions (7 ml) were

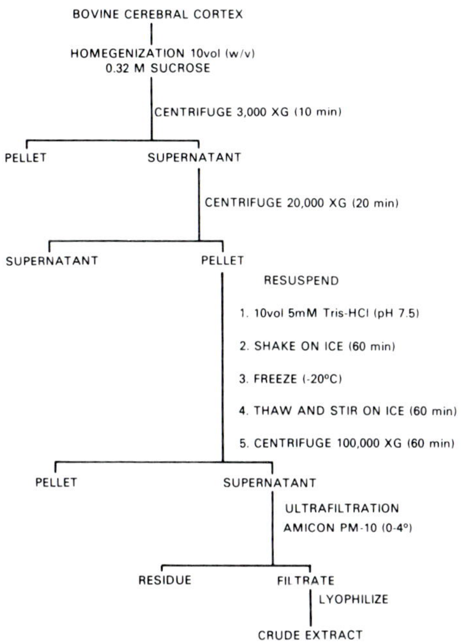

FIG. 1. Flow scheme for preparation of crude extract.

lyophilized and reconstituted in 0.5 ml of 50 mM Tris-HCl buffer (pH 7.4). Column fractions (0.1 ml) were assayed for activity as inhibitors of [^{3}H] diazepam binding to well washed (five times), freeze-thawed rat cortical membranes in the presence and absence of 1 μM GABA. The radioligand concentration ([^{3}H] diazepam) in these assays was 1 nM in an incubation volume of 1 ml. The conditions for assay of [^{3}H] diazepam binding have been described elsewhere (12).

Biogel P-6 fractions which inhibited [^{3}H] diazepam binding were further separated by high-pressure liquid chromatography (HPLC) using a Varian 5020 Liquid Chromatograph. Pooled fractions from the Biogel P-6 column (0.2-0.7 ml) were applied to a Varian TSK 2000 column and eluted with 50 mM sodium phosphate buffer (pH 7.0) at ambient temperature. Peaks were detected for UV absorbance at 206 nm and collected for assay as inhibitors of GABA-enhanced [^{3}H] diazepam binding as described (12).

Results

Examination of the Biogel P-6 eluates for their ability to

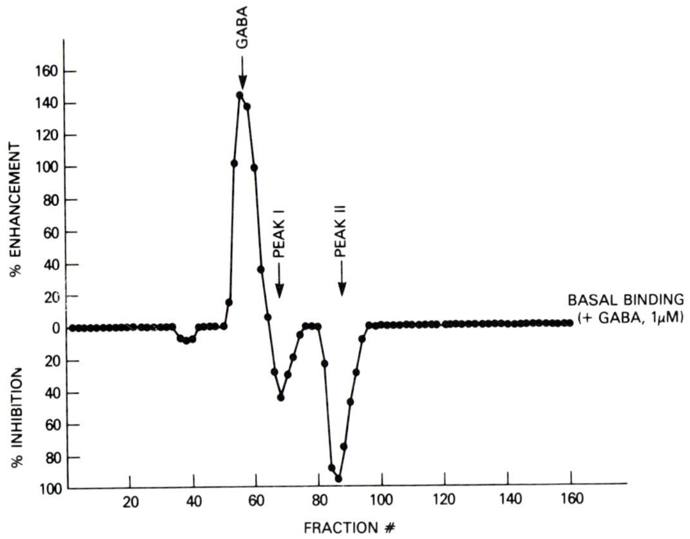

FIG. 2. Effects of Biogel P-6 on GABA-enhanced [^{3}H] diazepam binding. "Crude extract" was eluates prepared as described in Methods and applied to a Biogel P-6 column. The column was eluted as described and 7 ml fractions were collected, lyophylized, and resuspended in 0.5 ml of 50 mM Tris-HCl buffer (pH 7.4). Aliquots (0.1 ml) were assayed for their effects on [^{3}H] diazepam binding in the presence of 1 μM GABA. The % enhancement and inhibition refer to values obtained compared with GABA alone. Using well washed membranes, GABA (1 μM) elicited a 50-100% increase in [^{3}H] diazepam binding at a radioligand concentration of 1 nM. Results are from a typical elution profile.

effect GABA-enhanced [^{3}H] diazepam binding revealed two peaks of inhibitory activity (Peaks I and II) (Fig. 2) and one peak of stimulatory activity. In contrast, when GABA was omitted from the incubations, only an enhancement of [^{3}H] diazepam binding was observed (unpublished results). This increase in [^{3}H] diazepam binding seen in both the presence and absence of 1 μM GABA appears to be due to the presence of endogenous GABA, since application of authentic GABA to the Biogel P-6 column results in elution between tubes 50-65 (cf. Fig. 2). The potency of Peak II in inhibiting basal and GABA-enhanced [^{3}H] diazepam binding was then

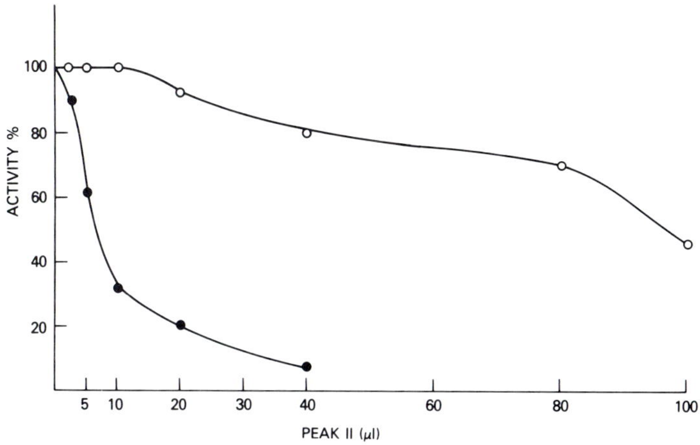

FIG. 3. Effects of Peak II on [^{3}H] diazepam binding. Aliquots of pooled fractions (Peak II) from the Biogel P-6 column were added to washed brain membranes containing 1 nM [^{3}H] diazepam with (●) or without (o) 1 μM GABA. % Activity refers to the amount of [^{3}H] diazepam binding per assay in the presence or absence of GABA. Values are from a representative experiment. The amount of active material extracted varied from perparation to preparation (e.g., compare Fig. 2 and 3).

examined (Fig. 3). Peak II is 10-20 fold more potent as an inhibitor of GABA-enhanced than basal [^{3}H] diazepam binding. The IC_{50} for inhibition of GABA-enhanced binding is approximately 7 μl in this preparation, while nearly 100 μl of Peak II is necessary to reduce basal binding by 50%. Since GABA has been demonstrated to increase [^{3}H] diazepam binding to brain membranes by increasing receptor affinity rather than receptor number, the antagonism of this effect by Peak II was then studied using Scatchard analysis. Addition of Peak II competitively antagonized the enhancement of [^{3}H] diazepam binding by GABA (Fig. 4) while the addition of this amount (10 μl) of Peak II to non-GABA stimulated membranes did not affect [^{3}H] diazepam binding. Chromatography of pooled fractions of Peak II on HPLC revealed several fractions containing uv absorbing material. One major fraction containing the inhibitor(s) of GABA-enhanced [^{3}H] diazepam binding was eluted with retention time of 19 min (Fig. 5).

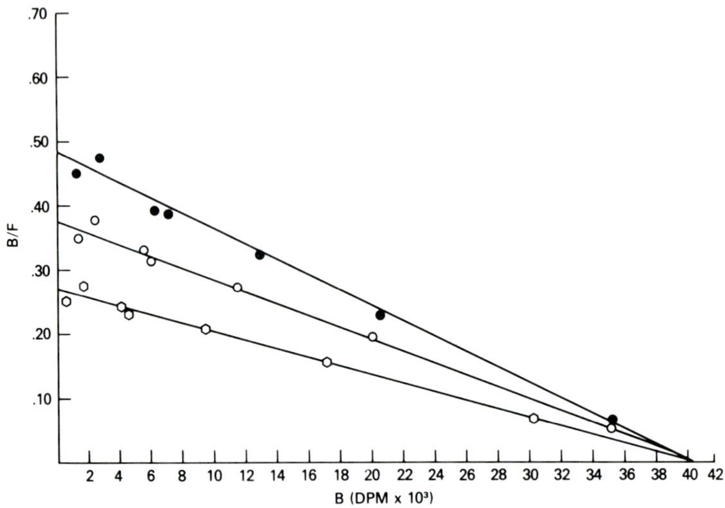

FIG. 4. Scatchard analysis of GABA-enhanced [^{3}H] diazepam binding. Radioligand concentrations ranged from 0.5 to 16 nM. Each point is the $\bar{X}$ of a triplicate determination.

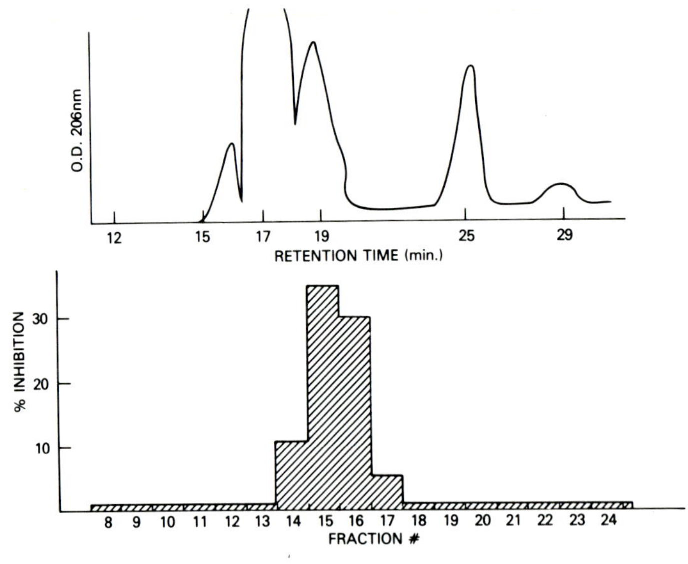

FIG. 5. HPLC characterization of Peak II. HPLC was performed using a Varian TSK 2000 column. Upper tracing: ordinate, absorbance at 206 nm. Abcissa: retention time in minutes. Lower tracing: ordinate, % inhibition of GABA-enhanced [^{3}H] diazepam binding. Abcissa: fractions collected (1 ml). Inhibition peak corresponds to a retention time of 19 min.

Discussion

The GABA mediated enhancement of benzodiazepine receptor affinity may represent an important means of expressing the actions of both pharmacologic agents and endogenous ligands. Recent observations that PTZ (Paul and Skolnick, in preparation) and Ro-5-3663 (11) can antagonize GABA-elicited increases in [^{3}H] diazepam binding and barbiturates can augment this effect (Skolnick, Paul, and Barker, in preparation) at concentrations lower than those needed to effect basal binding suggested that endogenous factors may also modify GABA-enhanced benzodiazepine binding. Using an aqueous extraction procedure, two peaks were eluted from a Biogel P-6 column which antagonized the GABA-enhanced increase in [^{3}H] diazepam binding. The substance(s) contained in one of the peaks (Peak II) proved to be far more potent in antagonizing this effect than in displacing [^{3}H] diazepam from non-GABA stimulated membranes, suggesting a specificity for the GABA-benzodiazepine coupling site rather than the benzodiazepine recognition site. Alternatively, in the presence of GABA, the affinity of this substance(s) (Peak II) may be selectively enhanced resulting in a decreased binding of radioligand. The mobility of this compound on HPLC suggests a molecular weight of between 300 and 1600 daltons. The factor(s) is heat stable, dialyzable, and not degraded by incubation with papain (Paul et al., unpublished observations), properties which differ substantially from other factors (e.g., GABA-modulin) which also appear to affect both GABA and benzodiazepine receptors. Future investigations will focus on the purification, identification, and determination of the physiologic role of this factor.

Acknowledgement

The authors thank Ms. B. Hulihan and Ms. M. Mattson for excellent technical assistance.

References

1. Asano, T., and Spector, S. (1979): Proc. Natl. Acad. Sci. (USA) 76: 977-981.
2. Colello, G.D., Hockenberry, D.M., Bosmann, H.B., Fuchs, S., and Folkers, K. (1978): Proc. Natl. Acad. Sci. (USA) 75: 6319-6323.
3. Davis, L.G., and Cohen, R.K. (1980) Biochem. Biophys. Res. Comm. 92: 141-148.
4. Fuxe, K., Andersson, K., Ogren, S.O., Perez de la Mora, M., Schwarcz, R., Hokfelt, T., Eneroth, P., Gustafsson, J.A., and Skett, P. (1979): In: GABA-Neurotransmitters: Pharmacochemical, Biochemical and Pharmacological Aspects, edited by P. Krogsgaard-Larsen, J. Scheel-Kruger, and H. Kofod, pp. 74-94. Academic Press, New York.

5. Guidotti, A., Toffano, G., and Costa, E. (1978): Nature 275: 553-555.
6. Lippa, A.S., Klepner, C.A., Younger, L., Sano, M.C., Smith, W.V., and Beer, B. (1978): Pharmacol. Biochem. Behav. 9: 853-856.
7. MacDonald, J.F., Barker, J.L., Paul, S.M., Marangos, P.J., and Skolnick, P. (1979): Science 205: 715-717.
8. Marangos, P.J., Clark, R., Martino, A.M., Paul, S.M., and Skolnick, P. (1979): Psych. Res. 1: 121-130.
9. Mohler, H., and Okada, T. (1977): Science 198: 849-851.
10. Mohler, H., Polc, P., Cumin, R., Pieri, L., and Kettler, R. (1979): Nature 278: 563-565.
11. O'Brien, R.A., and Spirt, N.M. (1980): Life Sci. 26: 1441-1445.
12. Paul, S., and Skolnick, P. (1978): Science 202: 892-894.
13. Paul, S.M., Syapin, P.J., Paugh, B., Moncada, V., and Skolnick, P. (1979): Nature 281: 688-689.
14. Skolnick, P., Marangos, P.J., Goodwin, F.K., Edwards, M., and Paul, S.M. (1978): Life Sci. 23: 1473-1480.
15. Skolnick, P., Syapin, P., Paugh, B., Moncada, V., Marangos, P., and Paul, S.M. (1979): Proc. Natl. Acad. Sci. (USA) 76: 1515-1518.
16. Squires, R., and Braestrup, C. (1977): Nature 266: 732-734.
17. Tallman, J.F., Paul, S.M., Skolnick, P., and Gallager, D.W. (1980): Science 207: 274-281.

GABA and Benzodiazepine Receptors,
edited by E. Costa et al.
Raven Press, New York © 1981.

Desensitization of GABA Receptors

K. Krnjević

Departments of Anaesthesia Research and Physiology, McGill University, McIntyre Medical Building, Montreal PQ Canada, Canada H3G 1Y6

That the inhibitory action of GABA tends to "fade" has been known since some of the earliest microiontophoretic studies on the mammalian central nervous system. Curtis et al. (10) and Krnjević and Phillis (22) noted that during a maintained iontophoretic application, the inhibitory effect was most pronounced initially and tended to diminish with time. Clearly, such a phenomenon might be due to a desensitization of GABA receptors, comparable to the desensitization of ACh-receptors at the neuromuscular junction proposed by Katz and Thesleff (18). Without more information about membrane changes, however, some alternative mechanisms could not be excluded.

In the present article, various possibilities will be considered and the likelihood that they can explain the observed experimental data.

A Diminished Cl^- Gradient

It is now well established that, in vertebrates, GABA acts predominantly by increasing Cl^- permeability (P_{Cl}). This appears to be true for both post-synaptic and presynaptic inhibition (20) - the only possible exception being the GABA-mediated presynaptic depression of Ca^{2+}-inward current recently described by Dunlap and Fischbach (14). The potential change evoked by GABA is thus a function of the transmembrane Cl^- gradient; so the large increase in P_{Cl} generated by GABA - and correspondingly large flux of Cl^- - must tend to bring the internal Cl^- concentration closer to equilibrium at the resting potential. Therefore GABA's hyperpolarizing post-synaptic action (or depolarizing presynaptic effect on primary afferent fibres) should diminish with time. If this were the only significant process, there would be no other major change in the membrane responses evoked by GABA. As discussed in the next section, however, the membrane conductance increase evoked by GABA also "fades" during a prolonged application.

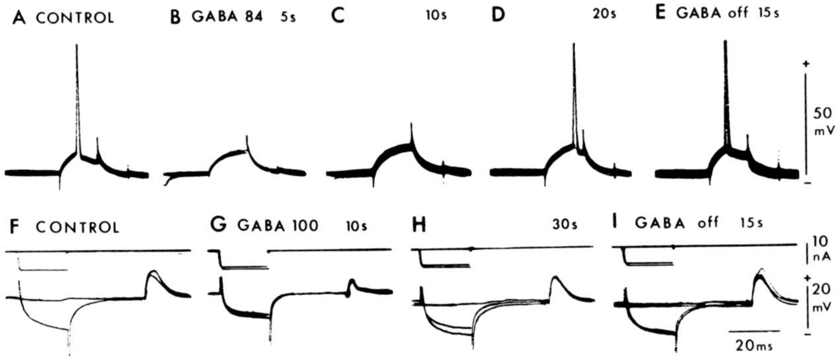

FIG. 1. Intracellular records from cat spinal motoneurons illustrating apparent desensitization to GABA. A-E: Direct stimulation by intracellular depolarizing pulse of constant intensity throughout. Steady iontophoretic application of GABA (84 nA) initially blocks firing (B) but after 10 s (C) subthreshold depolarization grows, and then (D) initiates delayed spike. E, post-GABA recovery. F-I: in another motoneuron, hyperpolarizing effect of constant current pulses (monitored in traces above), and partial antidromic spike were recorded before (F), during (G,H) and after (I) application of GABA (100 nA). Marked fall in membrane resistance in G is only transient. (Figure 2 from Krnjević et al. (23)).

Fading of GABA-evoked Conductance Increase

This was first reported in some detail by Dreifuss et al. (13). In their experiments on cortical neurons in cats, they observed a very pronounced increase in cell input conductance near the start of an iontophoretic injection; but within 10 sec, the conductance diminished to a lower plateau. This change was especially pronounced with larger applications of GABA when the initial peak of conductance was particularly high.

Comparable observations at a variety of sites have confirmed the widespread nature of this phenomenon: thus it has been seen in the Mauthner cell of fish (12); in mammalian sympathetic ganglia (2); dorsal root ganglia (11); spinal motoneurons (Fig.1) (23); and hippocampal pyramids (Fig. 5) (3).

Could the depression of the GABA-evoked conductance increase result from a significant depletion of Cl^- near the membrane? By reducing current flow through the open Cl^- channels this could result in a diminished *conductance*. Some reduction in external

Cl^- concentration is to be expected during inhibition by GABA; but in view of the relatively small difference between resting potential and the Cl^- equilibrium potential (V_{Cl}) the changes could only be small. Furthermore, fully comparable fading of GABA-evoked conductance is seen when V_{Cl} is relatively positive (Fig. 5) (2,3) and in spinal motoneurons, there is no fading of Cl^- conductance when this is raised by glycine rather than by GABA (23,37).

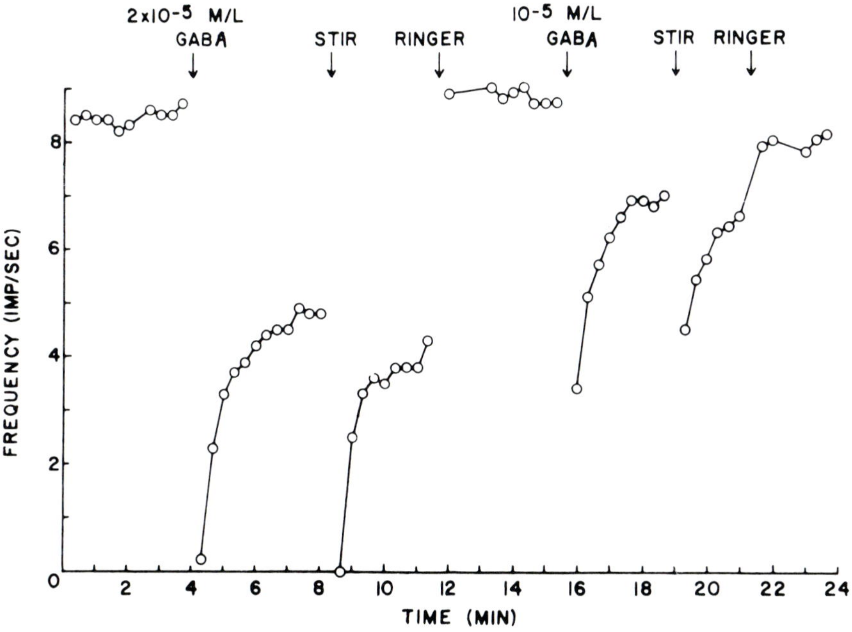

FIG. 2. Inactivation of GABA applied to crayfish stretch receptor neuron. Application of GABA at concentrations indicated cause only transient maximal inhibition of firing; but full inhibition is restored by stirring bathing solution (Fig. 10 from Kuffler and Edwards (25)).

Is Fading Due to GABA Uptake?

In their pioneering study of the inhibitory action of GABA in crustacean stretch receptor neurons, Kuffler and Edwards (25) made a striking observation. When enough GABA was applied in the bath, the neuron ceased firing; but the discharge resumed after a few sec (Fig. 2). At first, this seemed to indicate some form of desensitization; but it was then found that if the bathing medium was stirred the inhibition of firing returned (Fig. 2). The only reasonable conclusion was that, in the vicinity of the neuron, GABA must have been removed either by enzymatic action or by cellular uptake. GABA uptake is now widely recognized as the principal mechanism of removal of GABA from the synaptic space (15,27, 34). The uptake occurs both into nerve endings and satellite cells, and may be particularly effective at synaptic sites (cf.32).

Much emphasis has been placed on the Na^+ dependence of GABA uptake as a specific feature indicating its transmitter function (34); but Na^+-coupled transport is probably a universal feature of neutral amino acid (and sugar) uptake (17,33). Thus, GABA uptake may alter the membrane potential both in Aplysia and in cats. According to Kehoe (19), GABA (as well as other neutral amino acids) can produce significant depolarization by an effect that is independent of the GABA-synaptic receptors and which is most easily explained by a Na^+-coupled, electrogenic transport. A comparable process in cat spinal motoneurons may be indicated by a positive shift in the reversal potential for the effect of GABA observed during applications of GABA (23) as well as by the persistence of a depolarizing action of GABA after inactivation of GABA receptors by bicuculline (Fig. 4). There is at present no direct evidence that motoneurons are able to take up GABA, although Deiters' neurons - somewhat comparable non-inhibitory cells that also receive a GABA-ergic innervation - have been shown to contain a substantial amount of GABA (30), presumably because they take up GABA.

Further evidence that motoneurons may be able to transport GABA by an electrogenic mechanism is that intramotoneuronal injections of GABA have a hyperpolarizing action (Fig. 3) not associated with a conductance increase (6). This effect is consistent with an *outward* transport of Na together with GABA, driven by the unusually high outward gradient of GABA resulting from the intracellular injections. The possibility of such a reversal of the usual situation, where the neutral amino acid is transported *inward* along the Na electrochemical gradient, has been directly demonstrated in some other types of cells (26).

Why is there no comparable fading of the effect of glycine? One can presume that glycine is also actively transported out of the extracellular space; but perhaps not as rapidly as GABA and not into post-synaptic neurons. In keeping with this is the absence of any positive shift of reversal potential during applications of glycine (23) and the failure to evoke hyperpolarization by intramotoneuronal injections of glycine (6).

Active removal of GABA by cellular uptake is evidently also important for the maintenance of its normal very low extracellular concentration: and there are at least some indications that the uptake may be sufficiently rapid to reduce the effect of applied GABA and thus at least contribute to the observed fading of its action. But could any other processes also be important? For example, is there any evidence that Cl^- channels become inactivated or that GABA receptors are prone to desensitization?

Inactivation of Cl^- Channels

Changes in Cl^- channel permeability would not be readily distinguished from receptor desensitization, since Cl^- permeability cannot be studied independently of receptor activation. But fortunately, some cells, including spinal motoneurons, are at least as sensitive to glycine as to GABA, and both amino acids appear to induce a similar increase in membrane permeability, involving predominantly or exclusively Cl^- channels (9,23,37). As already mentioned, glycine's action shows no fading. Therefore, inactivation cannot be a general feature of Cl^- channels; and to explain the fading of GABA by this mechanism one would have to postulate

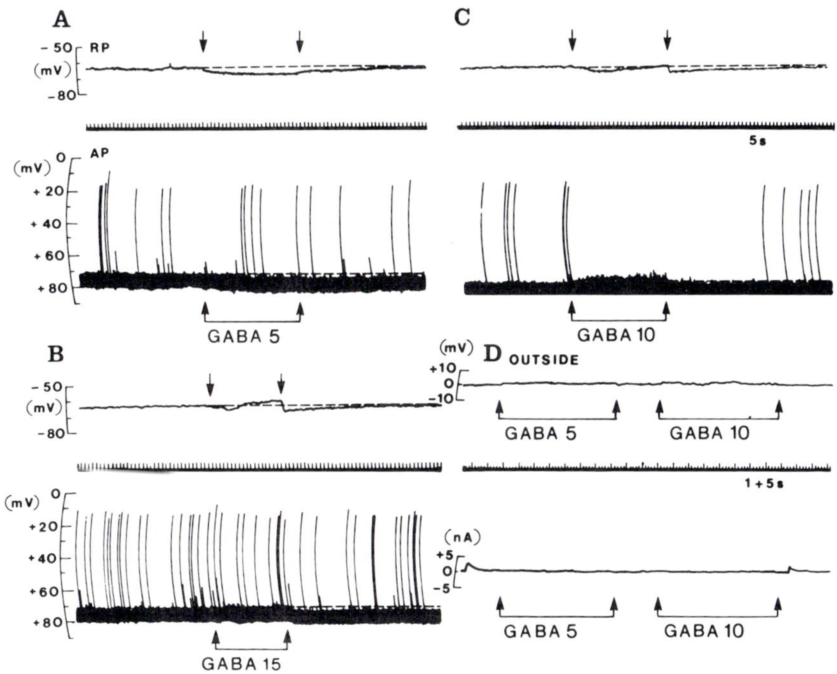

FIG. 3. Slow hyperpolarizing effect of injection of GABA into lumbar motoneuron in cat under Dial. A, B and C are intracellular records. In each case, upper trace shows resting potential (RP) and lower thick trace (AP) peak amplitude of action potential evoked by direct stimulation at 3/s; spike-like transients reflect spontaneous discharges. Intracellular injections of GABA are signalled by arrows; balanced iontophoretic currents are indicated in nA. D, control traces recorded after withdrawing electrode from motoneuron. (Figure 2 from Constanti et al. (6)).

a special property of the Cl^- channels that are controlled by GABA. Extensive tests on hippocampal pyramidal cells in rats (Y. Ben-Ari, K. Krnjević and W. Reinhardt, unpublished observations) have shown some dependence of IPSP-conductance increase (and the effects produced by GABA) on membrane potential; but the changes produced by even large potential shifts were too small to account for those seen during major fading.

Desensitization of GABA Receptors

It should not be taken for granted that desensitization is a universal property of chemical receptors. Apparent desensitization is a well-known characteristic of the nicotinic action of ACh, especially at the neuromuscular junction; but it is not conspicuous at muscarinic sites of action. In vertebrates, glutamate's excitatory action does not fade although it does in crustacean muscle (35). The reverse is seen with GABA, whose action fades in the vertebrate CNS but not in crustacean muscle (36). And of course there is little noticeable fading of glycine.

Even with nicotinic ACh, it is by no means certain that the observed fading of action is a true desensitization as proposed by Katz and Thesleff (18). There is some evidence that ACh receptors *in vitro* may exist in inactive ("desensitized") and active conformations (5); but it is not certain that these are relevant to the *in situ* observations. Other authors have proposed that the apparent loss of effectiveness of ACh may be due to positively charged molecules such as ACh itself entering and blocking the end-plate cationic channels(1).

In the case of GABA, no comparable mechanism of fading can be seriously envisaged, because neither extracellular cations nor GABA (which is practically neutral at a pH near 7) are likely to be attracted to Cl^- channels. On the other hand, it is increasingly evident from in vitro studies that GABA receptor sensitivity is markedly variable, depending on the methods of isolation and the presence or absence of an endogenous modulating factor (7). Thus, the affinity of membrane receptors for GABA is vastly increased by freezing and thawing or by treatment with detergents. Certain molecules have been extracted from the supernatants after such treatment which - when added to the membranes - can lower the receptor sensitivity. There is no consensus as yet concerning the identity of these inhibitory molecules - whether peptide or phospholipid, etc - but the concept of an endogenous modulator is now widely accepted.

Could such an endogenous modulator be "activated" by the binding of GABA to its receptor? Some pharmacological observations indicate that GABA-sensitivity is indeed susceptible to manipulation. It is known that at least two kinds of drugs enhance the action of GABA, barbiturates (29) and benzodiazepines (7), probably by somewhat different mechanisms. More recently, Nestoros (28) has obtained evidence that ethanol also increases the effectiveness of GABA.

A curious feature of fading is that it may disappear in the presence of certain GABA antagonists (24). Thus, as illustrated in Fig. 4, when a neuron recovers its sensitivity to GABA after an application of bicuculline, the GABA-evoked response shows little sign of the normal fading (cf. the control response obtained initially). In the same study, Na-benzyl penicillin - which is also a GABA antagonist, albeit weaker than bicuculline (8) - had only a marginal blocking effect when applied microiontophoretically to motoneurons; nevertheless it also clearly removed

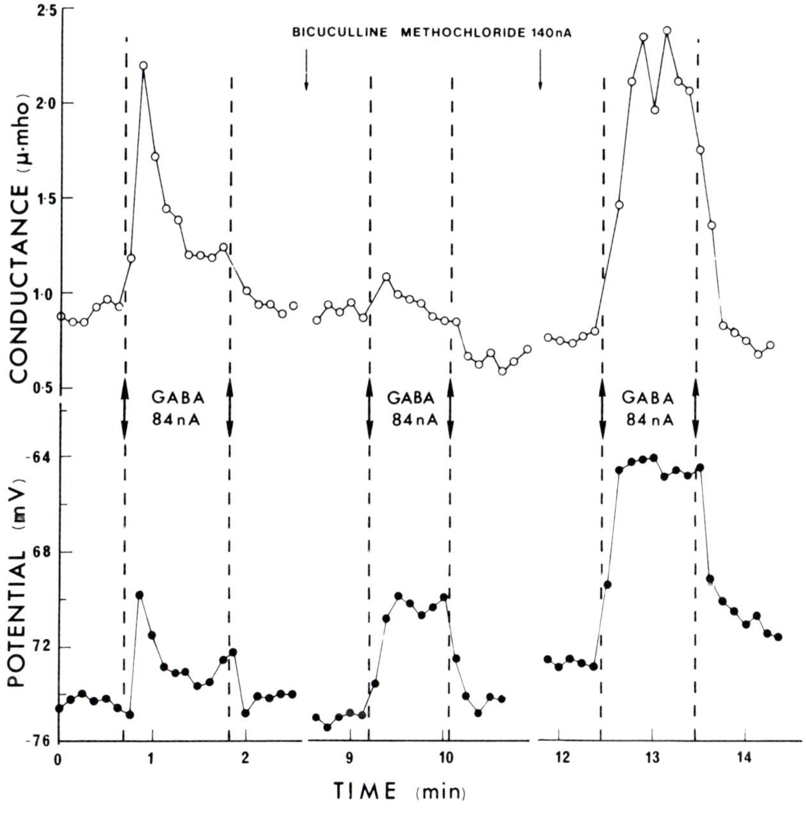

FIG. 4. Bicuculline methochloride eliminates GABA-evoked conductance increase, but not depolarization, and abolishes GABA "desensitization". Effects of GABA were recorded from motoneuron in spinal cord of cat before, during and 2 min after end of iontophoretic release of bicuculline (from left to right). (Figure 9 from Krnjević et al. (24)).

fading. Fading may thus be generated by a change in the conformation of the GABA receptor (presumably induced by the presence of GABA) that is prevented by a simultaneous interaction with antagonist molecules which can themselves bind to the GABA receptors.

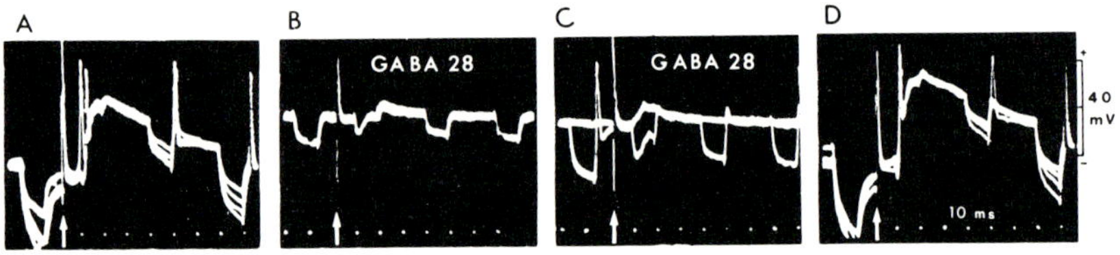

FIG. 5 Effects of GABA on hippocampal pyramidal neuron in rat under urethane. Traces A-D show superimposed IPSPs evoked by entorhinal stimulation. Input conductance was measured with hyperpolarizing pulses. In A, because of leakage of chloride from the microelectrode, IPSPs appear as large positive deflections (resting potential, -78 mV). Note large increase in conductance near peak of IPSP. B, 10 sec after start of GABA release (28 nA), there is a marked depolarization and large increase in resting conductance. C, 10 sec later, while maintaining same GABA release: traces show partial repolarization, clear fall in conductance, particularly at peak of IPSP, indicating not only desensitization to applied GABA but also to naturally released inhibitory transmitter. D, subsequent recovery 30 sec after end of GABA release. (From Fig. 2 in Ben-Ari et al. (3)).

Functional Significance of this Phenomenon

"Desensitization" to ACh at the neuromuscular junction has not been convincingly demonstrated as a consequence of neuromuscular transmission, even during tetanic stimulation (31); therefore it may well be of mainly pharmacological interest (16). This may not be the case with GABA. There are numerous examples of a post-inhibitory rebound of excitability in the CNS which could be accounted for at least partly by this phenomenon. An even more striking illustration may be the remarkable fall in inhibitory potency observed during quite low frequency activation of hippocampal inputs (3,4) resulting in a pronounced excitation of pyramidal cells (by disinhibition), which readily leads to electrical seizures. In this structure, disinhibition may be reinforced by large changes in extracellular ionic concentrations (21), consequent on strong cellular firing (thus acting in a positive feedback).

CONCLUSIONS

Several different mechanisms are probably involved in the "fading" that characterizes the inhibitory action of GABA: reduction in Cl^- gradient following the large Cl^- fluxes initiated by GABA; removal of extracellular GABA by active uptake, which is probably Na^+-coupled and therefore may have a significant depolarizing effect; and reduced affinity of GABA receptors, perhaps mediated by an endogenous modulator. All these mechanisms tend to limit the effectiveness of inhibitory control in the brain; at certain sites, as in the hippocampus, they provide a striking flexibility of synaptic action which may be largely responsible for the "plastic" properties of the neural processes.

Much of the experimental work described in this article was financially supported by the Medical Research Council of Canada.

REFERENCES

1. Adams, P.R. (1975): Pflugers Arch., 360:135-144.
2. Adams, P.R. and Brown, D.A. (1975): J. Physiol., 250:85-120.
3. Ben-Ari, Y., Krnjević, K. and Reinhardt, W. (1979): Can.J. Physiol. Pharmacol., 57:1462-1466.
4. Ben-Ari, Y., Krnjević, K. and Reinhardt, W. (1980): J.Physiol., in press.
5. Changeux, J.P., Benedetti, L., Bourgeois, J.P., Brisson, A., Cartaud, J., Devaux, P., Grünhagen, H., Moreau, M., Popot,J.L., Sobel, A. and Weber, M. (1975): Cold Spring Harbor Symposia on Quantitative Biology, 40:211-230.
6. Constanti, A., Krnjević, K. and Nistri, A. (1980): Can. J. Physiol. Pharmacol. 58:193-204.
7. Costa, E. and Guidotti, A. (1979): Ann. Rev. Pharmacol. Toxicol., 19:531-545.
8. Curtis, D.R., Game, C.J.A., Johnston, G.A.R., McCulloch, R.M. and MacLachlan, R.M. (1972): Brain Res., 43:242-245.
9. Curtis, D.R., Hösli, L., Johnston, G.A.R. and Johnston, I.H. (1968): Exp. Brain Res., 5:235-258.
10. Curtis,D.R., Phillis, J.W. and Watkins, J.C. (1959): J.Physiol. 146:185-203.
11. Deschênes, M., Feltz, P. and Lamour, Y. (1976): Brain Res., 118:486-493.
12. Diamond, J. and Roper, S. (1973): J. Physiol., 232:113-128.
13. Dreifuss, J.J., Kelly, J.S. and Krnjević, K. (1969): Exp.Brain Res., 9:137-154.
14. Dunlap, K. and Fischbach, G.D. (1978): Nature, 276: 837-839.
15. Elliott, K.A.C. and van Gelder, N.M. (1958): J. Neurochem. 3: 28-40.
16. Fiekers, J.F., Spannbauer, P.M., Scubon-Mulieri, B. and Parsons, R.L. (1980): J.Gen.Physiol., 75:511-529.
17. Johnstone, R.M. (1979): Can.J.Physiol.Pharmacol., 57:1-15.

18. Katz, B. and Thesleff, S. (1957): J. Physiol., 138:63-80.
19. Kehoe, J. (1975): Cold Spring Harbor Symposia on Quantitative Biology, 40:145-155.
20. Krnjević, K. (1976): In: GABA in Nervous System Function, edited by E. Roberts, T.N. Chase and D.B. Tower, pp.269-281. Raven Press, New York.
21. Krnjević, K., Morris, M.E. and Reiffenstein, R.J. (1980): Can. J. Physiol. Pharmacol., 58:579-583.
22. Krnjević, K. and Phillis, J.W. (1963): J. Physiol., 165: 274-304.
23. Krnjević, K., Puil, E. and Werman, R. (1977a): Can. J. Physiol. Pharmacol., 55:658-669.
24. Krnjević, K., Puil, E. and Werman, R. (1977b): Can. J. Physiol. Pharmacol., 55:670-680.
25. Kuffler, S.W. and Edwards, C. (1958): J. Neurophysiol. 21: 589-610.
26. Laris, P.C., Bootman, M. Pershadsingh, H.A. and Johnstone,R.M. (1978): Biochimica et Biophysica Acta, 512:397-414.
27. Neal, M.J. and Iversen, L.L. (1969): J. Neurochem., 16: 1245-1252.
28. Nestoros, J.N. (1980): Life Sci., 26:519-523.
29. Nicoll, R.A. (1981): This symposium.
30. Okada, Y. and Shimada, C. (1976): Brain Res., 107:658-662.
31. Otsuka, M. and Endo, M. (1960): Nature, 188:501-502.
32. Salpeter, M.M. and Faeder, I.R. (1971): Progr. Brain Res., 34:103-114.
33. Schultz, S.G. and Curran, P.F. (1970): Physiol. Rev., 50: 637-718.
34. Snyder, S.H., Young, A.B., Bennett, J.P. and Mulder, A.H. (1973): Federation Proc., 32:2039-2047.
35. Takeuchi, A. and Takeuchi, N. (1964): J. Physiol., 170: 296-317.
36. Takeuchi, A. and Takeuchi, N. (1965): J. Physiol., 177: 225-238.
37. Werman, R., Davidoff, R.A. and Aprison, M.H. (1968): J. Neurophysiol. 31: 81-95.

GABA and Benzodiazepine Receptors,
edited by E. Costa et al.
Raven Press, New York © 1981.

GABA Receptor Associated Drug Receptors

W. Sieghart, *P. Placheta, P. Supavilai, and M. Karobath

Psychiatrische Universitätsklinik, A-1090 Vienna, Austria; and Institute of Pharmacology, A-1090 Vienna, Austria

Benzodiazepines, drugs which are widely used because of their anxiolytic, anticonvulsant and hypnotic properties exhibit reversible stereospecific high affinity binding to membranes from mammalian brain, and the respective binding sites for ^{3}H-flunitrazepam most likely represent pharmacologically and clinically relevant receptors for benzodiazepines (12). Evidence from several laboratories based on electrophysiological and pharmacological studies suggests that benzodiazepines exert their action in the central nervous system by indirect potentiation of GABA neurons (3). Recent biochemical studies provided evidence that benzodiazepine and GABA receptors can be functionally linked together to form a GABA/benzodiazepine receptor complex (2, 4, 6, 12, 15). In addition, it has been shown that pyrazolopyridines (10, 13, 14) and chloride ions (6, 7, 10, 13) have important modulatory effects on GABA and benzodiazepine receptor binding. The effects of pyrazolopyridines appear to be mediated by a distinct new modulatory site of the GABA/benzodiazepine receptor complex. In the present study evidence for a molecular and pharmacological heterogeneity of this receptor complex is presented.

RESULTS

Heterogeneity of Benzodiazepine Binding Proteins Demonstrated by Irreversible ^{3}H-Flunitrazepam Binding.

Recently Möhler et al. (8) demonstrated that ^{3}H-flunitrazepam becomes irreversibly attached to a specific membrane protein with an apparent molecular weight of 50,000 daltons when incubations were exposed to UV light.

FIGURE 1. Fluorography illustrating the influence of several drugs on irreversible ^{3}H-flunitrazepam binding to membrane proteins from cerebellum and hippocampus[a]

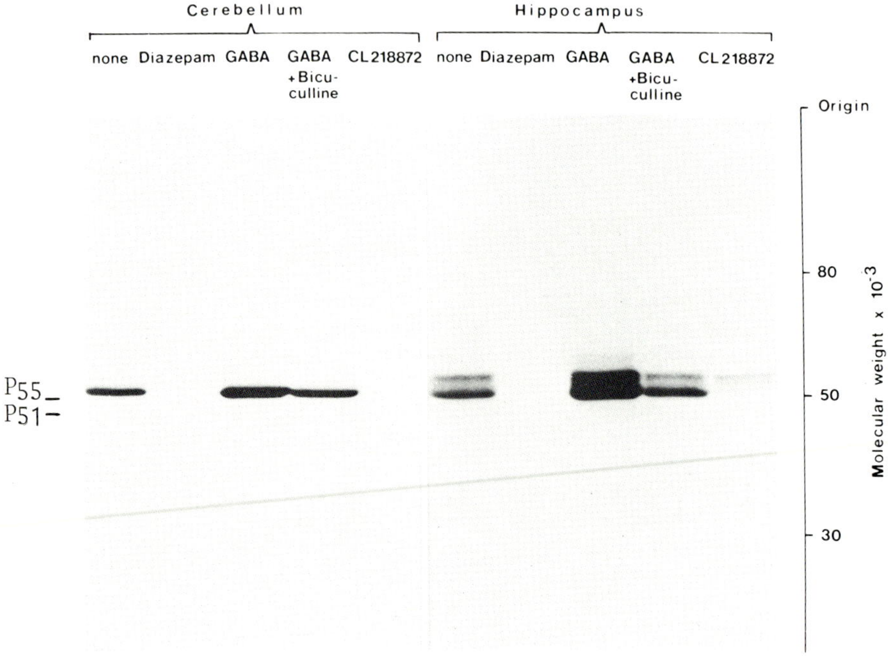

[a]Cerebellar or hippocampal membranes were incubated with 0.4 nM ^{3}H-flunitrazepam either without additions (lanes 1 and 6) or in the presence of 2 µM diazepam (lanes 2 and 7), 10 µM GABA (lanes 3 and 8), 10 µM GABA plus 10 µM bicuculline-methiodide (lanes 4 and 9), 1 µM Cl 218 872 (lanes 5 and 10) or 1 µM Ro 5-4864 (experiment not shown). Incubations were performed at 0° C for 90 min and the samples were then irradiated with UV light for 10 min. Membranes were centrifuged at 48,000xg for 10', resuspended in 100 µl H_2O and 50 µl SDS-stop solution (10 % SDS/w/v, Tris HCl 100 mM, pH 7.4, ß-mecaptoethanol 5 mM, sucrose 0.1 g/ml and bromophenol blue tracking dye 0.02 mg/ml) and placed in a boiling water bath for 5 min. Electrophoresis on 10 % SDS-polyacrylamide slab gels and protein staining of the gels was performed as described previously. After treatment with PPO, gels were dried and subjected to fluorography at - 70° C on Kodak X-Omat R film for 6 days.

Irreversible binding of ^{3}H-flunitrazepam had pharmacological properties similar to reversible benzodiazepine receptor binding indicating that ^{3}H-flunitrazepam is a photoaffinity label for the benzodiazepine receptor (8). We examined benzodiazepine binding proteins in different brain regions using this technique and subsequent electrophoretic separation of the labelled proteins in SDS-gels followed by fluorography (11).

In cerebellum ^{3}H-flunitrazepam irreversibly bound to a single protein band with an apparent molecular weight of 51,000 daltons (P_{51}). Similarly, most of the radioactivity bound to membranes from other brain regions was associated with a protein band with the same apparent molecular weight (P_{51}) which seems to be identical to the labelled benzodiazepine receptor described previously (8). However, in other brain regions several additional protein bands with apparent molecular weight of 53,000 (P_{53}), 55,000 (P_{55}), and 59,000 (P_{59}) were labelled with variable intensity (11). In hippocampus protein P_{55} was the most prominent of these additional bands (Figure 1). Irreversible binding of ^{3}H-flunitrazepam to P_{51} in cerebellum and to P_{51} and P_{55} in hippocampus was inhibited completely by diazepam but not by Ro 5-4864 (data not shown) which selectively inhibits binding to peripheral benzodiazepine binding sites (1). Furthermore, irreversible binding of ^{3}H-flunitrazepam to all binding proteins in cerebellum and hippocampus was stimulated by 10 μM GABA (Figure 1). This effect of GABA was antagonized by bicuculline-methiodide which suggests that the benzodiazepine binding proteins are associated with a GABA recognition site.

CL 218 872, a triazolopyridazine with anxiolytic but only weak sedative properties, has recently been shown to inhibit reversible benzodiazepine receptor binding with K_i values and Hill coefficients which differed in various brain regions (5). Based on these observations a heterogeneity of benzodiazepine receptors has been proposed (5). We therefore investigated a possible differential effect of CL 218 872 on the irreversible binding of ^{3}H-flunitrazepam to the different binding proteins. CL 218 872 inhibited irreversible binding to P_{51} more potently than binding to P_{55} (Figure 1).

Heterogeneity of the GABA/Benzodiazepine Receptor Complex Demonstrated by Reversible ^{3}H-Flunitrazepam Binding.

The evidence for a molecular heterogeneity of GABA receptor associated benzodiazepine binding proteins prompted us to investigate possible differences in the properties and in the modulation by GABA and the pyrazolopyridine etazolate (SQ 20009) of reversible ^{3}H-flunitrazepam binding in cerebellum and hippocampus.

Kinetic analysis of ^{3}H-flunitrazepam binding was performed using membranes from cerebellum and hippocampus which were prepared and assayed simultaneously in order to minimize variability. In hippocampus, the affinity for ^{3}H-flunitrazepam was consistently higher than in cerebellum (Table 1) suggesting that the additional benzodiazepine binding proteins (P_{53}, P_{55}, P_{59}) of this brain region exhibit higher apparent affinity than the cerebellar binding protein (P_{51}). These differences cannot be explained by variable contamination of the membranes by traces of endogenous GABA since ^{3}H-flunitrazepam binding to membranes from both regions was not significantly inhibited by bicuculline-methiodide (data not shown). The concentration of GABA necessary for half-maximal stimulation (EC_{50}) of ^{3}H-flunitrazepam binding was 3.3 times higher in hippocampus than in cerebellum, although the maximal stimulation by GABA and the change of affinity for ^{3}H-flunitrazepam (decrease of K_d values) was comparable in both regions (Table 1).

TABLE 1. Properties of basal, GABA or etazolate-stimulated ^{3}H-flunitrazepam binding to membranes from rat cerebellum and hippocampus[a]

Parameter	cerebellum	hippocampus
K_d(nM) control	2.2 ± 0.2 (5)	1.2 ± 0.1 (5)
K_d(nM) + 100 μM GABA	0.8 ± 0.1 (5)	0.5 ± 0.1 (5)
K_d(nM) + 10 μM etazolate	1.3 ± 0.1 (4)	0.9 ± 0.1 (4)
EC_{50} (μM) GABA	0.7 ± 0.1 (5)	2.4 ± 0.2 (5)
EC_{50} (μM) GABA + 1 μM etazolate	0.2 ± 0.0 (5)	1.0 ± 0.1 (5)

[a]Membrane preparations and binding assays were performed as described (14). For Scatchard analysis specific (total minus nonspecifically bound ^{3}H-flunitrazepam (83.4 Ci/mmol, New England Nuclear) in the presence of 2 μM diazepam) binding of 0.2 to 4.0 nM ^{3}H-flunitrazepam was determined in duplicate incubations containing 150 mM NaCl. The addition of GABA or etazolate did not alter the respective B_{max} values for ^{3}H-flunitrazepam (not shown). EC_{50} values were determined by incubating duplicate samples with 0.25 nM ^{3}H-flunitrazepam in the presence of 0 to 100 μM GABA and of 150 mM NaCl.

The pyrazolopyridine etazolate has been shown to have two distinct actions on benzodiazepine receptor binding in rat cerebellar membranes (14). Firstly, it directly stimulates binding by increasing the affinity for ^{3}H-flunitrazepam and, secondly, it has an indirect effect since it increases the potency of GABA-like drugs to stimulate ^{3}H-flunitrazepam binding. In hippocampus however, both effects of etazolate were much less pronounced than in cerebellum (Table 1).

Thus, the heterogeneity of benzodiazepine receptors appears to comprise differences in the composition of binding proteins and differences in the apparent pharmacological properties of the associated GABA recognition sites and the modulatory sites for the pyrazolopyridines.

Modulation of the GABA/Benzodiazepine Receptor Complex by Pyrazolopyridines - Evidence for a New GABA Receptor-Associated Drug Receptor.

Kinetic analysis revealed that the pyrazolopyridines cartazolate (Table 2) and etazolate (data not shown) increased the apparent number of GABA recognition sites (increase of the B_{max} value of ^{3}H-muscimol binding) without affecting the apparent affinity for the ligand (Table 2). There were striking similarities between the modulatory effects of pyrazolopyridines on GABA and benzodiazepine receptor binding: (i) only etazolate and cartazolate, but not their centrally inactive congener SQ 20006 displayed modulatory effects on both GABA (10) and benzodiazepine (14) receptor binding; (ii) the modulation of GABA (Table 2 and 3) and benzodiazepine (13, 14) receptor binding was halide ion dependent; (iii) both modulations were sensitive to pretreatment of the membrane fractions with Triton-X 100 (Table 4); (iv) the magnitude of the effect of etazolate on

TABLE 2. Effect of cartazolate and chloride ions on ^{3}H-muscimol binding[a]

Addition		^{3}H-muscimol binding	
Cl^- (mM)	cartazolate (μM)	K_d (nM)	B_{max} (pmol/mg protein)
--	--	9.6	2.7
--	30	9.7	4.2
100	--	9.5	2.7
100	30	9.5	6.1

[a]Scatchard analysis of the specific binding of ^{3}H-muscimol (0.5 - 50 nM) was performed in membranes from rat frontal cortex as described (10).

TABLE 3. Potentiation by anions of the effect of etazolate on Na^+-independent ^3H-GABA binding[a]

Addition			^3H-GABA binding (%)
none			100
etazolate (50 μM)			145
"	+ 30 mM	KF	148
"	"	KCl	191
"	"	KBr	260
"	"	KI	233
"	"	KNO_2	187
"	"	KNO_3	201
"	"	$NaClO_4$	173
"	"	KSCN	167

[a]The binding of 5 nM ^3H-GABA to membranes prepared from rat frontal cortex was determined in 50 mM Tris-citrate buffer, pH 7.2, as described (9). Results are the means of a typical experiment performed in triplicate with SEMs<4 %. The experiment was repeated with similar results. In the absence of etazolate, the ions listed above (all 30 mM) did not enhance ^3H-GABA binding.

TABLE 4. Effect of treatment of membranes with Triton-X 100 on the modulation by etazolate of ^3H-GABA and ^3H-flunitrazepam binding[a]

Addition	^3H-flunitrazepam binding in cerebellum (% of control)	
	control membranes	tritonized membranes
none (control)	100 ± 1	100 ± 1
etazolate 10 μM	140 ± 2	77 ± 1
GABA 1 μM	167 ± 3	146 ± 5
	^3H-GABA binding in frontal cortex (% of control)	
	control membranes	tritonized membranes
none (control)	100 ± 3	100 ± 4
etazolate 30 μM	192 ± 4	112 ± 3

[a]Membranes were pretreated with 0.05 % Triton-X 100 (9), binding assays were performed as described (9, 13) in the presence of chloride ions (150 mM) using 5 nM ^3H-GABA or 0.25 nM ^3H-flunitrazepam as ligands.

Na^+-independent GABA binding appeared to parallel the regional density of benzodiazepine receptors more closely than that of GABA recognition sites (9). These similarities suggest that the actions of pyrazolopyridines on GABA and benzodiazepine receptor binding are functionally linked together. Thus, the reversible anion sensitive "unmasking" of GABA recognition sites by pyrazolopyridines may lead to the increased potency of GABA like drugs to stimulate benzodiazepine receptor binding. This may be an important mechanism for the regulation of the sensitivity of those GABA recognition sites which are constituents of the GABA/benzodiazepine (P_{51}) receptor complex.

CONCLUSIONS

Recent evidence indicates that GABA receptors can be associated with drug receptors including a benzodiazepine binding site (2, 4, 6, 12, 15) and a modulatory site for pyrazolopyridines (10, 13, 14, 16). In addition, there is some evidence that at least in cerebellum GABA receptors may exist which are not associated with benzodiazepine binding sites (4, 9). In the present study we provide evidence for a heterogeneity of GABA receptors associated with drug receptors. Thus, at least two types of GABA/benzodiazepine receptor complexes appear to exist which differ with respect to the benzodiazepine binding protein. One type of complex which contains the benzodiazepine protein P_{51} occurs in all brain regions. Another receptor complex contains the benzodiazepine binding protein P_{55} and is found in hippocampus and other brain regions but not in cerebellum. This molecular heterogeneity of benzodiazepine binding proteins may be the cause of the observed differences in the modulation by GABA and pyrazolopyridines of benzodiazepine receptor binding in cerebellum and hippocampus. Alternatively, additional differences in the molecular properties of the GABA or pyrazolopyridine recognition sites or differences in the mode of coupling of the various constituents of the receptor complex might explain the observed regional pharmacological heterogeneity of the GABA/benzodiazepine receptor complexes.

Acknowledgements: We thank Martina Scherer and G. Drexler for excellent technical assistance and J. Reisenhofer for preparation of the manuscript. We thank Dr. S. J. Lucania for the donation of etazolate, cartazolate and SQ 20006. This work was supported by "Fonds zur Förderung der wissenschaftlichen Forschung in Österreich".

REFERENCES

1. Braestrup, C., and Squires, R.F. (1977): Proc. Natl.Acad.Sci.(USA), 74:3805-3809.
2. Briley, M.S., and Langer, S.Z. (1978): Europ.J. Pharmacol., 52:129-132.
3. Costa, E., Guidotti, A., Mao, C.C., and Suria, A. (1975): Life Sci., 17:167-186.
4. Karobath, M., and Sperk, G. (1979): Proc.Natl.Acad. Sci.(USA), 76:1004-1006.
5. Klepner, C.A., Lippa, A.S., Benson, D.I., Sano, M.C., and Beer, B. (1979): Pharmacol. Biochem. Behav., 11:457-462.
6. Martin, I.L., and Candy, J.M. (1978): Neuropharmacology, 17:993-998.
7. Martin, I.L., and Candy, J.M. (1980): Neuropharmacology, 19:175-179.
8. Möhler, H., Battersby, M.K., and Richards, J.G. (1980): Proc.Natl.Acad.Sci.(USA), 77:1666-1670.
9. Placheta, P., and Karobath, M. (1979): Brain Res., 178:580-583.
10. Placheta, P., and Karobath, M. (1980): Europ.J. Pharmacol., 62:225-228.
11. Sieghart, W., and Karobath, M. (1980): Nature (in press).
12. Speth, R.C., Wastek, G.J., Johnson, P.C., and Yamamura, H.I. (1978): Life Sci., 22:859-866.
13. Supavilai, P., and Karobath, M. (1979): Europ.J. Pharmacol., 60:111-113.
14. Supavilai, P.,and Karobath, M. (1980): Europ.J. Pharmacol., 62:229-233.
15. Tallman, J.F., Thomas, J.W., and Gallager, D.W. (1978): Nature, 274:383-385.
16. Williams, M., and Risley, E.A. (1979): Life Sci., 24:833-841.

GABA and Benzodiazepine Receptors,
edited by E. Costa et al.
Raven Press, New York © 1981.

GABA Receptors Regulate the Affinities of Anions Required for Brain Specific Benzodiazepine Binding

Richard F. Squires

Rockland Research Institute, Orangeburg, New York 10962

There is now excellent evidence for the existence of benzodiazepine (BZ)/ion/GABA receptor complexes in the central nervous system (2,3,5,6,7,8,9,14,19,20,21,22,23,24).

In particular, I have recently found that the specific binding of ^{3}H-flunitrazepam (^{3}H-FLU) to unwashed rat brain P2 membranes is almost entirely dependent on the addition of an anion to the incubation medium (20). The concentration of anion required to give 50% of maximum ^{3}H-FLU binding ("Kd" value) changes from one anion to another (in the range of 0.5 to 10 mM), but with all anions so far studied their "Kd" values are increased up to a factor of 12 by a group of GABA mimetics including THIP (4,5,6,7-tetrahydroisoxazolo 4,5c-pyridine-3-ol), IGV (isoguvacine) (15), P4S (piperidine-4-sulfonic acid) (16), in a GABA reversible way (20).

These effects of THIP and IGV on anion affinities provide a simple explanation for the earlier finding (22) of plateau inhibitions of ^{3}H-FLU binding by THIP and IGV. In addition, the failure of others to observe these inhibitory effects can be explained by the fact that they are used in high ion concentrations. (1,10,11,12,18).

P4S, like THIP and IGV, produces plateau inhibition of ^{3}H-FLU binding to unwashed P2 membranes, the magnitude of which is dependent on both the kind and the concentration of the buffer used (FIG. 1). In the 5 mM Tris HCl buffer pH 7.5, P4S produces 50% of its maximum inhibitory effect at a concentration near 2 μM.

Chloride ion promotes ^{3}H-FLU binding with a "Kd" value near 4 mM, and this is increased to 40 mM, by concentrations of P4S greater than 20 mM (FIG. 2, TABLE 1). The Hill coefficient for chloride is .72 ± .04 (n=8), significantly less than unity.

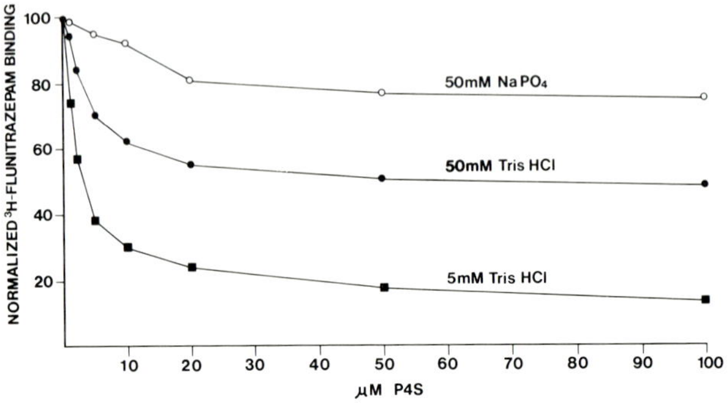

FIG. 1. Effect of varying P4S concentration on the specific binding of ^{3}H-FLU to unwashed rat brain P2 membranes (normalized) in 3 different buffers (all pH 7.5).

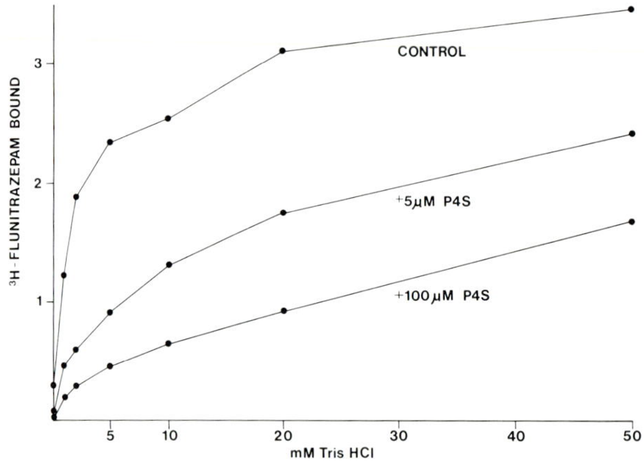

FIG. 2. Effect of varying Tris HCl, pH 7.5, (chloride ion) on ^{3}H-FLU binding without (control) and with P4S (5 and 100 μM).

TABLE 1. <u>The affinities of 15 anions in promoting ^{3}H-FLU (1 nM) to unwashed P2 membranes.</u>

	Control			+THIP 200 μM			Ratio $\frac{+THIP}{Control}$		
Anion (Tris salts)	"Kd" mM	Rel B_{max}	Hill Coeff α	"Kd" mM	Rel B_{max}	Hill Coeff α	"Kd"	B_{max}	α
Fluoride	3.5	85	0.81	31	72	0.86	8.8	0.84	1.06
Chloride	4.5	100	0.82	35	98	0.97	7.8	0.98	1.18
Bromide	4.2	105	0.74	40	125	0.97	9.5	1.19	1.31
Iodide	4.2	98	1.24	42	141	0.99	10.1	1.44	0.79
Citrate	1.2	82	1.65	5.4	74	1.28	6.5	0.90	0.77
Maleate	0.79	102	1.01	5.2	102	0.99	6.6	1.00	0.98
Sulphate	2.5	117	1.06	16	140	1.37	6.4	1.20	1.29
Phosphate	0.74	97	0.91	2.9	77	1.39	6.2	0.79	1.51
Na Phosphate	1.0	104	0.99	5.3	96	1.46	5.3	0.92	1.47
NH_4^+ Bicarbonate	1.5	70	0.62	12	80	0.86	7.6	1.14	1.39
Glutamate	14	110	0.83	129	101	0.78	9.2	0.92	0.94
Benzoate	2.2	73	1.20	12	48	1.00	5.4	0.65	0.83
Na EDTA	1.1	80	1.30	3.7	62	1.76	3.4	0.78	1.35
Succinate	2.2	95	1.00	15	100	1.10	6.8	1.05	1.10
Tartrate	1.4	101	1.60	10	131	1.30	7.1	1.06	0.81
Acetate	3.7	89	1.20	43	107	1.10	12	1.20	1.10

In most of the early experiments (results shown in TABLE 1) an unwashed P2 fraction from whole rat brain was used since this preparation seemed to contain substances or factors, in addition to GABA and ions, which affect ^{3}H-FLU binding to BZ receptors.

Addition of exogenous GABA to this preparation enhanced ^{3}H-FLU binding about 20% (22). However the omission of exogenous salts (buffers) from this unwashed preparation results in less than 10% of the specific ^{3}H-FLU binding obtained in the presence of 50 mM Tris HCl or Na phosphate buffers (pH 7.5).

TABLE 1 shows that: a) 15 anions enhance binding with apparent affinity constants ("Kd" values) ranging from 0.8 to 14 mM, b) THIP at 200 μM increases these "Kd" values from 3 to 12-fold, and can increase the Hill coefficient for some anions while decreasing it for others.

Tris-citrate has been used extensively for studying the enhancing effects of GABA or muscimol on BZ binding (1,10,17,19). Citrate has a high affinity for the anion recognition sites but the Bmax values obtained in the presence of citrate are lower than those obtained in the presence of chloride ions.

Tris maleate buffer which has been used in one study of anion effects on ^{3}H-diazepam binding (3) is also a potent activator of ^{3}H-FLU binding.

It is interesting to speculate that the potent activating effect ("Kd" ∿ 1 mM) of bicarbonate ion, after chloride the most abundant anion in blood, might be related to the anticonvulsant effect of the carbonic anhydrase inhibitors and of CO_2.

In the presence of THIP (200 μM) the halide ions exhibit a striking progression of Bmax values with I > Br > Cl > F.

In addition to the anions listed in TABLE 1, aspartate, borate, formate, molybdate, perchlorate, trichloracetate and vanadate were all found to enhance ^{3}H-FLU binding, and this enhancement could be inhibited by THIP. Thus, the anion recognition sites involved exhibit surprisingly little specificity. However, the results in TABLE 1 clearly show that enhancement of ^{3}H-FLU binding by anions is not related to ionic strength. Many monovalent, and at least one divalent ($CrO_4^{=}$), anions can substitute for chloride in reversing inhibitory post synaptic potentials (IPSPs) when injected intracellularly into cortical neurones (13). Many, especially larger, anions which potently activate ^{3}H-FLU binding may fail to substitute for chloride in reversing IPSPs because of their size, slow diffusion or action as chloride antagonists (4,13).

THIP (200 μM), P4S (50 μM) and IGV (200 μM) all increase the "Kd" value for chloride ion from about 4 mM to near 40 mM, while 3-amino propane sulfonate (200 μM) and imidazole acetic acid (500 μM) increase it to about 9 mM and 19 mM, respectively in a GABA reversible way (20).

Since there was a possibility that the inhibitory effects of this group of GABA mimetics was due solely to antagonism of endogenous GABA in the unwashed P2 preparation I retested P4S using an extensively dialyzed rat brain P2 fraction (4 changes of distilled water, 20 volumes, at least 2 hours between each change, over a 20 hour period). As shown in FIGs. 3 and 4, P4S (50 μM) in the absence of GABA, produces similar inhibitory effects on ^{3}H-FLU binding by reducing the affinities of chloride and bicarbonate ions which both promote binding in this system also. The inhibitory effects of P4S can be fully reversed either by increasing the anion concentration, or by adding GABA (200 μM). GABA has the double effect of increasing the affinities for both chloride and bicarbonate ions, and increasing the Bmax. A very similar pattern is obtained with varying phosphate concentrations (not shown). The low Hill coefficients (α) for chloride and bicarbonate suggest the presence of two or more populations of GABA/ion/BZ receptor complexes with different anion recognition sites having different affinities for some anions. Independent evidence also indicates the existence of two populations of BZ receptor complexes, one of which is selectively protected from heat inactivation at 60° by 50 mM Na phosphate buffer pH 7.5 (21).

It is interesting to note (FIGs. 3 and 4) that in the absence of added ions, GABA (200 μM) alone has very little enhancing activity on ^{3}H-FLU binding. In contrast, ions alone without GABA produce large increases in binding which can then be increased further by the addition of GABA.

Similarly, GABA alone cannot protect at all against the heat inactivation of ^{3}H-FLU binding sites (30 min, 60°C) while NaCl alone in concentrations above 5 mM provides considerable protection which is increased several fold by the addition of GABA (TABLE 2). In these heat inactivation experiments sodium phosphate buffer pH 7.5 and GABA were added after heat treatment and just before addition of ^{3}H-FLU for the usual binding assay to give final concentrations of 50 mM and 1 mM respectively. It therefore can be tentatively concluded that BZ receptors are indirectly coupled to GABA receptors through anion recognition sites. The BZ/ion/GABA receptor complex might then be visualized as an anionophore sandwiched between a GABA receptor on one side and a BZ recognition site on the other. It is interesting that P4S, in the heat protection situation behaves as a true GABA mimetic (TABLE 2).

The term "partial agonist", used by some investigators (1,10) to describe the interactions of THIP, IGV and P4S with the GABA/ion/BZ receptor complexes seems inadequate and misleading. Electrophysiologically (15,16) and behaviorally (J. Scheel-Kruger, A.V. Christensen, J. Arndt, personal communications) these substances behave as pure GABA agonists. It seems highly probable that they all open chloride channels on neuronal membranes, but the results presented here indicate that, at the same time, they reduce the affinity of chloride for the "channels" (chloride recognition sites) which would not be expected to greatly affect neuronal function because of the high (ca 100 mM) extracellular concentration of chloride compared to the "Kd" for chloride in the presence of THIP, P4S or IGV (near 40 mM). In reducing the affinities of anions required for BZ binding THIP, IGV and P4S behave as pure GABA antagonists.

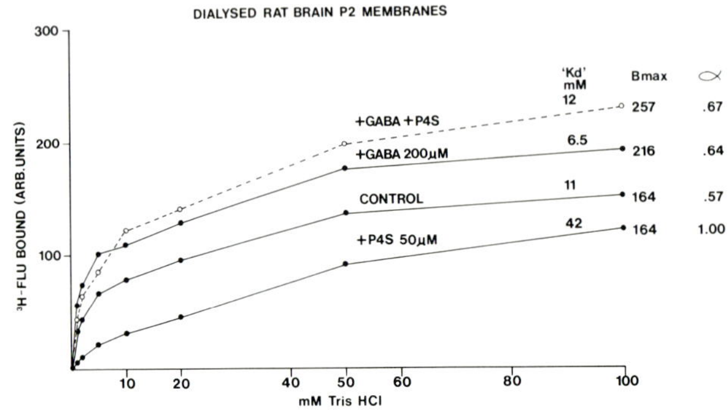

FIG. 3. Effects of GABA and P4S on the affinity of chloride in promoting ^{3}H-FLU (0.2 nM) binding to dialysed whole rat brain P2 membranes.

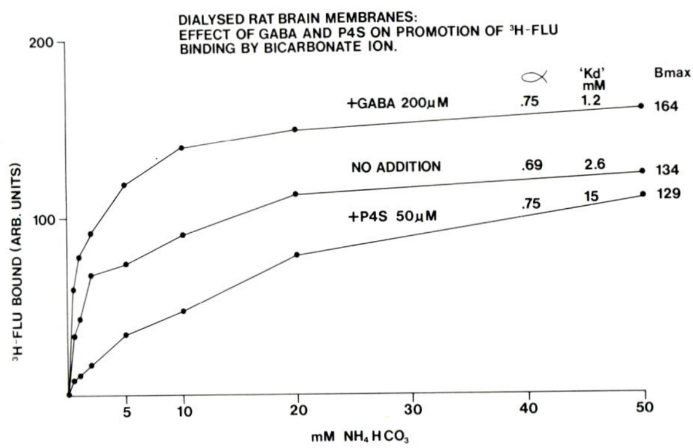

FIG. 4. Effects of GABA and P4S on the affinity of bicarbonate in promoting ^{3}H-FLU binding.

TABLE 2. Heat inactivation (30 minutes, 60°C) of ^{3}H-FLU binding sites on dialyzed rat brain P2 fractions. Protective effects of NaCl, GABA and P4S. ^{3}H-FLU binding in arbitrary units.

NaCl Added	Control	+GABA 200 μM	+P4S 50 μM	GABA + P4S
0	31	75	44	77
10 mM	28	361	60	232
20 mM	64	974	166	574
50 mM	709	3260	1609	3501
100 mM	1952	5493	3308	5610
200 mM	3348	6182	4966	6270

After heating, all assays in presence of 50 mM $NaPO_4$ + 1 mM GABA (final concentration).

Chloride ion also promotes ^{3}H-FLU binding to unwashed P2 membranes in three regions of calf brain with about twice the "Kd" value in cortex (4 mM) as in cerebellum and hippocampus (2 mM) (TABLE 3). THIP (200 μM) increases the "Kd" values 11-12 fold in cortex and cerebellum but only 6-fold in hippocampus. THIP also increases the Bmax in cortex and cerebellum about 20% while slightly lowering it in hippocampus. The Hill coefficient for chloride in hippocampus (0.72) is significantly less than unity and is increased by THIP (TABLE 3).

The inhibition pattern produced by beta carboline-3-carboxylate methyl ester (BCME) also demonstrates striking regional differences in calf brain with a "Ki" value of 2 nanomolar in cerebellum, 6 nM in cortex and 16 nM in hippocampus. In all three regions the Hill coefficient for BCME is in the range 0.6-0.7 suggesting heterogeneity of ^{3}H-FLU binding complexes. In whole rat brain unwashed P2 fractions, BCME inhibits ^{3}H-FLU binding with an IC_{50} ("Ki") value near 5 nM, and this value is not much affected by low ion concentrations, THIP or GABA. However, Ni^{++} ion selectively and dramatically antagonizes the inhibitory effect of BCME on ^{3}H-FLU binding: in the presence of 1-2 mM $NiCl_2$, the IC_{50} value for BCME is increased from 5 nM to 20-40 nM. The purine analogue SQ 20, 009 also produces a small (50-80%) but consistent increase in the IC_{50} value for BCME. Scatchard analysis of ^{3}H-FLU binding in the presence of 5 nM BCME reveals a straight line with Bmax reduced to 50% of control and the Kd for ^{3}H-FLU increased from 0.75 nM to 1.6 nM. Taken together these results strongly suggest that BCME does not compete directly with ^{3}H-FLU for its binding site, but instead binds to an allosteric site. Further, BCME discriminates between different BZ/ion/GABA receptor complexes. Taken together, the available evidence suggests that there are more than 2 such receptor complexes (8,21,22).

TABLE 3. Effect of THIP on affinity for chloride ion in promoting ^{3}H-FLU binding to membranes various regions of calf brain.

Brain Region	Control "Kd" mM	Control Rel Bmax	Control Hill Coeff. (α)	+ THIP 200 μM "Kd" mM	+ THIP 200 μM Rel Bmax	+ THIP 200 μM Hill Coeff. (α)	Ratio +THIP/Control "Kd"	Ratio +THIP/Control α
Cortex	3.9	100	0.92	42	123	0.92	11	1.00
Hippocampus	2.1	100	0.72	13	94	0.89	6.2	1.24
Cerebellum	2.0	100	0.88	23	117	0.94	12	1.07

TABLE 4. Inhibition of ^{3}H-FLU binding by beta carboline methyl ester in three regions of calf brain.

Brain Region	K_i nM	Hill Coeff. (α)
Cortex	5.6 ± .2 (n=2)	.62 ± .05
Hippocampus	16 ± 3	.64 ± .10
Cerebellum	2.1 ± 1	.74 ± .10

The pervasive effects of GABA mimetics on anion dependent ^{3}H-FLU binding suggests that virtually all BZ receptors are coupled to GABA receptors. This conclusion is also supported by light microscopic autoradiographic localization of ^{3}H-muscimol and ^{3}H-flunitrazepam binding sites, and these studies also suggest that many GABA receptors are not coupled to BZ receptors (24).

ACKNOWLEDGEMENTS

I thank Else Saederup for technical assistance and Sharon Marsico for typing the manuscript.

REFERENCES

1. Braestrup, C., Nielsen, M., Krogsgaard-Larsen, P., and Falch, E. (1979): Nature, 280:331-333.

2. Choi, D.W., Farb, D.H., and Fischbach, G.D. (1977): Nature, 269:342-344.

3. Costa, T., Rodbard, D., and Pert, C.B. (1979): Nature, 277: 315-317.

4. Eccles, J.C. (1964): Science, 145:1140-1147.

5. Gallager, D.W. (1978): Eur. J. Pharmacol., 49:133-143.

6. Geller, H.M., Taylor, D.A., and Hoffer, B.J. (1978): Naunyn-Schmiedenberg's Arch. Pharmacol., 304:81-88.

7. Guidotti, A. (1980): Adv. Biochem. Psychopharm., 21:271-275.

8. Guidotti, A., Gale, K., Suria, A., and Toffano, G. (1979): Brain Res., 172:566-571.

9. Haefely, W., Kulcsar, A., Mohler, H., Pieri, P., Polc, P., and Schaffner, R. (1975): Mechanisms of Action of Benzodiazepines, edited by E. Costa and P. Greengard, Raven Press, New York.

10. Karobath, M., and Lippitsch, M. (1979): Eur. J. Pharmacol., 58:485-488.

11. Karobath, M., Placheta, P., Lippitsch, M., and Krogsgaard-Larsen, P. (1979): Nature, 287:748-749.

12. Karobath, M., and Sperk, G. (1979): Proc. Natl. Acad. Sci., 76:1004-1006.

13. Kelly, J.S., Krnjevic, K., Morris, M.E., and Yim, G.K.W. (1969): Exp. Brain Res., 7:11-31.

14. Krnjevic, K. (1974): Physiol. Rev., 54:418-540.

15. Krogsgaard-Larsen, P., Johnson, G.A.R., Lodge, D., and Curtis, D.R. (1977): Nature, 268:53-55.

16. Krogsgaard-Larsen, P., Falch, E., Schousboe, A., Curtis, D.R., and Lodge, D. (1980): J. Neurochem., 34:756-759.

17. Martin, I.L., and Candy, J.M. (1980): Neuropharmacology, 19: 175-179.

18. Maurer, R. (1979): Neuroscience Letters, 12:65-68.

19. Supavilai, P., and Karobath, M. (1979): Eur. J. Pharmacol., 60:111-113.

20. Squires, R.F. (In press): Pharmacol. Drug Develop.

21. Squires, R.F., Benson, D.I., Braestrup, C., Coupet, J., Klepner, C.A., Myers, V., and Beer, B. (1979): Pharmacol. Biochem. & Behav., 10:825-830.

22. Squires, R.F., Klepner, C.A., and Benson, D.I. (1980): In: Receptors for Neurotransmitters and Peptide Hormones, edited by G. Pepeu, M.J. Kuhar and S.J. Enna, Raven Press, New York.

23. Tallman, J.F., Thomas, J.W., and Gallager, D.W. (1978): Nature, 274:383-385.

24. Young III, W.S., and Kuhar, M.J. (1979): Nature, 280:393-394.

I have recently found that a number of protein-containing materials of diverse origin, including casein, bacto-tryptose, dried yeast extract, dried liver extract, dried pituitary powder, and especially chicken feathers and sheep's wool (solutilized in thioglycollic acid, as sources of keratin) when heated in acid-ethanol, as described by Braestrup et al. (1980), PNAS 77:2288-2292 for the formation of beta-carboline-3-carboxylic acid ethyl ester, all yield material which strongly inhibits ^{3}H-FLU binding. Although the active substance(s) have not been identified, it seems likely that they are beta-carboline derivatives formed from tryptophan containing protein or peptides by a Bischler-Napieralski type reaction as described by Uphaus et al. (1959) Science, 129:641-643. Although beta-carboline-3-carboxylates may also be formed enzymatically from tryptophan-containing peptides the work of Uphaus shows clearly that they can be formed non-enzymatically. Assuming my ^{3}H-FLU displacing activity to be due to a beta-carboline ester, there would be at least several hundred times as much BCE per mg. dry material, as reported for brain tissue by Braestrup et al. (1980).

GABA and Benzodiazepine Receptors,
edited by E. Costa et al.
Raven Press, New York © 1981.

Benzodiazepine Receptors: Autoradiographical and Immunocytochemical Evidence for Their Localization in Regions of Gabaergic Synaptic Contacts

H. Möhler, *J.-Y. Wu, and J. G. Richards

*Pharmaceutical Research Department, Hoffmann-La Roche, CH-4002 Basle, Switzerland; and *Department of Cell Biology, Baylor College of Medicine, Houston, Texas 77020*

Benzodiazepines are widely used therapeutically as anxiolytics, hypnotics, anticonvulsants and spasmolytics. This group of drugs exerts its main pharmacological and therapeutic effects by interacting with a specific target structure in the central nervous system (CNS), the benzodiazepine receptor (BR) (2,5). The activation of BR triggers a complex series of events which finally results in the pharmacological and therapeutic drug response. The molecular events following BR activation are not well understood. In particular, it was not known on which types of cells and cellular elements BR are localized. Since knowledge of the cellular localization of BR is a key point for the understanding of the molecular mechanism of action of these drugs, we made an attempt to localize the BR autoradiographically on the electronmicroscopic (EM) level. A prerequisite for EM-autoradiography is the irreversible attachment of a radioactive ligand to the receptor. This was accomplished with a photoaffinity labeling technique, which enabled us to identify the cellular elements containing BR.

Since electrophysiological evidence indicated an interaction of benzodiazepines with GABAergic synaptic transmission in the CNS (1), a possible association of at least some BR with GABAergic synapses might be expected. In order to visualize GABAergic nerve terminals, we stained tissue sections with antibodies raised against glutamic acid decarboxylase (GAD) (7), the GABA-synthesizing enzyme. The EM localization of both the BR and the GABA nerve terminals in the same tissue section should allow us to determine if BR do occur in GABAergic synapses.

Photoaffinity labeling of BR

Fresh tissue

The benzodiazepine flunitrazepam (FNZP) binds reversibly and with high affinity to BR. On illumination with UV light, however, it is irreversibly linked to BR (3) : rat brain tissue was incubated with 3 nM ^{3}H-FNZP in the presence and absence of an excess of another benzodiazepine (10 μM diazepam) until binding equilibrium was reached (90 min, 4°C). The suspension was then illuminated with UV light for 4 min. After repeated rinses to remove free and reversibly bound ^{3}H-FNZP the radioactivity retained in the tissue was determined. The amount of radioactivity incorporated in the presence of diazepam was subtracted from that incorporated in the absence of diazepam ("total incorporation") in order to obtain the amount of ^{3}H-FNZP "specifically incorporated". Specific incorporation amounts to 85 % of total incorporation.

The conclusion that specific incorporation of ^{3}H-FNZP represents its covalent attachment to BR is based on several lines of evidence : 1) ^{3}H-FNZP is attached to the tissue by a heat-, light- and detergent-stable linkage which is apparently covalent. 2) Other benzodiazepines inhibit the irreversible incorporation of ^{3}H-FNZP with a potency corresponding to their apparent affinity to BR. 3) Photolabeling with FNZP reduces the number of BR subsequently accessible to other benzodiazepines, without altering the binding characteristics of the remaining BR. 4) Half maximal irreversible incorporation of ^{3}H-FNZP occurs at a concentration (1.2 nM) corresponding to the apparent dissociation constant of ^{3}H-FNZP in reversible binding experiments. Thus, FNZP is a photoaffinity label for the BR.

Fixed tissue

In order to visualize BR in tissue sections with a high ultrastructural integrity, we investigated whether photoaffinity labeling of BR could be performed in perfusion-fixed tissue. Generally, electronmicrographs with a high degree of ultrastructural preservation are obtained in tissue from animals killed by perfusion fixation with glutaraldehyde and formaldehyde (under ether anesthesia). First, it had to be established that the characteristics of reversible binding to BR are unaltered in fixed tissue. It was found that reversible BR-binding in homogenates of fixed rat brain tissue showed the same characteristics as in fresh tissue : both the apparent dissociation constant of ^{3}H-FNZP and the maximum amount of specifically bound ^{3}H-FNZP were similar in fresh and fixed tissue. Furthermore, the potency of various benzodiazepines in inhibiting reversible binding in fixed tissue corresponded to that in fresh tissue (Tab.1). Thus, the binding characteristics of BR seem to be unaltered by tissue fixation (4).

TABLE 1. Inhibition of ^{3}H-FNZP reversible binding in rat cerebral cortex

	IC_{50} (nM) Fresh tissue (P_2)	Fixed tissue (homogenate)
Clonazepam	1.8	1.2
Flunitrazepam	3.8	2.9
Diazepam	8.1	8.4
Bromazepam	18	12
Chlordiazepoxide	350	250
Ro 5-2181	$>$1000	$>$1000

Just as in fresh tissue, photolabeling with ^{3}H-FNZP was possible in fixed tissue. It was found that the potency of various benzodiazepines in preventing the specific incorporation of ^{3}H-FNZP in fixed tissue was the same as that found in fresh tissue (Tab.2). Furthermore, the specific incorporation of ^{3}H-FNZP reduced the number of BR without changing the apparent dissociation constant of the remaining BR. These results indicate that BR can be photolabeled with ^{3}H-FNZP in perfusion-fixed brain tissue (4).

TABLE 2. Inhibition of ^{3}H-FNZP photolabeling in rat cerebral cortex by benzodiazepines

	IC_{50} (nM) Fresh tissue (P_2)	Fixed tissue (homogenate)
Ro 11-7800	1.4	2.7
B1	2.6	4.0
B11(+)	6.6	7.7
B11(-)	320	340
B23	$>$1000	$>$1000

EM autoradiographic localization of BR

For the autoradiographic localization of BR, photolabeling was performed in brain slices. Rats were injected with ^{3}H-FNZP i.v. alone or together with a high dose of Ro 11-7800, a potent water soluble thienodiazepine. Two minutes later, the animals were decapitated, brain slices were prepared and exposed to UV light followed by fixation and preparation for autoradiography. Much better perservation of ultrastructure was obtained when the animals were killed by perfusion fixation followed by UV illumination of the fixed slices and their preparation for autoradiography. The results of the BR localization in fixed tissue were very similar to those obtained in fresh tissue (4).

Following injection of ^{3}H-FNZP alone, a selective accumulation of silver grains was found in synaptic contact regions (Tab. 3, Fig. 1a). This result which was found in slices from cerebral cortex, cerebellum and hippocampus, is consistent with a localization of BR on presynaptic and/or postsynaptic membranes without excluding the presence of BR on adjacent glial surfaces. The limited resolution of EM-autoradiography prevents a distinction between pre-, postsynaptic and adjacent glial structures. A glial localization of BR appears to be, however, unlikely since glial structures remote from synaptic contacts did not contain photolabeled BR.

In cerebellum, the nature of some synaptic contacts containing BR could be identified by their cytoarchi-

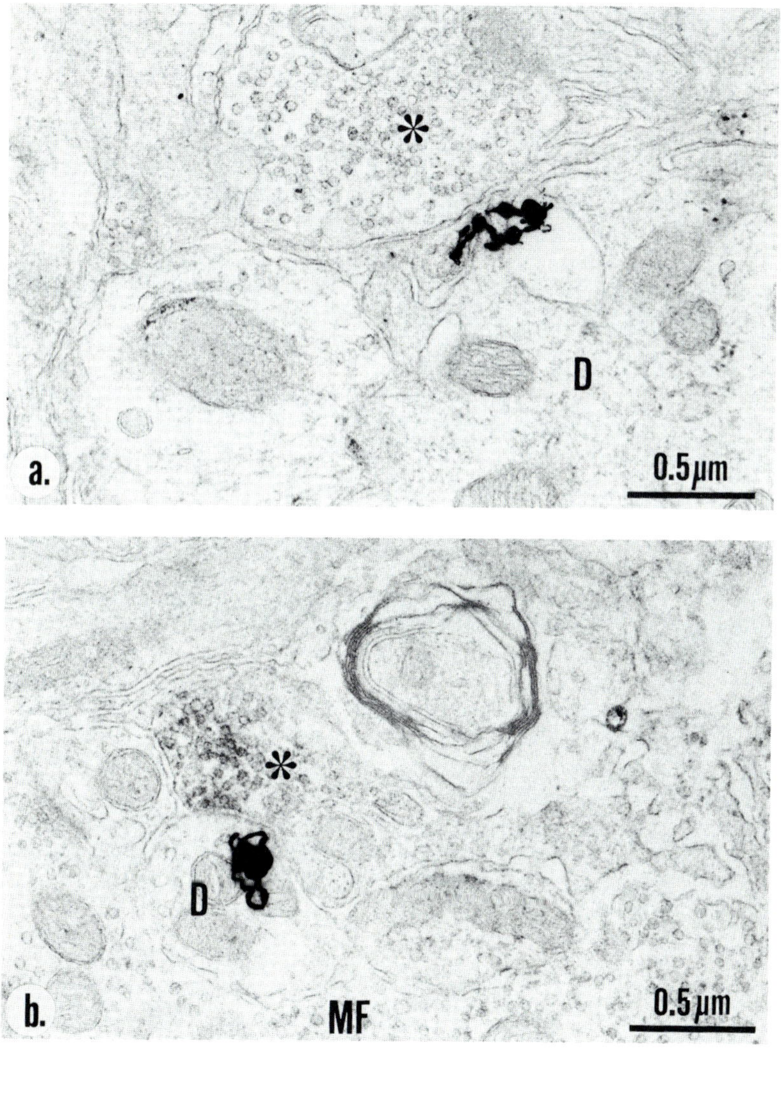

FIGURE 1. Ultrastructural localization of ^{3}H-FNZP in photolabeled rat cerebellar slices

A silver grain is associated a) with a region of contact between a nerve terminal (*) and a large dendrite (D), presumably of a Purkinje cell and b) with a region of contact between a Golgi nerve terminal stained for GAD (*) and a dendritic spine (D). MF, mossy fiber.

tecture. In cerebellar glomeruli synaptic contact regions of Golgi cells contained BR. Since Golgi cells are GABAergic, BR seem to occur at least in some GABA-ergic synapses.

TABLE 3. Semiquantitative analysis of silver grain distribution in EM autoradiographs of photolabeled rat cerebral cortex slices [a]

Drug co-injected	Grain density, grains/grid square[b]: Total	Regions of synaptic contacts[c]	Glia	Axon	Dendrite	Soma[d]	Unident. struct.
None	29.7± 2.0	16.4± 1.3	1.4± 0.3	0.5± 0.1	1.6± 0.3	4.3± 0.5	4.0± 0.5
Ro 11-7800	9.5± 0.6	3.5± 0.3	0.9± 0.2	0.4± 0.1	0.5± 0.1	0.7± 0.2	3.2± 0.3

[a]After injection of 100 μCi of ^{3}H-FNZP alone or in combination with 1 mg of Ro 11-7800 per rat, brain slices were photolabeled and prepared for autoradiography.

[b]Mean values ± SEM from 40 grid squares (1 grid square = 5776 μm^2).

[c]The 66 % probability circle around each grain contained at least part of a nerve ending or postsynaptic structure. Thus, the region of synaptic contacts comprises nerve endings and adjacent postsynaptic and glial structures (3).

[d]Grains localized intracellularly in the perikaryon.

Immunocytochemical identification of GABAergic synaptic contacts containing BR

In order to clearly identify GABAergic nerve terminals, brain slices in which BR had been photolabeled with ^{3}H-FNZP were stained with GAD antiserum (PAP Method, ref. 6). It should be noted that it is only in the outermost layer of a piece of tissue that nearly all the GABAergic nerve terminals present are stained immunocytochemically. With the concentration gradient of GAD antibodies and PAP complex decreasing towards the interior of the tissue, correspondingly less GABA-ergic nerve terminals are stained. The analysis of BR localization and GAD staining was therefore restricted to the 5 μm deep outer layer of the tissue.

In cerebellum it was found that about a third of the silver grains were associated with GAD-positive nerve endings, indicating that BR occur in GABAergic synaptic contacts (4). Among those were Golgi cell terminals (Fig. 1b). The association of silver grains with GAD-positive nerve terminals was not a random event, since in the presence of an excess of Ro 11-7800 no silver grains were found associated with GABAergic nerve terminals.

SUMMARY

The morphological demonstration of BR in GABAergic synapses is a major step forward in the understanding of the mechanism of action of benzodiazepines. It bridges the gap between the electrophysiological evidence stressing the involvement of GABAergic synaptic transmission in the action of benzodiazepines, and the biochemical evidence stressing BR as the site of action for this group of drugs.

At present we do not know in which types of synapses those BR are localized which were not associated with GAD positive terminals. At least some of the silver grains may nevertheless be localized in GABAergic terminals, since probably not all GABAergic terminals were stained immunocytochemically. However, it is also possible that some BR are localized in non-GABAergic synaptic contact regions. This possibility would open new concepts for our understanding of the mechanism of action of benzodiazepines and is presently under experimental investigation.

REFERENCES

1. Haefely, W., Polc, P., Schaffner, R., Keller, H.H., Pieri, L. and Möhler, H. (1978): In : GABA-Neurotransmitters, edited by O. Krogsgaard-Larsen, J. Scheel-Krüger and H. Kofod, pp.357-375. Munksgaard, Copenhagen.
2. Möhler, H. and Okada, T. (1977) : Science, 198:849-851.
3. Möhler, H., Battersby, M.K. and Richards, J.G. (1980) Proc. Nat. Acad. Sci. USA, 77:1666-1670.
4. Möhler, H. and Richards, J.G. (in preparation)
5. Squires, R.F. and Braestrup, C. (1977): Nature, 266: 732-734.

6. Sternberger, L.A. (1979): Immunocytochemistry, Wiley, New York, 2nd ed.
7. Wu, J.-Y. (1976): In : GABA in Nervous System Function, edited by E. Roberts, T.N. Chase and D.B. Tower, pp.7-55. Raven Press, New York.

GABA and Benzodiazepine Receptors,
edited by E. Costa et al.
Raven Press, New York © 1981.

β-Carboline-3-Carboxylates and Benzodiazepine Receptors

Claus Braestrup, *Mogens Nielsen, **Hanne Skovbjerg, and *Ole Gredal

*Research Laboratories, A/S Ferrosan, 5 Sydmarken, DK-2860 Soeborg, Denmark; *St. Hans Mental Hospital, DK-4000 Roskilde, Denmark; and **Panum Institute, Biochemical Department, C, 3 Blegdamsvej, DK-200 Copenhagen, Denmark,*

Putative endogenous ligands for brain benzodiazepine receptors have been pursued with appreciable effort since the discovery of benzodiazepine receptors in 1977 (for review see refs. 9, 20). It was argued that the presence of specific receptors for benzodiazepines on neuronal plasma membranes was not likely to be the consequence of mere chance. That some endogenous substance, a small neurotransmitter like molecule or a bigger neuromodulator like substance might reside in the brain, and participate in the perception of anxiety (an "anxiolytic" or "anxiogenic" substance) and which might be involved in regulation of seizure susceptibility.

It should not be overlooked, however, that at present the benzodiazepine receptors still assume status as drug receptors, as opposed to neurotransmitter receptors, which have identified neurotransmitters as ligands, with a more or less defined physiological function. The interaction between benzodiazepine receptor and other receptors, for example the GABA receptor, may provide the means for several of the pharmacological effects of benzodiazepines, without inferring the presence of endogenous ligands.

Several compounds and brain extracts have been proposed as endogenous ligands for benzodiazepine receptors, including hypoxanthine and inosine (2, 22), nicotinamide (22), GABA-modulin(14), an intestinal 15.800 dalton protein (25), and various unidentified extracts (10, 17). In this report, we present a compound (previously called the γ-fraction, ref. 24) which was obtained from human urine, and which possesses some interesting features.

ETHYL β-CARBOLINE-3-CARBOXYLATE

We have done extensive extraction and fractionation experiments using different tissues and biological fluids with the purpose of finding endogenous compounds with appreciable affinity for benzodiazepine receptors. We noted accidentally that one of the three fractions from urine on which we worked at that time (the α-, β- and γ-fractions) (24) was markedly augmented when the extract was heated at 60°C for a few hr. At first the heating seemed to cause break-down of urinary conjugates, but when it appeared that sulphatase and glucuronidase did not substitute for heating, and when optimizing revealed that alcohol was imperative, it became clear that ester formation occurred. The benzodiazepine receptor active product of the γ-fraction was identified as ethyl β-carboline-3-carboxylate (β-CCE, Fig. 1) by mass spectrometry, NMR-spectrometry and synthesis (8).

β-CCE is a potent and selective inhibitor of ^{3}H-flunitrazepam and ^{3}H-diazepam binding. The IC_{50} value for inhibition of benzodiazepine binding was about 7 nM in rat forebrain (Fig. 2 and ref. 8), and several other neurotransmitter receptors were not affected (8).

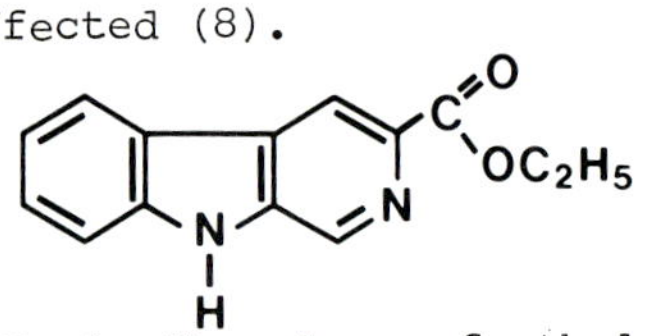

FIG. 1. Structure of ethyl β-carboline-3-carboxylate (β-CCE)

Ethyl esters are uncommon in the brain. Several reports, however, describe the preferential presence in CNS of methylase enzymes (11-13, 18). These methylases use S-adenosylmethionine as methyl donor and methylate acidic groups in proteins and peptides, for example the glutamate moiety of ACTH. However, we have not been able to extract methyl β-carboline-3-carboxylate or β-CCE from brain tissue (< 2 ng/g tissue). Also, methylation of β-carboline-3-carboxylic acid with brain enzymes and S-adenosylmethionine as methyl donor has not been demonstrated. Small amounts of β-CCE were obtained from brain tissue (≈ 20 ng/g tissue) only when the extracts were esterified during the isolation procedure (8).

Esters of β-carboline-3-carboxylic acid are therefore not likely candidates as ligands for brain benzodiazepine receptors. Other derivatives of β-carboline-3-carboxylic acid may be more relevant. Notably the amide and small "peptides" seem interesting.

The poorly defined biochemistry of β-carbolines is a matter of concern when evaluating their biological significance. It was shown already in 1961 that tryptamines and aldehydes readily react at physiological pH and temperature to form tetrahydro-β-carbolines (21), and it is well-known that β-carbolines easily show up as isolation artefacts (1). In several recent reports, however, where the presence of very small amounts of various β-carbolines in brain and peripheral tissues is described, attention was paid to the possible artefactual β-carboline formation (4, 5, 16, 26, 27).

β-CARBOLINE-3-CARBOXYLATE/BENZODIAZEPINE

RECEPTOR INTERACTIONS

Surprisingly it occurred that β-CCE was more potent in the cerebellum than in the hippocampus and several other brain regions (Fig. 2, and ref. 23). In addition, β-CCE exhibited mixed type competitive inhibition of ^{3}H-flunitrazepam binding in the hippocampus but pure competitive inhibition in cerebellum (23).

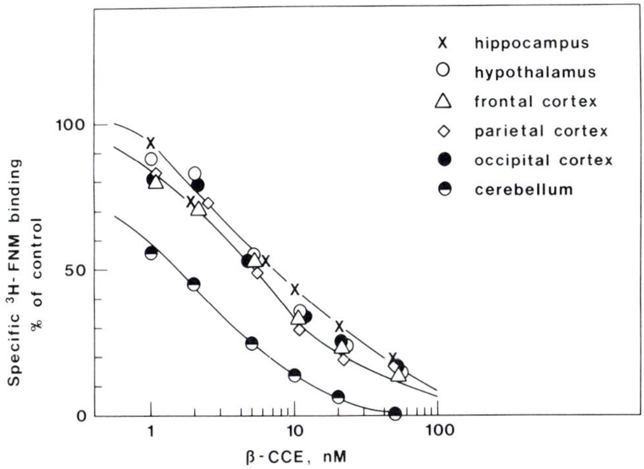

FIG. 2. Inhibition of specific ^{3}H-flunitrazepam binding to crude brain membranes by β-CCE (assay as described in legend to Table 2).

With the aim of investigating these findings in further detail, tritium labelled propyl β-carboline-3-carboxylate (^{3}H-PrCC) was synthesized for affinity binding experiments. ^{3}H-PrCC binds specifically to about the same number of binding sites as ^{3}H-flunitrazepam (40-80 pmol/g depending on the brain region); binding of the two ligands is mutually exclusive in the sense that binding of one ligand precludes the subsequent binding of the other; the regional distribution is similar except for a slight relative overweight of ^{3}H-PrCC binding in the cerebellum; and ^{3}H-PrCC can be displaced from specific sites in rat forebrain membranes only by those benzodiazepines and other agents which also inhibit the binding of ^{3}H-flunitrazepam and ^{3}H-diazepam (Nielsen and Braestrup, in preparation).

Furthermore, specific binding of ^{3}H-PrCC was sensitive to GABA receptor active agents. GABA and muscimol increased binding in a bicuculline, strychnine, and THIP sensitive fashion (Table 1). Similar results have been obtained with ^{3}H-diazepam (6, 7).

TABLE 1. Some GABA-ergic agents increase ^{3}H-PrCC binding *in vitro*

Addition (μM)	Specific ^{3}H-PrCC binding % of controls, ± SEM	p	N
None	100		8
GABA (100)	128 ± 2	0.001	4
Muscimol (10)	131 ± 2	0.001	8
Muscimol (3)	128 ± 3	0.001	8
THIP (100)	97 ± 5	n.s.	4
PSA (100)	76 ± 3	0.001	4
Bicuculline (10)	94 ± 2	n.s.	4
Bicuculline + GABA (100)	95 ± 4	n.s.	4
Strychnine (100)	73 ± 1	0.001	4
Strychnine + muscimol (3)	75 ± 3	0.001	4
THIP + muscimol (3)	105 ± 3	n.s.	4

Experiments were made using 5 times washed rat forebrain membranes as described in ref. (7), with the exception that ^{3}H-PrCC (0.28 nM) was used as ligand in place of ^{3}H-diazepam and that only 5 mg original tissue was used per assay. Control specific binding was 3590 ± 110 cpm/assay (mean ± SEM (8)). PSA is piperidine-4-sulfonic acid.

The available evidence thus suggests that ^{3}H-PrCC binds to the benzodiazepine receptors.

One attractive explanation for the observed regional selectivity of the effects of β-CCE using ^{3}H-FNM as ligand would be the presence of receptor heterogeneity. Circumstantial evidence, such as the presence of polyphasic heat inactivation curves and polyphasic receptor-ligand dissociation curves (29) as well as the more direct demonstration of two molecular species of receptors in the hippocampus (P_{51} and P_{55}) compared to only one species in the cerebellum (Sieghart and Karobath, personal communication) indicate the presence of multiple benzodiazepine receptors. The observed regional variation in IC_{50} values for β-carboline-3-carboxylates(23, Fig. 2) as well as the curvilinear Scatchard analysis (8,23) thus suggest that distinct benzodiazepine receptors occur in the hippocampus and some other brain areas. This group of receptors consist of at least one receptor with high affinity for β-carboline-3-carboxylates (the 'cerebellar type' receptor, possibly identical with the P_{51} molecular species) and another receptor type with low affinity for β-carboline-3-carboxylates. Benzodiazepines appear to be virtually nonselective because similar K_D values for ^{3}H-FNM were observed both in the cerebellum and in the hippocampus (23), and because cerebellar/hippocampal differences in IC_{50} values for several benzodiazepines (Table 2 and unpublished) were very small or absent.

Scatchard analysis, however, did not reveal the expected ca. 5 fold difference in K_D value for ^{3}H-PrCC between cerebellum and hippocampus. Slightly curvilinear Scatchard plots with affinity constants close to 1 nM were obtained for both regions (Fig. 3).

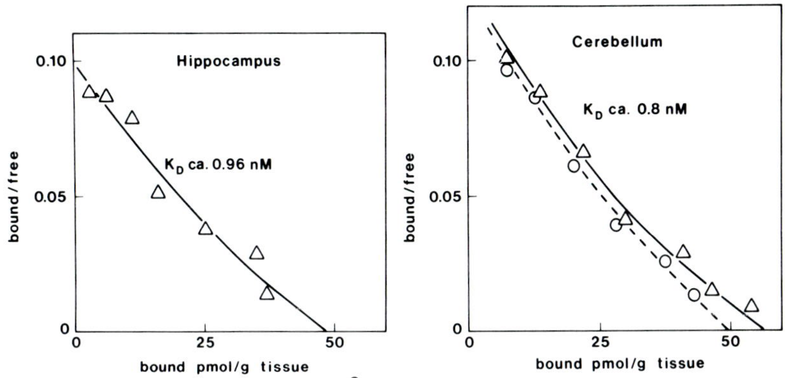

FIG. 3. Specific binding of ^{3}H-PrCC to crude rat brain membranes. Non-specific binding was estimated using diazepam (3 μM), circles; or using β-CCE (4 μM), triangles. See legend Table 2 for further details. K_D in hippocampus was 1.2 ± 0.3 nM (5); K_D in cerebellum was 0.9 ± 0.1 nM (7) (mean ± SEM of (N) values), calculated from 5 and 7 similar experiments by linear regression analysis.

Furthermore, it was also surprising that the ca. 5 fold difference in the IC_{50} values for β-CCE was only observed when ^{3}H-FNM was used as ligand, but not when ^{3}H-PrCC was used (Table 2).

TABLE 2. Inhibition of specific binding of ^{3}H-flunitrazepam (^{3}H-FNM) and ^{3}H-PrCC

Inhibitor	IC_{50}, nM			
	^{3}H-FNM		^{3}H-PrCC	
	hippocampus	cerebellum	hippocampus	cerebellum
Diazepam	11	11	15	15
Clonazepam	2.1	1.1	1.3	1.0
β-CCE	11	2.4	3.6	1.7
Methyl β-carboline-3-carboxylate	13	2.8	3.3	2.5

Each value in the table is the mean of two values, each obtained after addition of 3 concentrations of inhibitor in duplicate to assays. The proportion between first and second IC_{50} determination was 1.31 ± 0.35 (mean ± sd of 16 pairs). Assays consisted of crude rat brain membrane suspensions (homogenized by an Ultra Turrax homogenizer in 10 vol 25 mM KH_2PO_4, pH 7.1, pelleted once and resuspended). The resuspension was incubated with ^{3}H-FNM (1 nM, 2 mg tissue in 0.55 ml) or ^{3}H-PrCC (44.6 Ci/mmol, 0.28 nM, 5 mg tissue in 2.75 ml) for 60 min at 0°C before filtration through Whatman GF/C glass fibre filters, washing and counting. Blanks for ^{3}H-FNM (diazepam, 3 μM) amounted 5-7% of total binding and for ^{3}H-PrCC (β-CCE, 4 μM) 25-40%.

A simple explanation for these new findings (Fig. 3, Table 2) would be that the dissociation rate constant for the low affinity hippocampal site exceeds the limit for application of the filtration technique. Any bound ligand to the low affinity site would then be washed away during the filtration and washing procedures used to isolate free from bound ^{3}H-PrCC, and only the high affinity sites would be expressed in the assays. Further experimentation, however, is reguired to ascertain whether ^{3}H-PrCC can be useful as a selective ligand for the cerebellar type benzodiazepine receptor.

Alternatively, the lack of regional selectivity when ^{3}H-PrCC was used as ligand would be the presence of negative cooperativity among benzodiazepine receptors in the hippocampus. True negative cooperativity which was expressed only when both β-carboline-3-carboxylate and a benzodiazepine interact simultaneously with the receptors. More complicated models, such as mobile receptor models (15), might also be considered. There exists some indirect support for the proposal that site-site interaction among benzodiazepine receptors may occur. Irreversible photoaffinity labelling of benzodiazepine receptors with ^{3}H-flunitrazepam (3) causes more than one receptor site to disappear for each molecule of bound ^{3}H-flunitrazepam (H. Möhler, unpublished). In addition, removal of some benzodiazepine recognition sites with unlabelled flunitrazepam (photoaffinity labelling) transformed the mixed type competitive inhibition of ^{3}H-FNM binding by β-CCE in hippocampus (23) into pure competitive inhibition (Bræstrup and Nielsen, unpublished). Furthermore, the apparent molecular weight of the benzodiazepine receptor varies markedly with the procedure used for molecular weight determination. SDS-gel electrophoresis reveals molecular weights of ca. 50,000 daltons (3, Sieghart and Karobath, personal communication, Fig. 4). Sephadex G-200 gel filtration experiments of Lubrol-Px solubilized receptors (31) and ultracentrifugation (19) indicate molecular weights of 2-300,000 daltons. In the present study we used a carefully calibrated Ultrogel AcA-34 gel filtration column and found a molecular weight of ca. 110,000 daltons for photoaffinity labelled, Triton X-100 solubilized benzodiazepine receptors, both in hippocampus and cerebellum (Fig.4).

These results indicate that the photoaffinity labelled receptor may be solubilized as a dimer which is split into subunits upon SDS treatment. The presence of sharp, almost symmetrical peaks upon gel filtration do not indicate that the high molecular weight was obtained by unspecific formation of micelles containing the receptor and arbitrary proteins (however, one of the three major protein bands of synaptosomal plasma membranes, tubulin, has a molecular weight of 50,000 (28)). The possibility also exists of course that the second unit in the 110,000 daltons molecular species is the GABA receptor.

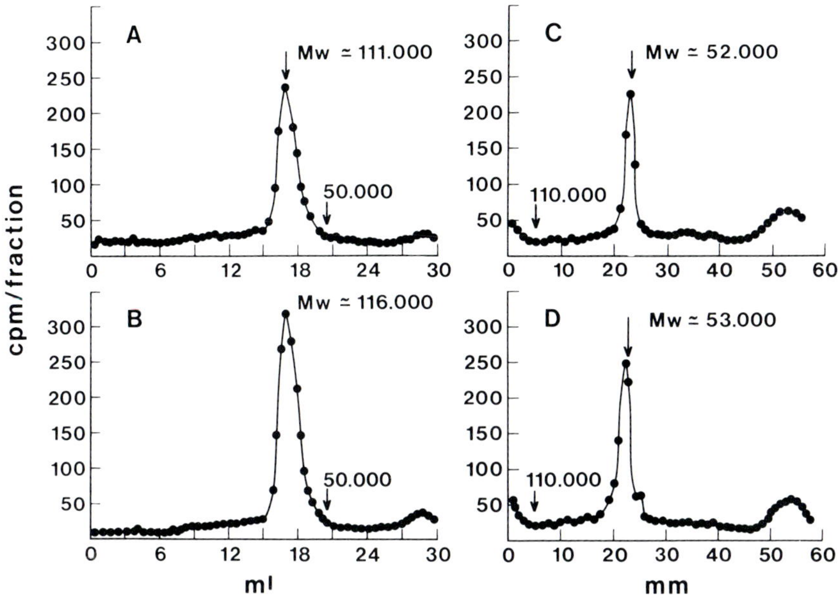

FIG. 4. Rat hippocampal (B and D) and cerebellar (A and C) membranes were homogenized in 100 mM TRIS,citrate, pH 7.1, and labelled irreversibly with ^{3}H-flunitrazepam (10 nM, 5 min UV-exposure, ^{3}H-FNM was incorporated corresponding to ca. 30% of Bmax). After 5 washings the membranes were divided into two parts and solubilized. Panels A and B, solubilization in Triton X-100 (0.7%) for AcA 34 gel filtration (column 0.9 x 44.5 cm, 0.42 ml/fraction, flow 3.6 ml cm^{-2}h^{-1}, equilibrated and eluted in 35 mM KH_2PO_4, pH 7.4, containing 150 mM KCl and 0.1% Triton X-100). The column was calibrated with (daltons), aminopeptidase M (280,000), albumin dimer (134,000), albumin (67,000), and ovalbumin (45,000). Panels C and D, solubilization in sodiumdodecylsulphate (SDS, 1.4%) and mercaptoethanol (0.02%) (boiling for 5 min) for SDS-electrophoresis according to Weber et al. (30) in 7.5 % polyacrylamide. External standards were (daltons), β-galactosidase (130,000), phosphorylase A (92,000), transferrin (77,000), albumin (67,000) and ovalbumin (45,000).

CONCLUSIONS

The studies with derivatives of β-carboline-3-carboxylic acid, which may well be part of an endogenous ligand for benzodiazepine receptors, suggest that ^{3}H-PrCC may be a selective ligand for subclasses of benzodiazepine receptors, in particular the P_{51} molecular species ('cerebellar type') demonstrated by Sieghart and Karobath. Alternatively, true negative cooperativity may exist in the hippocampus and the findings in the present study of complexes with molecular weight of ca..llo,ooo daltons may be relevant for the molecular arrangements responsible for these proposed site-site interactions.

Acknowledgement

^{3}H-Propyl β-carboline-3-carboxylate was synthesized by H. Schou, A/S Ferrosan, Denmark. The supply of THIP by Lundbeck and Co., Denmark and PSA (piperidine-4-sulfonic acid) by P. Krogsgaard-Larsen is highly appreciated.

REFERENCES

1. Abramovitch, R. A. and Spenser, I. D. (1964): In: Advances in Heterocyclic Chemistry, edited by A. R. Katritzky, A. J. Boulton, and J. M. Lagowski, pp. 79-210. Academic Press, New York.
2. Asano, T. and Spector, S. (1979): Proc. Natl. Acad. Sci. USA, 76:977-981.
3. Battersby, M. K., Richards, J. G., and Möhler, H. (1979): Europ. J. Pharmacol., 57:277-278.
4. Bidder, T. G., Shoemaker, D. W., Boettger, H. G., Evans, M., and Cummins, J. T. (1979): Life Sci., 25:157-164.
5. Dillon, J., Spector, A., and Nakanishi, K. (1976): Nature, 259:422-423.
6. Braestrup, C. and Nielsen, M. (1980): In: GABA and Other Inhibitory Neurotransmitters, edited by H. Lal, E. Usdin, and E. Roberts. Raven Press.
7. Braestrup, C., Nielsen, M., Krogsgaard-Larsen, P., and Falch Falch, E. (1979): Nature, 280:331-333.
8. Braestrup, C., Nielsen, M., and Olsen, C. E. (1980): Proc. Natl. Acad. Sci. USA, 77: 2288-2292.
9. Braestrup, C. and Squires, R. (1978): Brit. J. Psychiat., 133:249-260.
10. Colello, G. D., Hockenbery, D. M., Bosman, H. B., Fuchs, S., and Folkers, K. (1978): Proc. Natl. Acad. Sci. USA, 75:6319-6323.
11. Diliberto, E. J., and Axelrod, J. (1974): Proc. Natl. Acad. Sci., 71:1701-1704.
12. Diliberto, E. J. and Axelrod, J. (1976): J. Neurochem., 26: 1159-1165.
13. Gagnon, C. and Heisler, S. (1979): Life Sci., 25:993-1000.
14. Guidotti, A, Toffano, G., and Costa, E. (1978): Nature, 275: 553-555.
15. Hollenberg, M. D. (1979): Pharmacol. Rev., 30:393-410.
16. Honecker, H. and Rommelspacher, H. (1978): Naunyn-Schmiedeberg's Arch. Pharmacol., 305:135-141.
17. Karobath, M., Sperk, G., and Schöbeck, G. (1978): Europ. J. Pharmacol., 49:323-326.
18. Kim, S. and Li, C. H. (1979): Proc. Natl. Acad. Sci. USA,76: 4255-4257.

19. Lang, B., Barnard, E. A., Chang, L.-R., and Dolly, J. O. (1979): FEBS Letters, 104:149-153.
20. Marangos, P. J., Paul, S. M., and Goodwin, F. K., Life Sci.: 25:1093-1102.
21. McIsaac, W. (1961): Biochim. Biophys. Acta, 52:607-609.
22. Möhler, H., Polc, P., Cumin, R., Pieri, L., and Kettler, R.: (1979): Nature, 278:563-565.
23. Nielsen, M. and Braestrup, C.(1980): Nature. In press.
24. Nielsen, M., Gredal, O., and Braestrup, C. (1979): Life Sci., 25:679-686.
25. Nixon, J. C. and Woolf, J. H. (1979): Pharmacologist 21:242
26. Rommelspacher, H., Honecker, H., Barbey, M., and Meinke, B. (1979): Naunyn-Schmiedeberg's Arch. Pharmcol., 310:35-41.
27. Shoemaker, D. W., Cummins, J. T., and Bidder, T. G. (1978): Neuroscience, 3:233-239.
28. Smith, A. P. and Loh, H. H. (1979): Life Sci., 24:1-20.
29. Squires, R. F., Benson, D. I., Braestrup, C., Coupet, J., Klepner, C. A., Myers, V., and Beer, B. (1979): Pharmacol. Biochem. Behav., 10:825-830.
30. Weber, K., Pringle, J., and Osborn, M. (1972): Methods Enzymol., 26:3-27.
31. Yosufi, M. A. K., Thomas, J. W., and Tallman, J. F. (1979): Life Sci., 25:463-470.

GABA and Benzodiazepine Receptors,
edited by E. Costa et al.
Raven Press, New York © 1981.

GABA Autoreceptors: Structure-Activity Relationships for Agonists

M. J. W. Brennan, R. C. Cantrill, and *P. Krogsgaard-Larsen

*Brain Research Group, Department of Medical Biochemistry, School of Pathology, University of the Witwatersrand and South African Institute for Medical Research, Johannesburg 2001, South Africa; and *Department of Chemistry BC, Royal Danish School of Pharmacy, Universitetsparken, DK-2100, Copenhagen, Denmark*

There is considerable evidence, in both the peripheral and central nervous systems, that presynaptic α-adrenoreceptors modulate norepinephrine release induced by both electrical and potassium ion stimulation; α-agonists inhibit and α-antagonists facilitate this release (15,16,20,24,32). There is also evidence that similar control mechanisms occur in dopaminergic (14,22,28,29,32) and cholinergic (34) neurons. Classical postsynaptic receptor agonists and antagonists have varying degrees of affinity for the corresponding autoreceptors; such pharmacological differences may open up the possibility of selective activation or blockage of one or other class of receptor by drugs. The presence of autoreceptors capable of regulating the releaase of the important inhibitory transmitter γ-aminobutyric acid (GABA) from GABA-ergic neurons has recently been reported (10,11,27,31). At present the selectivity of the GABA autoreceptors for agonists and antagonists is unknown. In the experiments reported here we have examined the potency of a number of GABA agonists in inhibiting K^+-stimulated release of ^{3}H-GABA from preloaded rat cortical synaptosomes and compared and this with the potency of the drugs in inhibiting specific ^{3}H-binding to cortical synaptic plasma membranes. These studies were aimed at the elucidation of any pharmacological differences between the autoreceptors and the sites labelled with ^{3}H-GABA.

MATERIALS AND METHODS

Release of preloaded ^{3}H-GABA from rat cortical synaptosomes was monitored using a superfusion system described previously (7,8,9) Synaptosomes prepared from the cerebral cortices of adult male Wistar rats by a modification (5) of the method of Gray and Whittaker (21) were resuspended in 0,32M glucose to give a protein concentration (25) of about 5mg/ml and diluted 1:10 with ice-cold incubation medium (final concentration: 128mM NaCl; 5mM KCl; 2.7mM $CaCl_2$; 1.2mM $MgSO_4$; 0.1mM aminooxyacetic acid to prevent GABA catabolism; 10mM Tris-HCl buffer at pH 7.35). One ml aliquots of the suspension were preincubated at 37^{0}C for 15 minutes in a waterbath in an air atmosphere. 2,3-^{3}H-GABA of specific activity 65Ci/mmol (the Radiochemical Centre, Amersham) was diluted with unlabelled GABA to give a specific activity of

10Ci/mmol and a small volume (1% of the final volume) added to the incubation tubes to a final concentration of 0.5μM. Incubation was continued for a further 10 minutes after which the synaptosome suspensions were layered on Millipore filters (0.45μM pore) resting on filter supports constituting the bottoms of four parallel superfusion chambers (13) and thermostatically maintained at 37^{0}C. The chambers were connected to a multichanneled peri staltic pump, the excess medium drawn off at maximum flow rate, and the filters washed with 10ml of control medium (concentration as described above) containing 30mM glucose. The flow rate was adjusted to 0.5ml per minute and 1 minute fractions collected directly into scintillation counting vials. Superfusion was continued for 10 minutes with control medium to establish a baseline rate of GABA efflux; the control medium was then exchanged for the test medium containing the GABA agonists at various concentrations and superfusion continued for a further 15 minutes. Aquagel I liquid scintillant (Chemlab), 5ml, was added to each vial and the radioactivity of the vials counted in a Packard Tri-Carb 2660 Spectrometer with automatic quench correction. Filters were solubilized in 10ml of Aquagel I and counted in the same way. Stimulation of GABA release was calculated as the percentage increase in efflux over the baseline unstimulated level.

The sodium-independent binding of ^{3}H-GABA to rat cortical membrane was studied at 4^{0}C in Tris-citrate buffer by a modification (23) of the method of Enna and Snyder (18). Adult Wistar rats were decapitated and the cortices rapidly homogenized in 15 volumes of ice-cold 0.32M sucrose. The homogenate was centrifuged at 1 000g for 10 minutes, the pellets discarded, and the supernatant centrifuged at 20 000g for 20 minutes. A suspension of the crude mitochondrial pellet in distilled water was dispered with a Brinkman Polytron PT-10 (setting 6) for 30 seconds and centrifuged at 8 000g for 20 minutes. The supernatant fluid was collected and the pellet, a bi-layer with a soft, buffy coat, was carefully rinsed with the supernatant fluid to collect the upper layer. This suspension was centrifuged at 48 000g for 20 minutes. The final membrane pellets were submitted to two resuspensions in water and centrifugations at 48,000g for 20 minutes. The membranes were frozen rapidly at -70C and kept at -20C for at least 18 hours. Frozen pellets were resuspended in water, maintained at 25^{0}C for 20 minutes, and centrifuged at 48 000g for 10 minutes. This procedure was repeated once. For the standard ^{3}H-GABA binding assay, aliquots of these membranes (0.8-1.2mg of protein)were incubated in quadruplicate at 4^{0}C for 5 minutes in 2ml of 0.05M Tris-citrate buffer (pH 7.1) containing 5.8mM ^{3}H-GABA alone, or in the presence of 1mM unlabelled GABA or other agonist drugs at various concentrations.

After incubation, the tubes were centrifuged at 48 000g for 10 minutes, the supernatant fluid decanted, and the pellets rinsed superficially with two 5ml aliquots of ice-cold distilled water.

Bound radioactivity was extracted into 1ml of water, 10ml of scintillant added, and radioactivity measured in a scintillation counter. Total specific ^{3}H-GABA binding was obtained by subtracting from the total bound radioactivity the amount not displaced by 1mM unlabelled GABA. Using this procedure of extensive washing and very rapid freezing of the synaptic membranes, approximately 80% of the total binding represented specifically bound GABA. Estimates of the concentrations of the agonists producing 50% inhibition of specific ^{3}H-GABA binding (IC_{50}) were made by examining the displacements produced by at least 4 different concentrations of the drug and performing log-probit analyses of the results (1).

In addition to the above centrifugation procedure, rapid filtration through Millipore filters (0.45μM pore) was used in an attempt to select for high affinity binding sites in the synaptic membranes. After incubation, the reaction was terminated by filtration, and the filters washed with two 5ml aliquots of ice-cold Tris-citrate buffer. Filters were then solubilized in 10ml Aquagel I and counted for radioactivity.

RESULTS

The porphyrin precursor δ-aminolevulinic acid (δ-ALA) is an omega-amino acid with a 5-carbon chain similar in structure to GABA. The release of GABA from the nerve endings in response to K^{+}-depolarisation was reduced by δ-ALA in a dose-dependent fashion (Fig.1). This reduction was significant at a δ-ALA concentration of 1μM, and at a concentration of 100μM, 75% of the stimulated release was abolished. The concentration of δ-ALA which inhibited 50% of the K^{+}-stimulated release was approximately 10μM. At all concentrations the reduction was prevented by the GABA antagonists bicuculline and picrotoxin (1μM)(Table 1). δ-ALA at 1μM or 10μM exhibited no effects on basal release of GABA, although at 100μM, GABA efflux was slightly stimulated. Neither bicuculline nor picrotoxin alone (1μM or 10μM)modified the basal release of radioactivity in the conditions used here. This is expected, as we consider that any GABA released from the tissue is rapidly removed from the superfusion chamber by the flow of medium. The concentration of GABA in the medium does not therefore reach the levels necessary to stimulate presynaptic receptors and hence the bicuculline or picrotoxin has no negative feedback effect to antagonize.

Muscimol, piperidine-4-sulphonic acid (P4S), isoguvacine and 4,5, 6,7-tetrahydroisoxazolo 5,4-c pyridin-3-ol (THIP) are potent GABA receptor agonists (6,23). Again, all reduced the K^{+} (55mM)-stimulated release of preloaded ^{3}H-GABA from rat cortical synaptosomes in a dose-dependent fashion (Fig.2).

FIG.1.

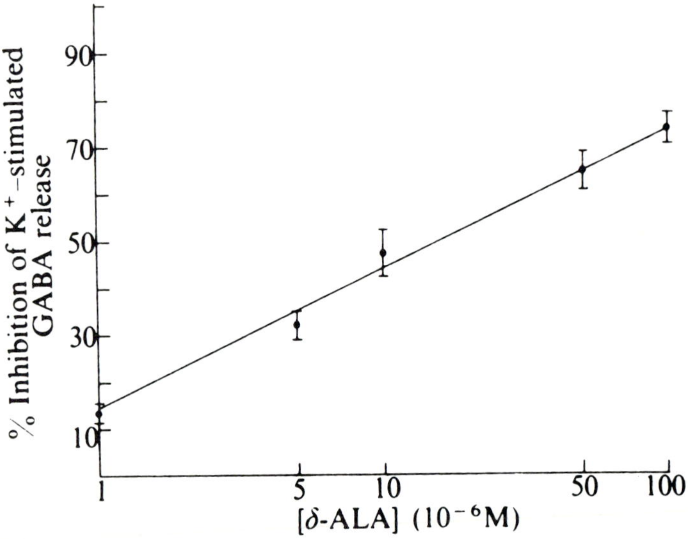

A dose-response curve for the inhibition of K^+-induced GABA release by δ-ALA. The horizontal axis gives concentration of δ-ALA ($x10^{-6}$M) on a logarithmic scale. Represented on the vertical axis is the % inhibition of K^+(55mM) GABA release. Each point is the mean % inhibition ± S.E.M. (n = 4). The curve is the best fit to the data by the method of least squares(r^2=0.97).

All the GABA agonists used in this study inhibited specific ^{3}H-GABA binding to high affinity receptor sites in synaptic membrane from rat cerebral cortex. The IC_{50} values for the compounds are listed in Table 2. The order of potency of the compounds in inhibiting GABA receptor binding was the same as that for inhibiting K^+-stimulated GABA release. In addition, with the exception of δ-ALA, there was a good absolute correlation between the potencies of the drugs in inhibiting binding and in inhibiting stimulated GABA release. Using the standard centrifugation assay for ^{3}H-GABA binding, δ-ALA appeared some 30 times more potent at the autoreceptor than at the sites labelled by ^{3}H-GABA. When ^{3}H-GABA binding was assayed using the filtration method, a single class of sites having a Kd of 7.5nM was detected. The binding of ^{3}H-GABA under these conditions was displaced by δ-ALA with an IC_{50}value of approximately 10μM.

TABLE 1.

Drug effects on the K^+-stimulated release of GABA from preloaded synaptosomes.

Drug present	Induced release (% increase over baseline control)	Mean drug effect on induced release
55mM K^+ alone (6)	188 ± 26.9*	
55mM K^+ + 10^{-5}M δ-ALA (4)	92 ± 13.5**	- 51.1%
55mM K^+ + 10^{-5}M δ-ALA + 10^{-6}M picrotoxin (4)	187 ± 10.2	- 0.5%
55mM K^+ + 10^{-8}M muscimol (4)	107 ± 11.1**	- 43.0%
55mM K^+ + 10^{-8}M muscimol + 10^{-6}M bicuculline (2)	194 ± 13.7	+ 3.0%
55mM K^+ + 5 x 10^{-8}M P4S (4)	86 ± 6.1**	- 54.0%
55mM K^+ + 5 x 10^{-8}M P4S + 10^{-6}M picrotoxin (2)	179 ± 12.1	- 5.0%
55mM K^+ + 10^{-7}M isoguvacine (4)	68 ± 7.8**	- 64.0%
55mM K^+ + 10^{-7}M isoguvacine + 10^{-6}M bicuculline (2)	184 ± 12.0	- 2.0%
55mM K^+ + 10^{-7}M THIP (4)	98 ± 5.0**	- 48.0%
55mM K^+ + 10^{-7}M THIP + 10^{-6}M picrotoxin (2)	177 ± 8.4	- 6.0%

Experiments were carried out as described in the test. The values in parentheses indicate the number of times the experimental conditions in the first columns were repeated. Baseline efflux was calculated as % total tissue stores released per fraction (0.57 ± 0.068%, n = 7). The second column refers to the % increase in efflux over this control baseline level; in each case the mean ± S.E.M. is given. Statistical significance was calculated using the two-sided Student t-test. The third column represents the average drug-induced change compared with the release caused by 55mM K^+ alone.

* Substitution of Mg^{2+} for Ca^{2+} in the medium did not significantly affect basal release of radioactivity, although 76 ± 2.2% (n = 4) of the K^+ (55mM)-induced release was Ca^{2+}-dependent.

** $P<0.001$, significant difference from 55mM K^+ alone.

It might therefore be that the filtration technique allows the selective labelling of a small number of high affinity binding sites which correspond to the autoreceptors.

FIG.2.

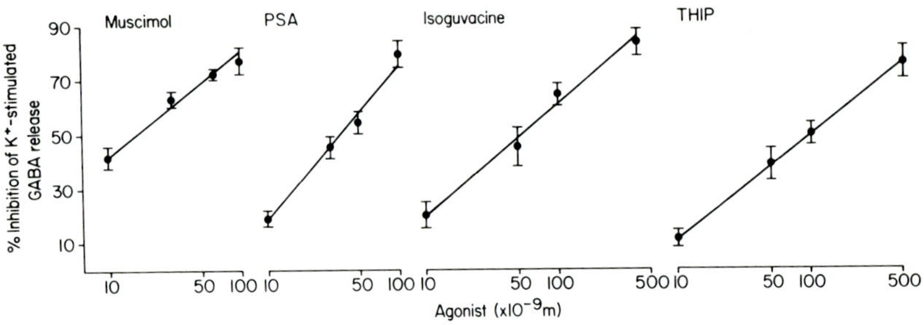

Dose-response curves for the inhibition of K^+-induced GABA release by GABA agonists. See legend to Fig.1.

In every case, at every drug concentration tested, the reduction in K^+-stimulated release was prevented by (+)bicuculline and picrotoxin at concentrations of 1μm (Table 1). P4S, isoguvacine and THIP, at concentrations up to 1μm, exhibited no effects on the basal release of GABA efflux in a dose-dependent fashion (Fig.3).

DISCUSSION

The data shown in Table 2 suggests that the GABA autoreceptors and the receptors labelled by ^{3}H-GABA in synaptic membranes show considerable pharmacological similarity. Many binding studies using ^{3}H-GABA or ^{3}H-muscimol as ligands have been published (18, 19,31,35). Our data suggest that the interpretation of these studies must consider the labelling of both pre- and postsynaptic GABA receptor sites. The autoreceptors might, however, represent only a very small percentage of the total binding.

Although the release studies and the binding studies were carried out in media of different ionic composition, there was a good absolute correlation between receptor occupancy by agonists and inhibition of stimulated GABA release. To date, strict quantitative comparison between the results of binding studies and neurophysiological data has proved difficult. This is due to the impossibility of precise regulation of drug concentrations in the extracellular fluid during microiontophoretic experiments. The results reported here thus provide the first direct correlation between a GABA receptor-mediated effect and receptor occupancy. It appears from these data that the autoreceptor is coupled directly to the effector mechanism (presumably a chloride channel since the inhibition of GABA release by agonist is picrotoxin-sensitive) and that there are no "spare" autoreceptors on the presynaptic terminal.

TABLE 2.

Inhibition of K^+(55mM)-stimulated ^3H-GABA release from synaptosomes and specific ^3H-GABA binding in synaptic plasma membranes by GABA agonists.

	IC_{50} (μM)	
	GABA release	GABA binding
Muscimol	0.016 ± 0.003	0.006 ± 0.002
P4S	0.036 ± 0.004	0.034 ± 0.002
Isoguvacine	0.049 ± 0.005	0.037 ± 0.003
THIP	0.110 ± 0.008	0.131 ± 0.005
δ-ALA	11.5 ± 0.87	> 300

Release experiments were carried out as described in the test. IC_{50} values for the inhibition of K^+-stimulated GABA release were calculated from a best fit line to the data by log-probit analysis. At every drug concentration tested, the inhibition of ^3H-GABA release was prevented by the GABA antagonists bicuculline and picrotoxin (10^{-6}M). Sodium-independent binding of ^3H-GABA to membranes isolated from rat cerebral cortex was studied at 4°C in Tris-citrate buffer using a centrifugation assay. The IC_{50} was estimated by varying the concentration over a range of values using 4 data points for each of 4 inhibitor concentrations and calculating the line of best fit for a log-probit plot. Results are means ± S.E.M. of 4 independent experiments.

Recently the existence of bicuculline-insensitive presynaptic GABA receptors which regulate the release of norepinephrine, dopamine and serotonin have been described in the mammalian peripheral and central nervous systems (3,4,12). Our results suggest that the autoreceptors are distinct from this second class of presynaptic GABA receptors and more closely resemble the classical postsynaptic GABA binding site.

The GABA agonist THIP has recently been introduced for clinical trial in a number of neurological and psychiatric conditions. It is apparent from our data that such a drug will act at both pre- and postsynaptic receptors and that these two actions will tend to produce different effects. The development of agonists and antagonists selective for one class of GABA receptor is therefore of prime importance for the successful manipulation of brain GABA systems by drugs.

It is interesting in this regard to consider a possible role for δ-ALA in the pathogenesis of the neural dysfunction characterzing acute attacks of the hereditary hepatic porphyrias. The presentation of nervous system involvement in acute porphyria varies; in decreasing order of frequency, there may be motor neuropathy, confusion, psychiatric manifestations, hyperexcitability and epileptic-type seizures (17). Psychiatric manifestations include depression, anxiety, insomnia and an organic brain syndrome. Although the aetiology of the neural dysfunction in the acute attack is unknown, several mechanisms have been suggested at a neurochemical level. It is possible that porphyrin precursors, which are produced in excess by the liver during acute episodes, gain access to the nervous system and exert direct neurotoxic effects (7,8); alternatively, a metabolic defect in heme biosynthesis in nerve cells might result in a functional hemoprotein deficiency which becomes critical at the time of the acute attack (30). δ-ALA exhibits various effects in mammalian central nervous tissue preparations. It inhibits high affinity uptake and increases efflux of GABA and L-glutamate in rat cortical synaptosomes (3,4); it also inhibits the ($Na^+ + K^+$) ATPase isolated from rabbit brain and red blood cells (2). These effects occur only at relatively high concentrations of δ-ALA (at least 100μM), and it is very unlikely that such concentrations are reached in the brain during acute porphyric attacks (30). Nevertheless, it has been demonstrated that δ-ALA can penetrate the blood-brain barrier of the rat at plasma concentrations known to occur in acute intermittent porphyria and appear in the cerebrospinal fluid in μM concentrations. In addition, cerebrospinal fluid levels of 16-20μM have been recorded in patients during acute attacks characterized by hyperexcitability and convulsions (33). In preliminary experiments conducted in our laboratory the intraventricular injection of 2-5μmoles of δ-ALA in rats caused jumping seizures. Injection of a larger dose (10μmoles) proved uniformly fatal within a few minutes. It is therefore conceivable that δ-ALA might be a relatively selective agonist for the GABA autoreceptors. We hope that this compound might serve as a parent structure for the development of more potent drugs acting selectively at GABA autoreceptors.

FIG.3.

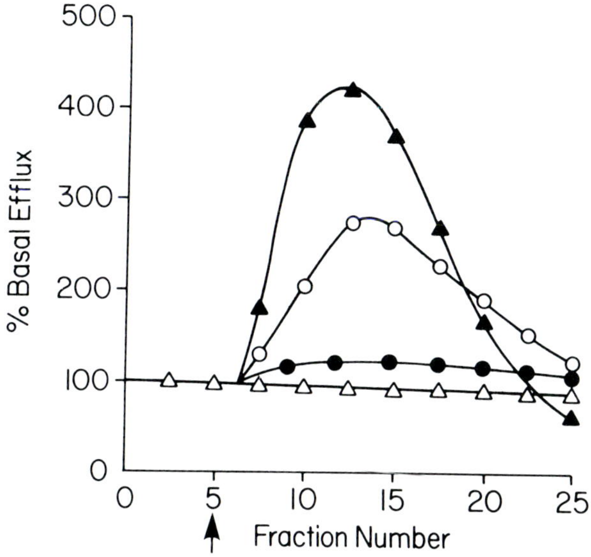

Stimulation of basal ^{3}H-GABA efflux from preloaded synaptosomes by muscimol. The superfusion technique is described in the text. Shown is the % change in efflux (baseline efflux + 100%) against fraction number. The arrow represents the changeover from control medium (Δ) to the test medium containing: O, 0.1μM muscimol; O, 1μM muscimol; Δ, 10μM muscimol. The first few fractions were very variable in each case and are now shown. Each curve is an average of 3 superfusion experiments. Variation between individual curves was less than 10% of the mean.

ACKNOWLEDGEMENTS

These studies were supported in part by grants from the Danish and South African Medical Research Councils and the Atomic Energy Board of South Africa. M.J.W.B. and R.C.C. are Mellor Research Fellows and M.J.W.B. is in receipt of a grant from the Loewenstein Research Foundation. We wish to thank Mrs. C. Parsons for preparation of the manuscript.

REFERENCES

1. Balcar, V.J., Johnston, G.A.R., and Stephanson, A.L. (1976): Brain Res., 102: 143-151.

2. Becker, D.M., Viljoen, J.D., and Kramer, S. (1971): Biochim. biophys. Acta, 225: 26-34.

3. Bowery, N.G., and Hudson, A.L. (1979): Br.J.Pharmac., 66: 108P.

4. Bowery, N.G., Hill, D.R., Hudson, A.L., Doble, A., Middlemiss, D.N., Shaw, J., and Turnbull, M. (1980): Nature, 283: 92-94.

5. Bradford, H.F., Bennett, G.W., and Thomas, A.J. (1973): J. Neurochem., 21: 495-505.

6. Braestrup, C., Nielsen, M., Krogsgaard-Larsen, P., and Falch, E. (1979): Nature, 280: 331-333.

7. Brennan, M.J.W., and Cantrill, R.C. (1978): J. Neurochem., 31: 1339-1341.

8. Brennan, M.J.W., and Cantrill, R.C. (1979): J. Neurochem., 32: 1781-1786.

9. Brennan, M.J.W., and Cantrill, R.C. (1979): J. Neurochem., 33: 721-725.

10. Brennan, M.J.W., and Cantrill, R.C. (1979): Nature, 280: 514-515.

11. Brennan, M.J.W., Cantrill, R.C., and Epstein, H. (1979): 4th Natn. Congr. S. Afr. Biochem. Soc., 102.

12. Brown, D.A., and Higgins, A.J. (1979): Br. J. Pharmac., 66: 108P-109P.

13. Cantrill, R.C., and Brennan, M.J.W. (1980): Experientia, 36: 141-142.

14. Carlsson, A. (1975): In: Pre- and Post-synaptic Receptors, edited by E. Usdin, and W.E. Bunney, pp.49-63. Marcel Dekker, New York.

15. DePotter, W.P., Chubb, I.W., Put, A., and DeSchaepdryver, A.F. (1974): Archs. int. Pharmacodyn. Ther., 193: 191-197.

16. Dismukes, R.K., and Mulder, A.H. (1976): Eur. J. Pharmac., 39: 383-388.

17. Eales, L. (1963): S. Afr. J. Lab. Clin. Med., 9: 151-162.

18. Enna, S.J., and Snyder, S.H. (1975): Brain Res., 100: 81-97.

19. Enna, S.J., and Snyder, S.H. (1977): Mol. Pharmac., 13: 442-453.

20. Farnebo, L.-O., and Hamberger, B. (1971): Acta Physiol. Scand. suppl., 371: 35-44.

21. Gray, E.G., and Whittaker, V.P. (1962): J. Anat., 96: 79-88.

22. Iversen, L.L., Rogawski, M.A., and Miller, R.J. (1976): Mol. Pharmac., 12: 251-262.

23. Krogsgaard-Larsen, P., Hjeds, H., Curtis, D.R., Lodge, D., and Johnston, G.A.R. (1979): J. Neurochem., 32: 1717-1724.

24. Langer, S.Z., Enero, M.A., Adler,Graschinsky, E., and Stefano, F.J.E. (1972): Vth Int. Congr. Pharmac., San Francisco, 134.

25. Lowry, O.H., Rosebrough, N.J., Farr, A.L., and Randall, R.J. (1951): J. Biol. Chem., 193: 265-275.

26. Meyer, U.A., and Schmid, R. (1974): In: Brain Dysfunction in Metabolic Disorders, edited by F. Plum, Res. Publs. Ass. Res. Nerv. Ment. Dis., 53: 211-223.

27. Mitchell, P.R., and Martin, I.L. (1978): Nature, 274: 904-905.

28. Roth, R.H., Walters, J.R., Murrin, L.C., and Morgenroth, V.H. (1975): In: Pre- and Post-synaptic Receptors, edited by E. Usdin, and W.E. Bunney, pp.5-46. Marcel Dekker, New York.

29. Seeman, P., and Lee, T. (1975): Science, 188: 1217-1219.

30. Shanley, B.C., Neethling, A.C., Percy, V.A., and Carstens, M. (1975): S. Afr. Med. J., 49: 576-580.

31. Snodgrass, S.R. (1978): Nature, 273: 392-394.

32. Starke, K., and Montel, H. (1973): Naunyn-Schmiedebergs Archs. Pharmak., 279: 53-60.

33. Sweeney, V.P., Pathak, A.M., and Asbury, A.K. (1970): Brain, 93: 369-380.

34. Szerb, J.C., and Somogyi, G.T. (1973): Nature new Biol., 241: 121-122.

35. Zukin, S.R., Young, A.B., and Snyder, S.H. (1974): Proc. Natl. Acad. Sci. U.S.A., 71: 4802-4807.

GABA and Benzodiazepine Receptors, edited by E. Costa et al.
Raven Press, New York © 1981.

Role of Membrane Lipids on the Regulation of GABA Recognition Sites

G. Toffano, C. Aldinio, M. Balzano, A. Leon, and G. Kirschner

FIDIA Research Laboratories, Via Ponte della Fabbrica, 3a-35031 Abano Terme, Italy

INTRODUCTION

An approach for understanding the pharmacology of GABAergic transmission and the mechanism of action of drugs that alter the GABAergic system at the post-synaptic level is the measurement of Na^+-independent ^{3}H-GABA binding to specific recognition sites on synaptic plasma membranes (5,18,11). The technique involves analysis of the binding to synaptic membranes that have been frozen, thawed and washed several times after Triton X-100 treatment. This procedure allows the removal of endogenous inhibitors and reveals a population of GABA recognition sites which becomes expressed only after such treatment (5,23). On the basis of pharmacological and biochemical data, the GABA receptor can be envisaged as a supramolecular unit in which a number of functionally related macromolecules, in the receptive zone of the neuronal membranes, form a cluster defined as GABA supramolecular receptor assembly. The GABA receptor unit is possibly composed of a GABA recognition site coupled with a Cl^- ionophore, a benzodiazepine receptor, one or more enzymes, and components which modulate the high-affinity GABA binding (23,24,-10,22).

Since GABA receptors are presumably inserted into the fluid lipid bilayer mosaic, with the recognition sites facing outward from the membrane, it is of interest to know whether the integrity of the lipid-protein complex might control the availability of the GABA binding sites. It is known that certain membrane bound phospholipids interact with noradrenaline (6), L-isoproterenol (12), acetylcholine (14) and morphine (1) which suggests a role for phospholipids in the control of synaptic membrane properties. Furthermore adrenergic and cholinergic drugs increase (7,13), while intracisternally administered GABA depresses (8), the incorporation of ^{32}Pi into rat brain phospholipids.

It has also been reported that phospholipase C increases ^{3}H-GABA binding (9,17) and that the addition of phosphatidylethanolamine to delipidated synaptic plasma membranes decreases the binding of ^{3}H-GABA to its recognition sites (9,15).

In the present work we have examined whether endogenous phospholipids are effective in the regulation of ^{3}H-GABA binding to synaptic receptors. For this purpose we have followed the classical procedures. Membrane preparations were treated with Triton X-100, or phospholipases, such as A_2, C and D, and then reconstitued by adding phospholipids back. ^{3}H-GABA binding was determined in both delipidated and reconstituted membranes. The results indicate that phospholipids are only minimally involved in the regulation of ^{3}H-GABA binding.

MATERIALS AND METHODS

Materials

Male adult Sprague-Dowley rats, 120-140 gr, were used throughout this work. ^{3}H-GABA, 40μCi/mmol, was purchased from New England Nuclear. Phosphatidylethanolamine, phosphatidylserine and phosphatidylcholine - were obtained from General Chemical and 1,2-dipalmitoylphosphatidylethanolamine from Sigma. All phospholipids used gave a single spot in thin layer chromatography with either a two-dimensional (20) or a one-dimensional (21) system. Phospholipase A_2 (from porcine pancreas, 600 U/mg), phospholipase C (from Bacillus cereus, 1000 U/mg) and phospholipase D (from cabbage, 0.3 U/mg) were from Boehringer.

Preparation of synaptic plasma membranes

Rats were decapitated and brains were rapidly dissected. Pooled cerebral cortices were homogenized in 10 vol of 0.31 M sucrose and synaptic plasma membranes (S.P.M.) were isolated and purified according to the combined sedimentation-flotation density gradient tecnique (16). Protein and phospholipid content (9) and (Na^+, K^+)ATPase were determined (25).

Binding of ^{3}H-GABA to synaptic plasma membranes

^{3}H-GABA binding was done in a Na^+-free medium. Frozen and thawed S.P.M. were incubated at 37°C for 30 min with or without Triton X-100 (0.18 mg/mg prot) and phospholipases, and washed three times with 50 mM Tris-citrate buffer, pH 7.4 as previously reported (23,24). ^{3}H-GABA binding was performed by using 0.2 - 0.3 mg protein per sample and an appropiate amount of radioactive ligand. Specific ^{3}H-GABA binding was calculated by correcting the binding occurring during incubation with ^{3}H-GABA for the binding occurring during incubation with ^{3}H-GABA plus 1 mM cold GABA.

Reassembly of delipidated membranes with exogenous phospholipids

Dry phospholipids were suspended in 0.25 M sucrose - 50mM Tris -HCl, pH 7.4 and sonicated for 10 min using a Branson sonifier (19). Liposomes of phosphatidylcholine required a longer sonication to yield vesicles of small diameter. 1 mg S.P.M. protein, previously treated with Triton X-100 or phospholipases, was reconstituted with 2 μmols sonicated liposomes in 50 mM Tris-citrate buffer pH 7.4. After incubation at 37°C for 10 min, samples were centrifuged at 97,000 g x 30 min on 0.31 M sucrose. The reconstituted membranes with bound phospholipids sedimented, whereas the unbound phospholipids remained in the supernatant. ^{3}H-GABA binding and phospholipids bound to the membranes were determined.

RESULTS

Effect of Triton X-100 on S.P.M.

A typical synaptic plasma membrane preparation, obtained according to the sedimentation-flotation tecnique, contains 3.42 mg protein per g fresh rat cerebral cortex and 36 μg lipidic phosphorus per mg protein with a phospholipid/protein ratio of about 0.9. Phosphatidylethanolamine, phosphatidylserine and phosphatidylcholine represent 34, 19.7 and 40 % of total phospholipids respectively. The specific activity of (Na^+, K^+)ATPase enzyme, a marker of plasma membrane, is 0.25 μmol ATP split per mg protein per min. The above values agree with the characteristics of S.P.M. preparations previously described (9,16,4,2).

Treatment of S.P.M. with 0.18 mg per mg protein Triton X-100 results in a marked decrease of both membrane-bound phospholipids and proteins with a concomitant increase of ^{3}H-GABA binding (Fig. 1). After the first detergent treatment both total proteins and phospholipids are reduced by about 35-40% and they continue to decrease until the last treatment. Furthermore after the first treatment, phosphatidylcholine and phosphatidylserine decrease by about 20%, and phosphatidylethanolamine by about 50%. ^{3}H-GABA binding increases by about 100% after the first treatment, and maximal binding capacity is obtained at the third treatment (+ 180% with respect to untreated S.P.M.).

Reassembly of Triton X-100 treated S.P.M. with exogenous phospholipids

The reconstitution of delipidated membrane preparations with exogenous phospholipids is a crucial point. Triton X-100 treatment produces an unknown membrane rearrangement while the addition of phospholipids back to membrane is difficult to achieve and bound exogenous phospholipid would not necessarily be associated with GABA-binding sites. We have used the method of Palatini et al. (19) which allows restoration of (Na^+, K^+)ATPase and 30-40% incorporation of sonicated phospholipids in delipi-

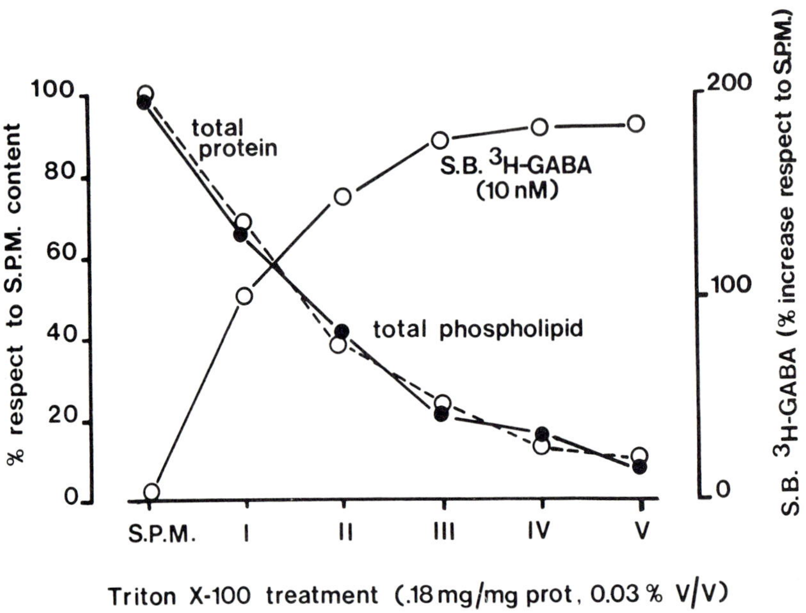

FIG. 1 -Effect of Triton X-100 treatment on ^{3}H-GABA binding, phospholipid and protein content in S.P.M. Frozen and thawed membranes were incubated at 37°C x 30 min with Triton X-100 (0.18 mg/mg protein). After three washes with 50 mM Tris - citrate buffer pH 7,4, membranes were frozen overnight and then the procedure was repeated four times. ^{3}H-GABA binding phospholipid and protein content were determined after each Triton X-100 treatment. Control values : protein 3.42 mg and phospholipid 3.08 mg per gr fresh tissue, ^{3}H-GABA binding, measured with 10 pmol/ml, was 390 nmol/mg protein. The standard error mean is less than 10 per cent.

dated membranes (19). When sonicated phospholipids are added back to Triton X-100 treated S.P.M., only phosphatidylethanolamine is capable of partially reversing the effect of the detergent on ^{3}H-GABA binding (Tab. 1). Natural phosphatidylethanolamine decreases the specific ^{3}H-GABA binding by about 30-35%, while synthetic 1,2 dipalmitoylphosphatidylethanolamine is less active. In contrast phosphatidylserine and phosphatidylcholine do not produce significant changes.

Effect of phospholipases on ^{3}H-GABA binding in S.P.M. preparations

Due to the specificity of the enzymatic attack, the incubation of

PHOSPHOLIPID ADDED (μmol/mg prot)	S.B. ^{3}H-GABA (fmol/mg prot)			
	1st TRITON	△%	2nd TRITON	△%
none	830 ± 38	----	1440 ± 86	----
Phosphatidylethanolamine (prepared)	564 ± 31	- 32	1051 ± 72	- 27
Phosphatidylethanolamine (commercial)	553 ± 27	- 34	1010 ± 49	- 30
Phosphatidylethanolamine (dipalmitoyl)	710 ± 41	- 17	1252 ± 79	- 13
Phosphatidylserine	760 ± 37	- 9	1296 ± 102	- 10
Phosphatidylcholine	815 ± 25	- 2	1500 ± 131	+ 4

TABLE 1 - Effect of various phospholipids on ^{3}H-GABA binding in Triton X-100 treated S.P.M. Incubation of sonicated phospholipids with delipidated S.P.M. (2μmol phospholipid/mg protein) was carried out as reported in "materials and methods". ^{3}H-GABA binding (10 nM) was assayed with 0.3 mg protein.

Samples	S.B. ^{3}H-GABA fmol/mg prot	Δ%	Total phospholipid mg/ml	PE	PS	PC	L-PE	L-PS	L-PC
				(% of total phospholipids)					
Control	370 $\pm$ 20	----	0.71 $\pm$ 0.03	34.0	19.7	40.0	--	----	----
Phospholipase A_2 (50 μg/ml)	230 $\pm$ 15	- 38	0.63 $\pm$ 0.02	20.5	8.4	24.3	12	14.5	16.6
Phospholipase C (10 μg/ml)	519 $\pm$ 32	+ 40	0.14 $\pm$ 0.01	33.3	25.0	12.5	--	----	----
Phospholipase D (100 μg/ml)	335 $\pm$ 30	- 10	0.69 $\pm$ 0.03	33.2	19.2	36.5	--	----	----

TABLE 2 - Effect of phospholipase treatment on ^{3}H-GABA binding and phospholipid content in S.P.M. Samples were incubated with or without phospholipases at 37°C x 30 min, and centrifuged at 48,000 g x 20 min. ^{3}H-GABA binding (10 nM) and phospholipid content were determined on the pellet.

membranes with phospholipases may provide more precise information as to the role of endogenous phospholipids on the regulation of ^{3}H-GABA binding. The effect of phospholipase A_2, C and D on phospholipid content and on ^{3}H-GABA binding is reported in Table 2.

Phospholipase A_2 (50 μg/ml) splits phosphatidylethanolamine, phosphatidylserine and phosphatidylcholine by about 40, 58 and 40% respectively and reduces ^{3}H-GABA binding by about 40%. The effect of phospholipase A_2 might be due to the splitting products of the enzyme treatment possessing detergent properties. Lyso-phosphatidylcholine has been used for solubilizing ^{3}H-GABA receptors (3).

Phospholipase C (10 μg/ml) produces an extensive splitting of endogenous phospholipids, reducing their total content by about 80%, and an increased ^{3}H-GABA binding by about 40%. This suggests that removal of the polar heads affects the binding of ^{3}H-GABA to its recognition sites.

The effect of phospholipase C on the kinetics of ^{3}H-GABA binding, in the high affinity range, is reported in Fig. 2. Scatchard analysis indicates

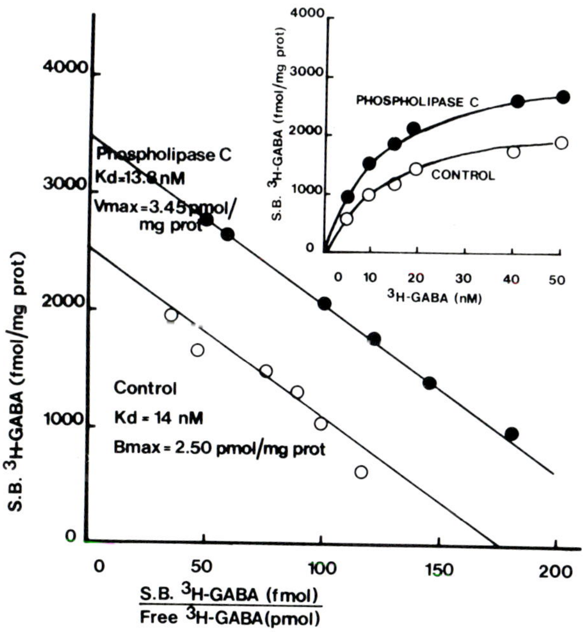

FIG. 2 - Scatchard's plot of ^{3}H-GABA binding in S.P.M. Effect of 10 μg/ml phospholipase C. Frozen and thawed membranes were incubated at 37°C x 30 min with or without phospholipase C and centrifuged at 48,000 g x 20 min. ^{3}H-GABA binding was assayed with 0.2 mg protein.

that the enhancement of ^{3}H-GABA binding is due to an increase of the apparent Bmax (3.45 pmol/mg prot versus 2.50 pmol/mg prot of control preparation) rather than a change of the apparent Kd (13.8 nM versus 14 nM of control preparation). The reassembly of phospholipase C -treated S.P.M. preparations with exogenous phosphatidylethanolamine, phosphatidylserine, phosphatidylcholine or with O-phosphoethanolamine and 1,2-dipalmitoyl-glycerol, which are the resulting products of phospholipase C cleavage, does not result in significant changes.

Comparison between the effect of phospholipase C and Triton X-100 on ^{3}H-GABA binding, protein and phospholipid content

The removal by phospholipase C of the polar heads is accompanied by extensive phospholipid depletion and increased ^{3}H-GABA binding. Triton X-100 reproduces the same effect on the phospholipid content but causes a more marked enhancement of ^{3}H-GABA binding (Fig. 3). Maximal ^{3}H-

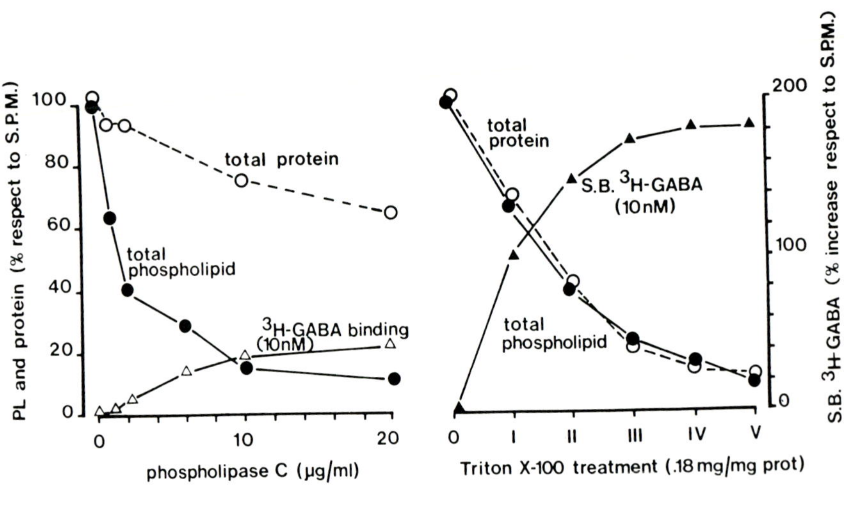

FIG. 3 - Comparison between the effect of phospholipase C and Triton X-100 treatment on phospholipid, protein and ^{3}H-GABA binding in S.P.M. For explanation see legends of Fig. 1 and 2.

GABA binding is obtained with 10 μg/ml of phospholipase C (+ 40 % with respect to control) or with three Triton X-100 washes (+ 200 % with respect to control).

Amounts of 1 μg/ml phospholipase C and one Triton X-100 treatment have the same effect on phospholipid content, although only after Triton

X-100 treatment does the ^{3}H-GABA binding increase. This suggests the absence of correlation between amounts of membrane bound phospholipids and ^{3}H-GABA binding.

Triton X-100 also removes membrane bound protein, while phospholipase C is capable of releasing protein only at high doses presumably because of its effects on lipid-protein complexes.

CONCLUSION

The hypothesis that endogenous phospholipids have a physiological role in the modulation of ^{3}H-GABA binding to synaptic receptor has been reexamined. Triton X-100 and phospholipase C have been found to increase ^{3}H-GABA binding in both crude and purified synaptic plasma membranes (5,23,24,9) while phosphatidylethanolamine decreases ^{3}H-GABA binding (9,15). The results, reported here, suggest that endogenous phospholipids have only a modest indirect effect on the regulation of ^{3}H-GABA binding.

Triton X-100 treatments deplete synaptic plasma membranes of proteins and phospholipids and increase ^{3}H-GABA binding. Only phosphatidylethanolamine added back to delipidated membranes causes a 35% inhibition of ^{3}H-GABA binding which does not account completely for the impressive increase of ^{3}H-GABA binding. Also the removal of polar heads by phospholipase C-attack results in a 35-40% increase of ^{3}H-GABA binding presumably due to enhanced availability of binding sites. Amounts of phospholipase C causing a reduction of the phospholipid content of 40% have no effect, while one Triton X-100 treatment, causing the same effect on phospholipid content, increases the binding 100%. In previous work (23,24) we have demonstrated that by reconstituting Triton X-100 treated synaptic plasma membranes with a supernatant devoid of both phospholipids and endogenous GABA, it is possible to completely inhibit the specific ^{3}H-GABA binding. This indicates that the most important endogenous inhibitory factor is present in the supernatant fraction.

It is unlikely (9,15) that the phosphatidylethanolamine polar head directly competes with endogenous GABA for binding to the protein receptor. The asymmetric phospholipid distribution (26), predicts that the phosphatidylethanolamine polar head faces the cytosol space while presumably the GABA recognition sites face the interstitial space. Assuming that phosphatidylethanolamine controls the availability of the GABA binding sites, it may be calculated that only 20-25 % of the effect of Triton X-100 on ^{3}H-GABA binding could be ascribed to phospholipid depletion, while the remaining part could be an effect on the proteic part of the membrane.

REFERENCES

1. Abood, L.C., and Hoss, W. (1975): Europ. J. Pharmacol. 32: 66-75.

2. Breckenridge, W.C., Gombos, G., and Morgan, I.C. (1972): Biochim. Biophys. Acta 266: 695-707.

3. Chude, O. (1979): J. Neurochem. 33: 621-629.

4. Cotman, C.W., and Mattews, D.A. (1971): Biochim. Biophys. Acta 249: 380-394.

5. Enna, S.J., and Snyder, S.H. (1977): Mol. Pharmacol. 13: 442-453.

6. Farmby, B. (1967): Molec. Pharmacol. 3: 284-289.

7. Friedel, R.O., Johnson, J.R., and Schamberg, S.M. (1972): J. Pharm. Exp. Ther. 181: 583-588.

8. Friedel, R.O., Slotmik, R.N., and Bombardt, P.A. (1977): Life Sci. 20: 235-242.

9. Giambalvo, G.T., and Rosemberg, P. (1976): Biochem. Biophys. Acta 436: 741-756.

10. Guidotti, A., Toffano, G., and Costa, E. (1978): Nature (London) 275: 553-555.

11. Guidotti, A., Gale, K., Suria, A., and Toffano, G. (1979): Brain Res. 172: 566-571.

12. Hirata, F., Strittmatter, W.J., and Axelrod, J. (1979): Proc. Natl. Acad. Sci. USA 76: 368-372.

13. Hokin, M.R. (1969): J. Neurochem. 16: 13-19.

14. Izumi, F., and Freed, S. (1974): FEBS Letters 42: 319-322.

15. Johnston, G.A.R., and Kennedy, S.M.E. (1978): In : Amino Acids as Chemical Transmitters, edited by F. Fonnum, pp. 507-516. Plenum Press, New York.

16. Jones, D.H., and Matus, A.I. (1974): Biochim. Biophys. Acta 356: 276-287.

17. Lloyd, J.G., and Davidson, L. (1979): Science 205: 1147-1149.

18. Olsen, R.W., Ticku, M.K., Van Ness, P.C., and Greenlee, D. (1978): Brain Res. 139: 277-294.

19. Palatini, P., Dabbeni-Sala, F., Pitotti, A., Bruni, A., and Mandersloot, J.C. (1977): Biochim. Biophys. Acta 466: 1-9.

20. Rauser, G., Kritchvesky, G., Yamamoto, A., Simon, G., Galli, C., and Bauman, A.J. (1969): Meth. Enzymol. 14: 272-317.

21. Skipski, V.P., and Barclay, N. (1969): Meth. Enzymol. 14: 530-597.

22. Tallman, J.F., Thomas, J.W., and Gallager, D.W. (1978): Nature (London) 274: 383-385.

23. Toffano, G., Guidotti, A., and Costa, E. (1978): Proc. Natl. Acad. Sci. USA 75: 4025-4028.

24. Toffano, G., Leon, A., Massotti, M., Guidotti, A., and Costa, E. (1980): In: Receptors for Neurotransmitters and Peptide Hormones, edited by G. Pepeu, M.J. Kuhar and S.J. Enna, pp. 133-142, Raven Press, New York.

25. Wallick, E.T., Dowd, F., Allen, J.C., and Schwartz, A. (1974): J. Pharmacol. Exp. Ther. 189: 434-444.

26. Zwaal, R.F.A. (1978): Biochim. Biophys. Acta 515: 163-205.

GABA and Benzodiazepine Receptors,
edited by E. Costa et al.
Raven Press, New York © 1981.

Chronolgy of Neurochemical Alterations Induced by GABA Agonist Administration

S. J. Enna, J. W. Ferkany, and I. J. Butler

Departments of Pharmacology, Neurobiology, Anatomy, and Neurology, University of Texas Medical School at Houston, Houston, Texas 77025

INTRODUCTION

Because of the data indicating that underactive GABAergic systems may be responsible for the symptoms of a variety of neuropsychiatric disorders (4,7), a number of approaches are now being taken to develop drugs which will activate these neurotransmitter pathways (7). Two classes of these agents are the GABA transaminase (GABA-T) inhibitors (13,20), drugs which will inhibit GABA metabolism thereby raising the brain level of this amino acid, and the direct acting GABA receptor agonists (9,14).

Since, if clinically effective, these drugs will be used to treat chronic disorders of the central nervous system, patients will receive these medications for long periods of time. Accordingly, in order to better understand the basic pharmacology of GABA agonists as it may relate to clinical therapy, it is important to investigate the neurochemical changes which may occur as a result of chronic administration of these drugs. The value of such a study is supported by the reports indicating that many, if not all, psychoactive compounds induce lasting neurochemical alterations following chronic, but not acute, administration (3,16, 17,21). In addition to yielding information about possible clinical effects of these agents, chronic studies may also give insights into the basic mechanism of action of the drug under investigation.

In a series of recent reports (5,6,9,11), data have been presented showing that chronic (15 days) administration of either GABA-T inhibitors or direct acting agonists induces an increase in dopamine receptor binding and function and a decrease in GABA receptor binding in the rat corpus striatum. These findings imply that chronic GABA agonist therapy may result in the development of extrapyramidal side effects. In the present study, the time-course and reversibility of these receptor alterations are explored in an attempt to better understand this phenomenon. The results indicate that the GABA receptor binding changes precede the dopamine receptor alterations and that both receptor changes are completely reversible following cessation of treatment. In addition, the data reveals that the time course of the receptor changes observed does not correlate with the elevation in brain GABA content induced by the GABA-T inhibitor. Furthermore, other findings suggest that tolerance may develop to some of the neurochemical changes induced by acute treatment with GABA agonists.

MATERIALS AND METHODS

Male Sprague-Dawley rats (Charles Rivers) were used in all experiments. For chronic studies, the animals weighed 90-100 gm at the initiation of treatment and 200-250 gm at the time of death. During chronic treatment, animals were housed normally and allowed access to food and water ad libitum. In acute experiments, animals weighed 90-120 gm.

In chronic studies, rats were injected with γ-acetylenic GABA (GAG), a GABA-T inhibitor (20), twice daily with a dose of 10 mg/kg. Animals were decapitated at various times during the chronic treatment period and in all cases the animals were sacrificed 16 hrs following the last injection of drug. The GAG was administered in saline and control animals received an equivalent volume of vehicle twice daily. Following decapitation, the brains were rapidly removed, dissected on ice, then stored at -20°C until assayed. For acute experiments, animals were treated with a single dose of either THIP, a direct acting GABA receptor agonist (14), at 12 mg/kg, or GAG, 100 mg/kg, and were decapitated 30 min after the former and 4 hr after the latter compound. Control animals received an equivalent volume of saline. All injections were made intraperitoneally.

In some experiments, the GABA content of cisternal cerebrospinal fluid (CSF) was measured as an index of the brain GABA concentration. For these studies, the rats were lightly anesthetized with chloral hydrate and a midline incision made over the occipital protruberance. Following the incision, the animals were placed in a lateral position with the head flexed downward at the neck. A 25 gauge Butterfly intravenous needle was prepared by reducing the length of the bevel, removal of the plastic wings and shortening the connected tubing to about 5 cm. The needle was inserted into the cisternal space and CSF collected by gravity into ice-cold glass centrifuge tubes containing a small amount of ascorbic acid. Approximately 100-150 μl of CSF was collected over a period of 30-45 min., then stored at -80°C until assayed. Blood contaminated fluid was discarded. For the chronic studies, repeated cisternal punctures were performed on the same animal and the wound closed by metal clips. The CSF GABA content was analyzed by combined gas chromatography/mass spectrometry (GC/MS) using a deuterated internal standard (10). Striatal dopamine receptor binding was studied using ^{3}H-spiroperidol (23.1 Ci/mmole, New England Nuclear) as a ligand and (+)-butaclomol as a blank (19). GABA receptor binding was quantified using ^{3}H-muscimol

(13 Ci/mmole, New England Nuclear) as a ligand and unlabeled bicuculline as a blank (2). High affinity choline uptake was examined by the procedure of Atweh et al (1) using ^{3}H-choline (8.3 Ci/mmole, Amersham Searle) as a substrate and unlabeled choline as a blank. Protein was measured using the method of Lowry et al (15). Levels of significance between groups were determined using a student's two-tailed t-test.

THIP was generously supplied by Dr. A. V. Christensen of H. Lundbeck and Co., and GAG by Dr. Paul Schechter of Merrell International. All other chemicals and reagents were obtained from commercial suppliers.

RESULTS

CSF GABA Content During Chronic Treatment with GAG

Since the chronic dose of GAG employed in this study was one-tenth the acute dose normally given to raise brain GABA levels, it was important to determine whether the treatment employed was sufficient for elevating the brain content of this amino acid.

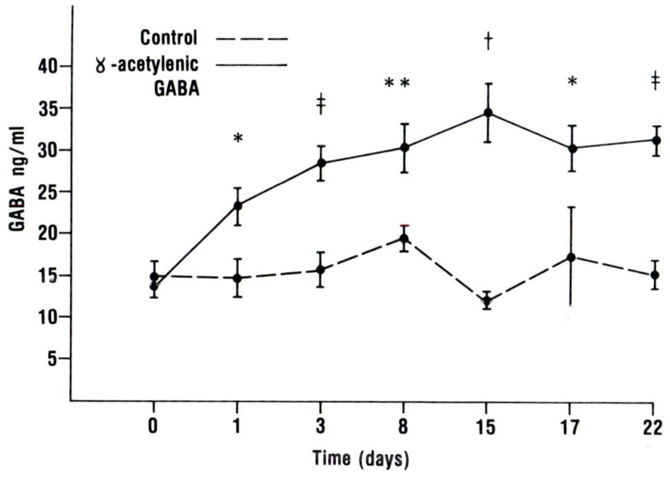

FIG. 1. GABA concentration of rat cisternal CSF during chronic treatment and after withdrawal of GAG. Animals were treated with 10 mg/kg GAG twice daily and CSF collected before (day 0), during (to day 15) and after cessation (day 15 to 22) of drug administration. Control animals received an equivalent volume of saline. Each point is the mean ± s.e.m. of 3-7 separate animals.

* $p < 0.05$
‡ $p < 0.025$
† $p < 0.005$
** $p < 0.001$

To this end, cisternal CSF samples were collected from GAG-treated and control animals at various times throughout the treatment period and the GABA content of this fluid analyzed (Fig. 1). Following the administration of GAG, the CSF GABA content was significantly greater than control animals as early as day 1, and continued to slowly rise throughout the treatment period (14 days) then leveled off at about 30 ng/ml, which is some two-fold greater than control values. Following the last drug administration, cisternal CSF GABA content remained elevated and relatively constant for up to one week.

Time Course of GABA and Dopamine Receptor Alterations

Animals were treated with 10 mg/kg GAG twice daily and, after various treatment times, a group of treated and control animals were decapitated and striatal GABA receptor binding quantified. No significant change in GABA receptor binding was noted after the first day of treatment, but by day 7, GABA receptor binding was reduced and remained significantly less than the corresponding control up to one day (day 15) following the last injection of drug (Table 1). On day 17, three days after the final dose of

TABLE 1. Chronology of striatal GABA and dopamine receptor alterations following chronic administration of GAG*

Time (days)	Receptor Binding (% of control) ^3H-Spiroperidol		^3H-Muscimol
1	112		93
7	105		80 †
14		Treatment Ends	
15	120 †		76 †
17	60 †		166 †
22	88		97
30	102		90

* Rats were injected i.p. with 10 mg/kg GAG twice daily for 14 days and at various times during the treatment period animals were killed and striatal dopamine and GABA receptor binding measured and compared to a saline treated control group. Each value represents the percentage difference between the mean of the treated and control groups, with each group having 4-6 animals, each analyzed in triplicate.

† $p < 0.05$

GAG, GABA receptor binding was significantly elevated, being over 60% greater than control animals at this time. By day 22, eight days following the last injection, striatal GABA receptor binding had returned to control levels.

With regard to striatal dopamine receptor binding, no changes in this parameter were noted after up to 7 days of GAG administration (Table 1). However, between days 7 and 15, dopamine receptor binding significantly increased relative to control levels, being some 20% higher on day 15. Three days following the last injection of GAG (day 17), dopamine receptor binding was 40% less than control values and by day 22, eight days after the last injection, dopamine receptor binding had returned to normal.

TABLE 2. Effect of chronic treatment with THIP or γ-acetylenic GABA on high affinity ^{3}H-choline transport into rat striatal synaptosomes

Treatment	Dose (mg/kg)	Net ^{3}H-Choline Uptake (pmoles/mg protein/4 min)
Saline		6.3 ± 0.2
Saline + acute THIP	12	7.5 ± 0.3[†]
Saline + acute γ-acetylenic GABA	100	7.3 ± 0.3[†]
Chronic THIP + acute THIP	8 ± 12 (b.i.d.)	7.0 ± 0.6
Chronic γ-acetylenic GABA + acute γ-acetylenic GABA	10 ± 10 (b.i.d.)	6.0 ± 0.3
Chronic γ-acetylenic GABA + acute γ-acetylenic GABA	10 ± 100 (b.i.d.)	6.5 ± 0.5

* For acute experiments, animals were treated with the dose indicated and were killed 30 min after THIP or 4 hr after GAG administration. Following decapitation, the corpus striatum was rapidly dissected, synaptosomes prepared, and high affinity choline uptake measured by the method of Atweh et al (1). For chronic studies, animals were treated for 14 days and 16 hrs following the last injection they were challenged with a single dose of drug and high affinity choline uptake measured. Each value is the mean ± s.e.m. of 6-10 animals, each analyzed in triplicate.

* $p < 0.05$

Effect of Chronic Treatment with GABA Agonists on Striatal High Affinity Choline Uptake

Previous reports have indicated that acute administration of GABA agonists induces an increase in high affinity choline uptake into striatal synaptosomes (5,9). In the present study, this phenomenon was investigated after both acute and chronic treatment with these agents. As shown previously, acute administration of either GAG or THIP resulted in a significant 20% increase in choline transport (Table 2). However, following chronic administration (15 days) of either THIP or GAG, an acute, previously effective dose of either of these agents no longer elicited a significant rise in ^{3}H-choline transport.

DISCUSSION

The results of the present study confirm and extend previous observations that chronic administration of GABA agonists causes significant changes in striatal GABA and dopamine receptor binding. While the precise mechanism of these changes is unknown, an hypothesis can be proposed which is consistent with the current theories relating to the functional interactions between the various neurotransmitter systems in basal ganglia. Thus, numerous anatomical and pharmacological investigations have provided evidence to indicate that there exists a striatonigral GABA pathway which synapses upon and regulates the nigrostriatal dopamine system (Fig. 2)(12,18). This GABA pathway appears to have an inhibitory influence on the dopamine cells. Thus it is conceivable that chronic activation of the nigral GABA receptors, either directly with GABA receptor agonists such as THIP or indirectly by elevating GABA levels with agents such as GAG, causes a prolonged inhibition of the nigrostriatal dopamine pathway which ultimately leads to an increase in the number, and therefore the sensitivity, of the striatal dopamine receptors. In contrast to this indirect modulation of dopamine receptor binding by GABA agonists, the decrease in striatal GABA receptor binding noted after chronic treatment with these agents is most likely due to a direct and prolonged activation of these sites by GABA itself or by THIP (9). In addition, the present results support the hypothesis that the nigrostriatal dopamine pathway exerts an inhibitory influence on the striatal cholinergic system (Fig. 2) since high affinity choline uptake, a measure of cholinergic cell activity(1), is enhanced after acute treatment with these agents.

In the present study, data is obtained to indicate that the dose of GAG used for chronic treatment is sufficient to raise and maintain GABA levels above control values throughout, and in fact beyond, the duration of treatment. However, while brain GABA levels are elevated after the first dose of GAG, no receptor changes occur until sometime during the first week of treatment when GABA receptor binding is reduced. Assuming that the CSF GABA content is an accurate reflection of brain GABA levels, as has

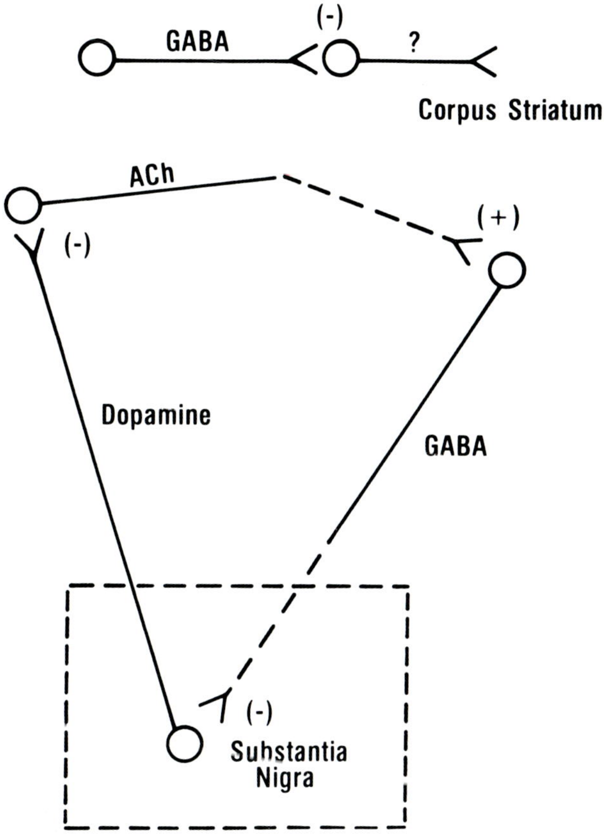

FIG. 2. Proposed functional interrelationships between the GABA, dopamine and cholinergic systems in the basal ganglia. This illustration is not intended to be an accurate anatomical chart, but rather indicates the apparent functional relationships between these systems.

- - -

been suggested (8), and that there is a fairly uniform elevation of this amino acid in the various brain regions, this finding would suggest that the changes in GABA receptor binding noted are not simply due to the presence of more GABA in the assay tubes, but probably reflects a change in receptor number. This is further supported by kinetic studies indicating that the changes in GABA binding are due to a decrease in receptor number, with no significant change in affinity. Furthermore, the finding that

GABA receptor binding actually increases above control values 3 days following the withdrawal of drug, while GABA levels are still elevated, is further proof that the receptor changes noted are not due to interference by endogenous ligand. Indeed, the increase in GABA receptor binding above control values followed by a return to normal levels, at a time when brain GABA content remains elevated, suggests that brain GABA levels alone are very poor indicators of the increase in functional activity of the GABA system in response to GABA-T inhibitors. While the precise reason for this poor correlation is unclear, one possibility would be that the turnover of neuronal GABA-T is more rapid than in nonneural tissue and that the majority of the GABA measured after GABA-T inhibition reflects extraneuronal stores of this amino acid.

With regard to the dopamine receptor changes observed, again there is no simple correlation between brain GABA content and the level of dopamine receptor binding. Thus, the increase in dopamine receptor binding develops later than the change in GABA receptor binding, possibly because the dopamine receptor change is secondary to GABA receptor activation. Furthermore, like the GABA receptor, there appears to be a rebound in the dopamine receptor system following termination of GAG administration, but at a time when GABA levels are still elevated. Again, this phenomenon would indicate that the GAG-induced elevation in brain GABA content outlasts the GAG-induced increase in GABAergic activity. Neither the mechanism, nor the functional consequences, of the rebound in GABA and dopamine receptor binding is as yet known. However, the results do indicate that the GABA agonist-induced changes in striatal GABA and dopamine receptor binding are readily reversible, at least in rat.

Finally, the results relating to high affinity choline uptake suggest that tolerance develops to this phenomenon during prolonged treatment with GABA agonists. From the present results it is unclear whether this tolerance is due to the change in dopamine and/or GABA receptor sensitivity, or to an adaptation of the uptake process itself. Nevertheless, this finding suggests that certain biochemical, and therefore perhaps behavioral, responses to GABA agonists may diminish with time.

ACKNOWLEDGEMENTS

Supported in part by USPHS grants NS-13803, a Research Career Development Award NS-00335 (S.J.E.) and an NIMH predoctoral fellowship MH-07688 (J.W.F.). We thank Dr. W. Seifert and Ms. N. Vernon for their assistance in this study.

REFERENCES

1. Atweh, S., Simon, J.R. and Kuhar, M.J. (1975): Life Sciences, 17:1535-1544.
2. Beaumont, K., Chilton, W.S., Yamamura, H.I. and Enna, S.J. (1978): Brain Res., 148:153-162.
3. Burt, D.R., Creese, I. and Snyder, S.H. (1977): Science, 196: 326-328.
4. Enna, S.J. (1979): Ann. Rep. Med. Chem. 14:41-50.
5. Enna, S.J. and Ferkany, J.W. (1980): IN: Psychopharmacology and Biochemistry of Neurotransmitter Receptors, edited by H. Yamamura, E. Usdin and R. Olsen, in press. Elsevier-North Holland, New York.
6. Enna, S.J., Ferkany, J.W. and Strong, R. (1980): IN: Receptors for Neurotransmitters and Peptide Hormones, edited by G. Pepeu, M.J. Kuhar and S.J. Enna, pp. 253-263. Raven Press, New York.
7. Enna, S.J. and Maggi, A. (1979): Life Sciences 24:1727-1738.
8. Ferkany, J.W., Butler, I.J. and Enna, S.J. (1979): J. Neurochem. 33:29-33.
9. Ferkany, J.W. and Enna, S.J. (1980): Life Sciences, in press
10. Ferkany, J.W., Smith, L.A., Seifert, W.E., Caprioli, R.M. and Enna, S.J. (1978): Life Sciences, 22:2121-2128.
11. Ferkany, J.W., Strong, R. and Enna, S.J. (1980): J. Neurochem. 34:247-249.
12. Javoy, R., Euvard, C., Herbert, A. and Glowinski, J. (1977): Brain Res., 126:382-386.
13. Jung, M.J. and Metcalf, B.W. (1975): Biochem. Biophys. Res. Comm. 67:301-306.
14. Krogsgaard-Larsen, P., Honore, T. and Thyssen, F. (1978): IN: GABA-Neurotransmitters, edited by P. Krogsgaard-Larsen, J. Scheel-Kruger and H. Kofod, pp. 201-216. Munksgaard, Copenhagen.
15. Lowry, O.H., Rosebrough, N.J., Farr, A.L. and Randall, R.J. (1951): J. Biol. Chem., 193:265-275.
16. Maggi, A. and Enna, S.J. (1980): J. Neurochem. 34:888-892.
17. Maggi A., U'Prichard, D.C. and Enna, S.J. (1980): Europ. J. Pharmacol. 61:91-98.
18. Perez de la Mora, M. and Fuxe, K. (1977): Brain Res., 135: 107-122.
19. Reisine, T.D., Fields, J.Z., Yamamura, H.I., Bird, E.D., Spokes, E., Schreiner, P.S. and Enna, S.J. (1977): Life Sciences 21:335-344.
20. Schechter, P.J., Tranier, Y., Jung, M.J. and Sjoerdsma, A. (1977): J. Pharmacol. Exptl. Therap. 201:606-612.
21. Sulser, F. (1978): Pharmakopsychiatry 11:43-51.

GABA and Benzodiazepine Receptors,
edited by E. Costa et al.
Raven Press, New York © 1981.

Barbiturates and GABA Receptors

G. A. R. Johnston and M. Willow

Department of Pharmacology, University of Sydney, New South Wales, 2006, Australia; and Department of Pharmacology, Australian National University, Canberra City, ACT, 2601, Australia

There is good evidence that pentobarbitone enhances synaptic transmission mediated by the inhibitory neurotransmitter GABA (15, 18, 21) but the detailed mechanism of such enhancement is uncertain. Attempts to demonstrate enhancement by pentobarbitone of the binding of GABA to synaptic membranes have been thus far unsuccessful (4, 19, 20). We have used a relatively crude membrane preparation isolated from rat brain, after gentle homogenization and repeated washing, to show a dose-dependent enhancement of GABA binding by pentobarbitone which involved an increased affinity of GABA for the higher affinity of the two apparent binding sites. The kinetics of GABA binding to rat brain membranes are dependent on the methods used to prepare the membranes due to the presence of endogenous inhibitors of GABA binding which are normally found in association with GABA binding sites (9). In the previous studies where pentobarbitone failed to influence GABA binding, certain endogenous inhibitors had been removed from the membranes by high frequency homogenization, freezing and thawing, and/or detergent extraction. One of the endogenous inhibitors of GABA binding appears to be a phosphoethanolamine derivative (9), the absence of which may underlie the apparent supersensitivity of certain GABA receptors in Huntington's disease (13). It seemed possible that a lipophilic drug such as pentobarbitone could interact with this endogenous phospholipid inhibitor of GABA binding sites and thus we have investigated a membrane preparation designed to preserve interaction between endogenous inhibitors and GABA binding sites as far as is consistent with measureable and reproducible binding of GABA.

METHODS

Membrane Preparations

Crude synaptic membranes were prepared from the P2 mitochondrial pellet of whole brain homogenized in a glass homogenizer with a Teflon pestle (0.22 mm clearance in diameter) in 0.32 M sucrose as described by Gray and Whittaker (6). This P2 pellet, obtained by centrifugation of the 'nuclear' supernatant at 14,500 g average for 20 min, was washed 8 to 10 times by careful resuspension in ice-cold 50 mM Tris-citrate buffer at pH 7.1, centrifugation at 14,500 g average for 20 min and the supernatant removed. Preliminary subcellular fractionation studies suggested that most of the GABA binding was to lysed synaptosomal membranes. Furthermore, when supernatants from each washing of the P2 mitochondrial pellet were tested for their ability to displace radioactive GABA from Triton-treated membranes, the supernatant from the final wash failed to displace any radioactive GABA suggesting that most of the free endogenous GABA had been removed by the washing process.

Experiments were also carried out on membranes prepared by extraction with 0.5% Triton X-100 at 37°C for 30 min, followed by centrifugation and extensive washing by suspension in buffer, centrifugation and removal of the supernatant.

Enhancement of GABA Binding by Pentobarbitone

The effects of pentobarbitone on the binding of radioactive GABA to the above membrane preparations were studied by incubating the resuspended membrane material (0.5 mg protein in 2.0 ml of Tris-citrate buffer at pH 7.1) for 5 min at 4°C with 2.3 nM tritiated GABA (specific activity 60 Ci/mmol, prepared by The Radiochemical Centre, Amersham) in the presence of varying concentrations of pentobarbitone (0-400 μM). This was followed by centrifugation for 10 min at 48,000 g average, removal of the supernatant and superficial rinsing of the pellet with 2 x 5 ml ice-cold distilled water. Non-specific binding was assessed in the presence of 1 mM GABA. Typically, specific and non-specific binding under these conditions were 3000 and 500 CPM respectively. Binding experiments were also carried out using a range of GABA concentrations (0.00625 - 10 μM) in the presence and absence of 100 μM pentobarbitone in order to assess the kinetic parameters of GABA binding.

RESULTS

Pentobarbitone enhanced GABA binding to the crude membranes in a dose-dependent manner. Maximal enhancement varied from 30-50% of specific binding depending on the membrane preparation and occurred at 100 μM pentobarbitone. Log-probit analysis indicated that half-maximal enhancement occurred at 38 ± 2 μM pentobarbitone.

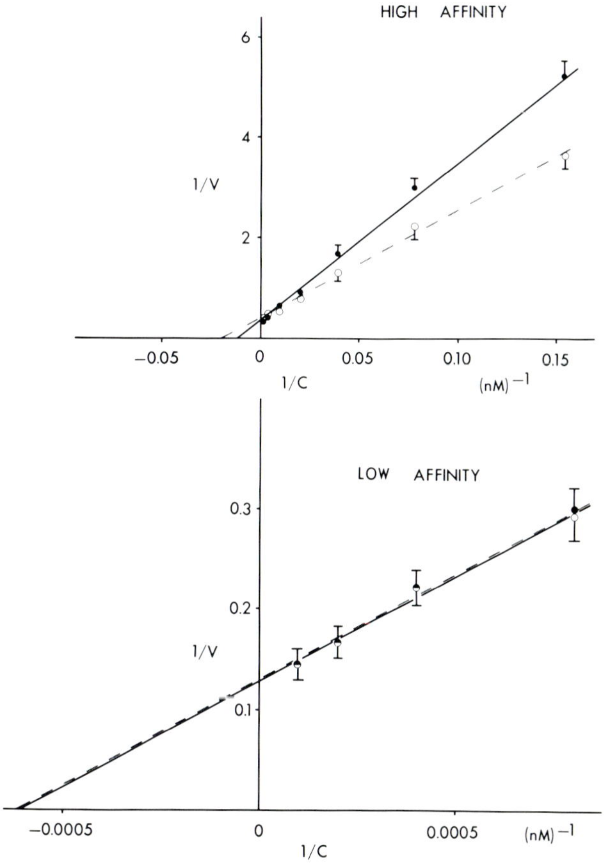

FIG. 1. ANALYSIS OF GABA BINDING TO CRUDE RAT BRAIN MEMBRANES IN THE PRESENCE (OPEN SYMBOLS, BROKEN LINES) AND ABSENCE (CLOSED SYMBOLS, SOLID LINES) OF 100 μM PENTOBARBITONE. THE VALUES ARE MEANS OF 6 EXPERIMENTS ± STANDARD ERRORS. V IS THE AMOUNT OF GABA BOUND IN PMOLES/MG PROTEIN. C IS THE FREE nM CONCENTRATION OF GABA. THE LINES WERE COMPUTER FITTED BY LINEAR REGRESSION ANALYSIS.

Kinetic analysis of the enhancement of GABA binding by pentobarbitone, 100 μM, using the Klotz plots in Fig.1. showed the binding could be described by a two site model with pentobarbitone significantly altering the affinity of the higher affinity component. The stepwise equilibrium analysis of Klotz (12) appears to be superior to Scatchard analysis for the determination of multicomponent binding data (6) and has been used for the analysis of the binding of L-glutamate to rat brain membranes (16).

TABLE 1. Enhancement of GABA binding by pentobarbitone

	Affinity	K_D	B_{max} (pmole/mg)
Control	high	89±8 nM	2.74±0.18
	low	1.60±0.16 μM	7.70±0.88
Pentobarbitone (100 μM)	high	54±4 nM*	2.53±0.11
	low	1.62±0.10 μM	7.74±0.80

* significantly different from control at $P<0.05$

Picrotoxinin (1-100 μM) completely blocked the potentiation of GABA binding by 100 μM pentobarbitone, but was without effect on GABA binding in the absence of pentobarbitone.

Diazepam (0.1 μM) also enhanced GABA binding to a similar extent to pentobarbitone, an effect also blocked by 10 μM picrotoxinin. Log-probit analysis indicated that half-maximal enhancement occurred at 13 + 1 nM diazepam.

GABA binding to the crude membranes could be inhibited by the GABA receptor antagonist bicuculline, 50 μM bicuculline producing 50% inhibition of GABA binding. Similar inhibition by bicuculline was observed in the presence of 100 μM pentobarbitone.

Pentobarbitone, 100 μM, did not influence GABA binding to membranes treated with 0.5% Triton X-100.

GABA enhanced the binding of radioactive diazepam (measured at 4°C for 15 min), by increasing binding affinity without significantly altering binding capacity, in both the crude P2 membrane preparation and membranes treated with 0.5% Triton X-100.

DISCUSSION

The concentrations of pentobarbitone which enhance GABA binding in the present study are comparable with those measured in the brain during surgical anaesthesia in laboratory animals (22). Similar concentrations of pentobarbitone have been shown to enhance GABA-mediated postsynaptic inhibition in tissue cultured mouse spinal neurones (21), and GABA-induced depolarization of frog sympathetic ganglion cells (18) and dorsal root fibres in the immature rat spinal cord in vitro (5).

Pentobarbitone is known to inhibit the binding of dihydropicrotoxinin to fresh rat brain membranes, 50% inhibition occurring at 50 μM pentobarbitone, without influencing the binding of GABA to these membranes (19). Dihydropicrotoxinin binding is considered to reflect binding to chloride ionophores normally linked to GABA receptors, but GABA does not influence dihydropicrotoxinin binding (19). Picrotoxinin inhibited the binding of dihydropicrotoxinin by 50% at 0.4 μM, similar to the concentration of picrotoxinin which abolished the enhancement of GABA binding by pentobarbitone in the present study.

The finding that high affinity GABA binding is enhanced by pentobarbitone in crude rat brain membranes is in contrast to results obtained in other laboratories (4, 19, 20). Our membrane preparation differed from most other preparations used for GABA binding studies in three respects: high frequency homogenization as with a Polytron was not employed, nor was detergent extraction e.g. with 0.05% Triton X-100, and the preparation was washed extensively before freezing. The extended washing regime did influence apparent GABA binding, probably by removing endogenous GABA from mitochondria present in the membrane preparation. After the extended washing regime, GABA binding was not influenced by freezing and thawing, but could be enhanced appreciably by extraction with 0.5% Triton X-100.

The crude membrane preparation which showed the enhancement of GABA binding by pentobarbitone appeared to retain the integrity of some of the GABA receptor-ionophore complexes which is lost in other preparations, thus representing a situation closer to that pertaining in vivo, and enabling links between receptors and ionophores to be studied in more detail. Picrotoxinin and dihydropicrotoxinin are considered to interact with the GABA-linked

ionophore without altering the binding of GABA to its recognition site. Pentobarbitone antagonizes the binding of dihydropicrotoxinin at concentrations similar to those which enhance GABA binding in the present study. Furthermore, picrotoxinin abolished the enhancement of GABA binding yet alone did not influence the binding of GABA.
Pentobarbitone and picrotoxinin may thus interact at the same site related to GABA-linked ionophores in an analogous manner to agonists and antagonists: pentobarbitone acting as an 'agonist' indirectly enhancing GABA binding, while picrotoxin may 'antagonise' this action of pentobarbitone without influencing GABA binding. This is consistent with the antagonism by picrotoxin of pentobarbitone-induced changes in membrane conductance of neurones in tissue culture (3).

Preliminary experiments with other barbiturates, including convulsant barbiturates, indicate that the ability to enhance GABA binding in these crude membranes may be a general property of barbiturates. This would be consistent with the ability of most barbiturates to inhibit the binding of dihydropicrotoxinin to rat brain membranes (19), and the potentiation of GABA-induced inhibition of spinal neurones by the convulsant 5-ethyl 5-(3-methylbut-2-enyl)barbiturate (14). The lack of differentiation between anaesthetic and convulsant barbiturates in their actions on GABA and dihydropicrotoxinin binding is in sharp contrast to their different effects on amino acid release and on the activity of synaptosomal calcium-dependent ATPase. Convulsant barbiturates stimulate D-aspartate release from rat brain slices and inhibit calcium ATPase activity, whereas anaesthetic barbiturates inhibit D-aspartate release and enhance calcium ATPase activity (23, 24). The effects of these barbiturates on D-aspartate release are unlikely to be due to any effects on GABA receptors since GABA does not influence D-aspartate release (10).

Chronic administration of phenobarbitone or diazepam to rats leads to a decrease in the number of high affinity GABA binding sites in the striatum (17). This decrease in the number of sites appears to be due to the loss of a regulatory component that can be removed from the control membrane preparations by extraction with 0.05% Triton X-100. In the present experiments, pentobarbitone does not influence the number of GABA binding sites, but alters the affinity of binding as though pentobarbitone was displacing an endogenous competitive inhibitor of GABA binding. The action of pentobarbitone enhancing GABA binding appears to differ from that of diazepam, which acts in a non-competitive manner with GABA binding (8). There is much evidence for a multiplicity of GABA binding sites (2) and that not all GABA binding sites can be influenced by benzodiazepines such as diazepam (11). Since barbiturates and benzodiazepines stimulate GABA binding in different ways, it is possible that these classes of drugs act on different populations of GABA binding sites. It should be emphasized that not all GABA binding sites are necessarily associated with synaptic GABA receptors. Indeed, recent studies have suggested that the binding sites found in most membrane preparations have a structural specificity analogous to that of GABA receptors on non-myelinated nerve fibres rather than synaptic GABA receptors (1).

GABA-receptor-ionophore complexes appear to be composed of a number of interacting domains. Depending on the rat brain membrane these domains may be studied in relative isolation or in varying degrees of interaction. The present study describes a membrane preparation which appears to preserve links between some GABA binding sites and certain pentobarbitone binding sites such that pentobarbitone enhances GABA binding, a mechanism that may underlie one aspect of barbiturate anaesthesia.

REFERENCES

1. Allan,R.D., Evans,R.H., and Johnston,G.A.R. (1980): Brit. J. Pharmac., in press.
2. Andrews,P.R., and Johnston,G.A.R. (1979): Biochem. Pharmac., 28:2697-2702.
3. Barker,J.L., and Ransom,B.R. (1978): J. Physiol. (Lond.), 280:355-372.
4. Enna,S.J., and Snyder,S.H. (1976): J. Neurochem., 26:221-224.
5. Evans,R.H. (1979): Brain Res., 171:113-120.
6. Fletcher,J.E., Spector,A.A. and Ashbrook,J.D. (1970) Biochemistry, 9:4580-4587.
7. Gray,E.G., and Whittaker,V.P. (1962): J. Anat. (Lond.), 96:79-87
8. Guidotti,A., Toffano,G., and Costa,E. (1978): Nature (Lond.) 275:553-555

9. Johnston,G.A.R., and Kennedy,S.M.E. (1978): In: Amino Acids as Chemical Transmitters, edited by F. Fonnum, pp. 507-516. Plenum Press, New York.
10. Johnston,G.A.R., Hailstone,M.H., and Freeman,C.G. (1980): J. Pharm. Pharmac., 32:230-231.
11. Karobath,M., Placheta,P., Lippitsch,M., and Krogsgaard-Larsen,P. (1979): Nature (Lond.), 278:748-749.
12. Klotz,I.M. (1946): Arch. Biochem., 9:109-117.
13. Lloyd,K.G., and Davidson,L. (1979): Science, N.Y., 205:1147-1149.
14. Lodge,D. (1979): Clin. Exp. Pharmac. Physiol., 6:686.
15. Lodge,D., and Curtis,D.R. (1978): Neuroscience Letters, 8:125-129.
16. Michaelis,E.K., Michaelis,M.L., and Boyarsky,L.L. (1974): Biochim. Biophys. Acta, 367:338-348.
17. Möhler,H., Okada,T., and Enna,S.J. (1978): Brain Res., 156:391-395.
18. Nicoll,R.A. (1978): Science, N.Y., 199:451-452
19. Olsen,R.W., Ticku,M.K., Greenlee,D., and Van Ness,P. (1979): In: GABA-Neurotransmitters, edited by P. Krogsgaard-Larsen, J. Scheel-Kruger, and H. Kofod, pp. 165-178. Munksgaard, Copenhagen.
20. Peck,E.J., Miller,A.L., and Lester,B.R. (1976): Brain Res. Bull., 1:595-597.
21. Ransom,B.R., and Barker,J.L. (1976): Brain Res., 114:530-535.
22. Richards,C.D. (1972): J. Physiol. (Lond.), 227:749-767.
23. Willow,M., and Johnston,G.A.R. (1979): Neuroscience Letters, 14:361-364.
24. Willow,M., Bornstein,J.C., and Johnston,G.A.R. (1980): Neuroscience Letters, in press.

GABA and Benzodiazepine Receptors,
edited by E. Costa et al.
Raven Press, New York © 1981.

The Role of GABA Mediated Neurotransmission in Convulsive States

*K. G. Lloyd, **C. Munari, *P. Worms, *L. Bossi, **J. Bancaud, †J. Talairach, and *P. L. Morselli

**Research Department, Synthélabo-LERS, Paris 75013, France; and **Unité 97 INSERM and †Service de Neurochirurgie Fonctionnelle, Hôpital Ste Anne, Paris, France*

INTRODUCTION

The evidence for the assumption that a dysfunction of gamma-aminobutyric acid (GABA)-utilizing neurons in the brain is fundamental to at least certain types of epilepsy has been reviewed in depth frequently during the past years (Refs 23, 37). The evidence is mainly circumstantial and rests chiefly on the observations that inhibition of GABA neuron function results in a convulsive state. Thus, in man, a deficiency of pyridoxine (a substance necessary for GABA synthesis) results in convulsions, which are rapidly terminated by pyridoxine administration (37). Furthermore, blockade of GABA receptors by bicuculline (cf. ref. 11) or of GABA-mediated chloride channels by picrotoxin (35), penicillin (19) or bicyclic phosphates (27) always leads to the production of a convulsive state. In a similar manner inhibition of GABA synthesis by allylglycine (28) or isonicotinic acid hydrazide (36) readily results in seizures. Other convulsant substances, for example metrazole (12, 20) have been suggested to act via GABA-mediated mechanisms. However, it is clear that convulsions can be induced by mechanisms other than those involving a dysfunction of GABA neurons, for example the convulsive state induced by strychnine, an inhibitor of glycine receptors (7).

Some anticonvulsant drugs have also been suggested to act by GABAergic mechanisms. Thus, for the barbiturates (20, 27), diphenylhydantoin (20) and dipropylacetate (18, 30) there is evidence (but no definitive proof) that an augmentation of GABA synaptic activity is responsible for the anti-epileptic action of these drugs.

The present article will consider the anticonvulsant actions of drugs which are known to augment GABA synaptic activity either by being GABA receptors agonists (SL 76 002 and muscimol (ref. 11) or relatively specific inhibitors of GABA metabolism (gabaculine (31) ; amino-oxyacetic acid, AOAA (29)). Furthermore new evidence that GABA neurons are dysfunctional in human epilepsy will be presented as ascertained from the study of brain material removed during surgical resection for intractable epilepsy.

METHODS

For the animal models (Swiss albino mice, 18-22 g weight), convulsions were induced by bicuculline, picrotoxinin, metrazol, strychnine or electroshock as previously described (15, 40). For the human studies (temporal cortex material removed at surgical resection for intractable epilepsy), published methods were used for GAD (5), GABA-T (41), ^{3}H-GABA binding (16) and ^{3}H-kainic acid binding (4, 17).

RESULTS AND DISCUSSION

As several aspects of this study rely on the GABA receptor agonist spectrum of SL 76 002 (PROGABIDE®), a brief review of the supporting evidence is required. This compound is a lipophilic benzophenone attached to a GABAmide chain (13) which readily penetrates the brain where it forms the GABA-benzophenone derivative (SL 75 102) and, more slowly, GABA itself (3). Both SL 76 002 and SL 75 102 are direct agonists as suggested by their displacement of ^{3}H-GABA from its binding site to rat brain or human cerebellar membranes (3). Furthermore, and most conclusively, SL 75 102, when applied to the rat dorsal root ganglion "in vitro", has the same effect on chloride conductance as does GABA itself ; this effect is blocked by bicuculline and shows cross-desensitization with GABA : additionally, and most importantly GABA and SL 75 102 have the same reversal potential (8,9).

As can be seen in Table 1, increasing GABA synaptic activity reverses the effect of a broad range of convulsant agents. Thus, the GABA receptor agonist SL 76 002 is effective against all of the convulsive challenges whether it be by a blockade of GABA synaptic effects (bicuculline, picrotoxinin, metrazol), via a blockade of other receptors (strychnine), or by unknown mechanisms (electroshock). Furthermore, this compound blocks the EEG alterations related to an epileptic focus induced by intracortical or intraamygdala injection of penicillin in the cat (14). The other GABA receptor agonist studied (muscimol) was less effective than SL 76 002. There are likely several contributing factors for this : (i) muscimol is rapidly metabolized to unknown compounds (2, 21), some of which are possibly antagonistic to the action of muscimol ; inhibition of muscimol metabolism enhances its anticonvulsant effect (10) ; (ii) muscimol is too toxic to allow the necessary dose levels required (13) ; (iii) muscimol may be a partial agonist for GABA receptors (40). Muscimol has previously been reported to be active against audiogenic seizures (1) and isoniazid-induced convulsions (26).

Apart from the GABA agonists, increasing GABA synaptic activity by other means also reduces convulsive behaviour. Thus, inhibitors of GABA-transaminase (Table 1, and ref. 33, 34) exhibit anti-convulsant activity. Moreover, dipropylacetate, a clinically-proven anticonvulsant (30), inhibits bicuculline, strychnine and metrazole effects in mice (40). Although the relevance of GABA-T inhibition by this compound to its anticonvulsant effect is disputed (22, 33), this drug apparently augments GABA synaptic activity at anticonvulsant doses (18).

TABLE 1. Anticonvulsant Effects of GABAergic Compounds.

Convulsant (Dose mg/kg)	ED50 (mg/kg, i.p.) SL 76 002	Muscimol	AOAA	Gabaculine
Bicuculline (0.45 i.v.)	20 ± 3 (3)	0.25 ± 0.11 (3)	8 ± 1.0 (3)	15 ± 1.6 (3)
Picrotoxinin (2.0 i.v.)	105 ± 12 (2)	1.5 ± 0.14 (3)	25 ± 1 (2)	35 ± 6 (2)
Metrazol (35, i.v.)	30 ± 3.8 (4)	1.0 ± 0.24 (3)	11 ± 1.0 (2)	13 ± 1.7 (2)
Strychnine (0.5, i.v.)	75 ± 19 (3)	0.90 ± 0.14 (3)	26 ± 4 (3)	-
Electroshock (Cornea, 10 mA, 50 Hz, 0.5 sec)	75 ± 8 (3)	> 2 (3)	-	-

Data from Refs 15, 39, 40.
Results are expressed as mean with S.E.M. The number of experimental groups (10 animals per dose, 3-5 doses per dose-response curve) in parentheses. ED50 is the dose necessary to reduce the number of convulsions of lethality (strychnine) by 50 percent.

Until recently clinical confirmation of the anticonvulsant activity of GABA receptor agonists was not available. Muscimol is too toxic in man for prolonged use (6) and others such as GABA itself and imidazole-acetic acid cross the blood-brain barrier only to a very limited extent (cf. ref. 37). At the present time sufficient preliminary clinical results with SL 76 002 are available to assess this compound with respect to its antiepileptic potential. Thirty-six epileptic patients with diverse etiologies, all of whom were refractory or uncontrolled by conventional medication (eg. barbiturates, benzodiazepines, diphenylhydantoin, dipropylacetate), have completed 1-3 month trials with this compound (24). Of these, 17 responded with a marked-major maintained improvement of their clinical status. Side effects were limited to 3 cases involving sedation and/or gastric upset. In view of the severity of these cases, our findings must be considered clinical evidence for the anti-epileptic efficacy of SL 76 002. Furthermore, they suggest that GABA receptor agonists may form an apparent lack of toxicity for clinical studies.

A direct verification of the GABA hypothesis would be to examine material removed from the brains of epileptic patients either at the time of surgical resection for uncontrolled epilepsy, or post-mortem. Some initial studies have been performed (cf. ref. 35) but the results have been equivocal. However in monkeys with epileptic foci induced by alumina gel application, a large decrease in GAD-containing nerve terminals was observed (32), supporting earlier observations of a GABA and GAD loss in epileptic foci (38). We have presently re-examined the question of GABA neuron dysfunction using material obtained at surgical resection from epileptic patients with previous stereo-EEG analysis by means of deep-implanted electrodes (25). Furthermore, for many samples a neuroanatomical analysis of the tissue has been made. Neurochemical parameters examined have been : GAD activity, to identify GABA cell bodies and terminals ; ^{3}H-GABA binding, for GABA receptive neurons ; and GABA-T activity, as a non-specific marker related to GABA. In addition to these GABA-related parameters, ^{3}H-kainic acid binding has been performed on a few samples, in order to have an impression of the possible changes in the sub-group of glutamate receptors labelled by this ligand (17).

The major findings to date from the study are shown in Table 2. GAD activity was found to be decreased in epileptic regions as compared to non-epileptic regions of the same brains : this is true whether the reference criterion was a neurophysiological parameter (stereo-EEG recordings from depth electrodes) or neuro-anatomical parameters. When the GAD activities were analyzed for individual patients (data not shown), several further conclusions can be drawn : (1) all patients with epilepsy due to the presence of a tumour showed a marked reduction in GAD activity in the affected areas ; (2) for patients with epilepsy not associated with the presence of a tumour, GAD activity in epileptic regions varied greatly between patients. In those patients with a reduced GAD activity this was true for all epileptic regions. This suggests that some epileptic states are associated with a decreased GABA neuron activity.

The binding of ^{3}H-GABA was studied with respect to two parameters : the affinity for the binding site (Kd) and the amount bound at a single concentration (25 nM) of ^{3}H-GABA. At present only the results for stereo-EEG analysis of non-tumour patients are available for comparative analysis. When the data from all of the patients are globally analyzed (Table 2) the Kd and amount bound in the epileptic regions are not different from that observed for the non-epileptic areas. However when the cases are analyzed individually it is apparent that there is a marked patient-to-patient variation in both parameters. Together with the large inter-individual variations in the loss of GAD activity in the epileptic zones, this may explain why different blood concentrations (and therefore probably brain levels) of SL 76 002 are needed to obtain an antiepileptic action. If this is correct, patients with fewer functional GABA terminals and/or receptors

TABLE 2. Neurochemical Alterations Observed in Samples from Surgically Resected Temporal Cortex From Epileptic Patients[1]

	Glutamic Acid Decarboxylase nmol CO_2/mg protein/hr	^{3}H-GABA Binding Kd nM	^{3}H-GABA Binding Bound H-GABA fmol/mg Protein	GABA Transaminase nmol succinate/ mg protein/15 min	^{3}H-Kainic Acid Bound fmol/mg protein
Regions without EEG or Neuroanatomical Abnormalities	79 ± 9 (23)	89 ± 5 (7)	139 ± 20 (11)	2.0 ± 0.2 (22)	123 ± 21(4)
Epileptogenic Brain Regions[2]					
Tumour Patients	33 ± 8 (5)***	-	-	2.6 ± 0.3 (5)	-
Non-Tumour Patients	53 ± 4 (18)**	101 ± 10 (7)	104 ± 13 (11)	2.4 ± 0.2 (17)	103 ± 12(4)
Anatomopathological Brain Regions[3]					
Tumour Patients	30 ± 5 (5)***	-	-	2.6 ± 0.4 (5)	-
Non-Tumour Patients	57 ± 5 (18)*	-	-	2.4 ± 0.7 (17)	-

1. Results expressed as mean with S.E.M. Number of patients in parentheses.
2. As defined from depth electrodes.
3. As defined from gross microscopy studies (scarring,malformation, gliosis, etc)

* $p < 0.05$; ** $p < 0.01$; *** $p < 0.001$ vs control regions

would need higher doses of GABA agonists than those with more normal GABA synapses.

GABA-transaminase activity was not significantly altered in these brain regions (Table 2). This was the case when either tumour or non-tumour patients were examined ; when the patients were individually examined only one of 22 cases showed a low GABA-T activity in epileptic regions. This finding tends to confirm the hypothesis that the alterations in GAD activity and GABA binding are specific for GABA synapses and are not generally a result of a non-specific tissue loss.

The binding of ^{3}H-kainic acid was also determined in brain material from 4 patients with non-tumoural epilepsy. In 3 of the 4 patients ^{3}H-kainic acid binding in epileptic areas was normal ; in the fourth case it was significantly lower. The overall result is a non-significant trend to a decrease in ^{3}H-kainic acid binding. Although there are too few cases to make any firm conclusions, it could be hypothesized that in epilepsy there is not a generalized increase in the pool of glutamate receptors labelled by ^{3}H-kainic acid.

CONCLUSIONS

Changes in GABA-mediated neurotransmission likely play a role not only in certain animal models of epilepsy, but also in the underlying neurochemical pathology of tumour-related epilepsy and other human epileptic conditions. Thus, glutamic acid decarboxylase activity and ^{3}H-GABA binding sites are decreased in epileptic regions of many patients, as compared to non-epileptic brain regions.

Increasing GABA-mediated neurotransmission also plays a role in the mechanism of action of numerous anticonvulsants, either by direct GABA receptor stimulation (e.g. with SL 76 002 or muscimol) or by inhibition of the metabolism of GABA (by GABA transaminase inhibitors). This is directly translated into the clinical efficacy of new antiepileptics as has been shown from the results of clinical trials with SL 76 002.

REFERENCES

1. Anlezark, G., Collins, J. and Meldrum, B. (1977): Neurosci. Letts, 7:337-340.
2. Baraldi, M., Grandison, L. and Guidotti, A. (1979): Neuropharmacology, 18:57-62.
3. Bartholini, G., Scatton, B., Zivkovic, B. and Lloyd, K. G. (1979): In : GABA-Neurotransmitters, edited by P. Krogsgaard-Larsen, J. Scheel-Kruger and H. Kofod, pp. 326-339. Munksgaard, Copenhagen.
4. Beaumont, K., Maurin, Y., Reisine, T. D., Fields, J. Z., Spokes, E., Bird, E. D. and Yamamura, H. I. (1979): Life Sci., 24: 809-816.
5. Bird, E. D. and Iversen, L. L. (1974): Brain, 97:457-472.

6. Chase, T. N. and Tamminga, C. A. (1979): In : GABA-Neurotransmitters, edited by P. Krogsgaard-Larsen, J. Scheel-Kruger and H. Kofod, pp. 283-294. Munksgaard, Copenhagen.
7. Curtis, D. R. and Johnston, G. A. R. (1974): Ergebn. Physiol. 69: 97-188.
8. Desarmenien, M., Feltz, P., Headley, P. M. and Santangelo,F. (1980): Brit. J. Pharmacol. in press.
9. Desarmenien, M., Headley, P. M., Santangelo, F. and Feltz,P. (1980): Brain Res. Bull. in press.
10. Enna, S. J., Maggi, A., Worms, P. and Lloyd, K. G. (1980): Brain Res. Bull. in press.
11. Johnston, G. A. R. (1976); In : GABA in Nervous System Function, edited by E. Roberts, T. N. Chase and D. B. Tower, pp. 395-411. Raven Press, New York.
12. Johnston, G. A. R. and Mitchell, J. F. (1971): J. Neurochem. 18: 2442-2446.
13. Kaplan, J. P., Raizon, B. M., Desarmenien, M., Feltz, P., Headley, P. M., Worms, P., Lloyd, K. G. and Bartholini, G. (1980): J. Med. Chem. in press.
14. Lloyd, K. G. Unpublished results.
15. Lloyd, K. G., Worms, P., Depoortere, H. and Bartholini, G. (1979): In : GABA-Neurotransmitters, edited by P. Krogsgaard-Larsen, J. Scheel-Kruger and H. Kofod, pp. 308-325. Munksgaard, Copenhagen.
16. Lloyd, K. G., Shemen, L. and Hornykiewicz, O. (1977): Brain Res., 127: 269-278.
17. London, E. D. and Coyle, J. T. (1979): Molec. Pharmacol., 15: 492-505.
18. Löscher, W. (1980) Personal Communication.
19. MacDonald, R. A. and Barker, J. L. (1978): Neurology, 28: 325-330.
20. MacDonald, R. A. and Barker, J. L. (1979): Brain Res., 167: 323-336.
21. Maggi, A. and Enna, S. (1979): Neuropharmacology, 18: 361-366.
22. Maitre, M., Ossola, L. and Mandel, P. (1979): In : GABA-Biochemistry and CNS Functions, edited by P. Mandel and F. De Feudis, pp. 3-20, Plenum Press, New York.
23. Meldrum, B. S. (1975): Int. Rev. Neurobiol. 17: 1-36.
24. Morselli, P. L., Bossi, L., Henry, J. F., Zarifian, E. and Bartholini, G. (1980): In : GABA and Other Inhibitory Neurotransmitters, edited by H. Lal and S. Fielding. In Press. Ankho, Fayetteville.
25. Munari, C., Rovei, V., Lloyd, K. G., Talairach, J., Sanjuan, M., Vendrenne, C., Bancaud, J. and Morselli, P. L. (1979): Abstracts, Eleventh Epilepsy International Symposium, p.138.
26. Naik, S. R., Guidotti, A. and Costa, E. (1976): Neuropharmacology, 15:479-484.
27. Olsen, R. W., Ticku, M. K., Van Ness, P. and Greenlee, D. (1979): Brain Res., 139:277-294.
28. Orlowski, M., Reingold, D. F. and Stanley, M. E. (1977):

J. Neurochem., 28: 349-353.
29. Perez de la Mora, M. and Tapia, R. (1973): Biochem. Pharmacol., 22: 2635-2639.
30. Pinder, R. M., Brogden, R. N., Speight, T. M. and Avery, G.S. (1977): Drugs, 13:81-123.
31. Rando, R. R. (1979): In : GABA-Neurotransmitters, edited by P. Krogsgaard-Larsen, J. Scheel-Kruger and H. Kofod, pp. 228-235, Munksgaard, Copenhagen.
32. Ribak, C. E., Harris, A. B., Banhan, J. E. and Roberts, E. (1979): Science, 205: 211-214.
33. Schechter, P. J., Trainier, Y. and Grove, J. (1979): In : GABA-Biochemistry and CNS Functions, edited by P. Mandel and F. V. De Feudis, pp. 43-58. Plenum Press, New York.
34. Schechter, P. J., Trainier, Y., Jung, M. J. and Bohlen, P. (1977) : Europ. J. Pharmacol., 45: 319-328.
35. Takeuchi, A. (1976): In : GABA in Nervous System Function, edited by E. Roberts, T. N. Chase and D. B. Tower, pp. 255-267, Raven Press, New York.
36. Tapia, R. (1974): In : Neurohumoral Coding of Brain Function, edited by R. D. Myers and R. R. Drucker, pp. 3-26. Plenum Press, New York.
37. Tower, D. B. (1978): In : GABA in Nervous System Function, edited by E. Roberts, T. N. Chase and D. B. Tower, pp. 461-478, Raven Press, New York.
38. Van Gelder, N. and Courtois, A. (1972): Brain Res., 43: 477-484.
39. Worms, P. and Lloyd, K. G. Unpublished results.
40. Worms, P., Depoortere, H. and Lloyd, K. G. (1979): Life Sci., 25: 607-614.
41. Wu, J-Y (1976): In : GABA in Nervous System Function, edited by E. Roberts, T. N. Chase and D. B. Tower, pp. 7-55, Raven Press, New York.

GABA and Benzodiazepine Receptors,
edited by E. Costa et al.
Raven Press, New York © 1981.

GABA-Agonists as Anti-Epileptic Agents

Brian Meldrum

Department of Neurology, Institute of Psychiatry, London SE5 8AF, United Kingdom

The term 'GABA agonist' is used to describe a compound that acts at a GABA recognition site in the neuronal membrane to reproduce the action of GABA at that site.

The term 'GABA mimetic' is used here to describe compounds that can mimic or enhance the effect of GABA in pharmacological test systems by a means other than action as a direct GABA agonist (such as augmenting the physiological release of GABA, acting allosterically to increase the affinity of the recognition site for GABA, augmenting inhibitory potentials by an action on the Cl^- ionophore, or by inhibiting the reuptake of synaptically released GABA).

GABA agonists merit investigation as antiepileptic agents because (i) impairment of GABA-mediated inhibition is associated with convulsions (20) and (ii) several clinically useful anticonvulsant drugs are GABA mimetics (12).

This paper summarises studies on the anticonvulsant action of GABA agonists. It reports the paradoxical epileptogenic action of classical GABA agonists (i.e. those acting on post-synaptic inhibition that is bicuculline-sensitive and strychnine-insensitive). The question whether this effect is due to action on other GABA receptors or is a consequence of diffuse action on classical GABA receptor sites is evaluated.

DIVERSITY OF GABA RECEPTORS

Systemically administered GABA agonists may modify brain function by acting not only at GABA receptors that are pre- or post-synaptic but also at extra-synaptic neuronal membrane sites and at non-neuronal sites (such as glia, vascular smooth muscle, etc). Information suggesting a diversity of GABA receptors comes from iontophoretic experiments, pharmacological studies *in vitro* and radioactive ligand studies with brain membrane preparations. At present it is not possible to integrate this information into a unified account.

Iontophoretic studies have defined a post-synaptic receptor that is bicuculline-sensitive and strychnine-insensitive. This appears to be the physiological receptor for the major intrinsic inhibitory systems in many regions of the mammalian brain (7). Bicuculline-insensitive receptors at which GABA acts in a folded conformation have been demonstrated in several invertebrate preparations (29). Recently in mammalian preparations, both from the peripheral and the central nervous system, a receptor has been identified at which GABA acts to diminish the release of noradrenaline, dopamine and 5-hydroxytryptamine (4). This action of GABA is not bicuculline sensitive. It is weakly reproduced by muscimol; 3-aminopropane sulphonic acid is completely inactive. In contrast, (-)baclofen and 4-hydroxybutyrate are potent agonists. The endogenous agonist and its physiological role remain to be defined.

Binding studies with radioactive ligands and membrane preparations have provided evidence for a diversity of GABA receptors. Thus there are both high and low affinity Na-independent binding sites, which vary independently in their regional density in the brain (11). There are twice as many high-affinity GABA binding sites as there are muscimol binding sites (1). This suggests that there is a high affinity GABA binding site that is not the muscimol (and bicuculline) sensitive receptor. Binding studies also suggest that some but not all GABA receptors are contiguous to benzodiazepine binding sites.

CLASSIFICATION OF GABA AGONISTS (Table 1)

The above observations provide the basis for a classification of GABA agonists (25). There is an unequivocal differentiation between the Types I-III, and Type IV. Type IV agonists are distinctive in terms of pharmacological responses, binding studies and molecular structure. Types I, II and III act identically on bicuculline-sensitive post-synaptic inhibition and in binding studies employing GABA or bicuculline as ligands (15). However, Type I agonists mimic the action of GABA in facilitating the binding of labelled benzodiazepines to membrane preparations, whereas Type III agonists do not, but act as antagonists to muscimol in this system (5,19). Type II GABA agonists are partial agonists and antagonists in the GABA-mediated facilitation of benzodiazepine binding. This classification into Types I-III does not necessarily involve more than one type of GABA receptor. It is probable that following combination of an agonist with the GABA recognition site there is a change in molecular conformation that involves the receptor, the agonist and the benzodiazepine binding site. Type III agonists have a double ring structure and a highly restricted conformation of the charged groups. Thus any change in conformation following combination with the GABA recognition site might be impeded.

ANIMAL MODELS OF EPILEPSY

Previous reports of the anticonvulsant action of GABA agonists

TABLE 1. A classification of GABA agonists (data from 4,5,14,15)

	TYPE I	TYPE II	TYPE III	TYPE IV
AGONISTS	muscimol dihydromuscimol	3-APS isoguvacine	THIP P-4-SA	(-)baclofen 4-hydroxy-butyrate
GABA binding	6		131	0
IC_{50} nM (Na. Indep.)	9	37	40	0
BZD binding facilitation	0.6	±	- -	
ED_{50} μM	1.9	±	- -	
Bicuculline-sensitive	+++	+++	++	0
Post-syn. Inhib.	+++	+++	++	0
GABA binding Calf ganglia IC_{50} μM	0.1	1 10		>1000
Inhibition of N-A release mouse v.d. ED_{50} μM	23	>1000		2.9

have primarily concerned the effect of muscimol in rodent test systems, utilising either seizures induced by electroshock, by sound stimulation (in genetically susceptible mice) or by the administration of convulsant drugs (isoniazid, metrazol, bicuculline) (2,16,18,27). The effect of 3-aminopropane sulphonic acid in various models of focal epilepsy has also been reported (9).

Rodent test systems, particularly the maximal electroshock test and threshold metrazol seizures, are of particular value as screening tests in the evaluation of new compounds. However, they do not establish that a compound is an anticonvulsant that will be effective against natural syndromes of epilepsy. They can be misleading, and as will be shown, this appears to be significantly so for the evaluation of GABA agonists.

We have compared the apparent anticonvulsant efficacy of GABA agonists belonging to all the Types discussed above in a rodent and a primate model of epilepsy - audiogenic seizures in DBA/2 mice and photically-induced seizures in Senegalese baboons, *Papio papio*.

These models avoid the problem of possible effects of the test substance on the absorption or metabolism of convulsant compounds that arises with drug-induced seizures.

The photosensitive baboons provide the closest natural animal model to any syndrome of epilepsy occurring in man (28). They have been used for the evaluation of many established and potential anticonvulsant drugs (21,24). Toxic side effects are observed in baboons that correspond closely to those seen in man after a wide range of drugs.

Results obtained with compounds representative of each Type of GABA agonist are summarised here. The molecular structures of the compounds discussed are shown in Figure 1.

Muscimol (Type I)

In DBA/2 mice, muscimol protects against sound-induced seizures. Figure 2 shows that the ED_{50} for abolition of the clonic phase of the response is approximately 0.4 mg/kg. Complete protection occurs after muscimol 1-2 mg/kg, but is associated with ataxia, ptosis and piloerection (2). Muscimol 2 mg/kg produces a 30% mortality (LD_{50} by this route is 2.5 mg/kg). These results compared with an ED_{50} of 0.25 mg/kg against bicuculline-induced seizures and of 1.1 mg/kg against picrotoxin convulsions in mice (16).

In photosensitive baboons, muscimol 0.25-1.0 mg/kg, intravenously, failed to protect against photically-induced myoclonus or seizures (30). In contrast, spontaneous paroxysmal EEG abnormalities appear within a few minutes of the injection, become maximal after 30-60 minutes and persist for 3-5 hours. This activity is sometimes associated with a diffuse myoclonus of the limbs. Pretreatment with a transaminase inhibitor (γ -acetylenic GABA) which slows the conversion of muscimol to 3-hydroxy-

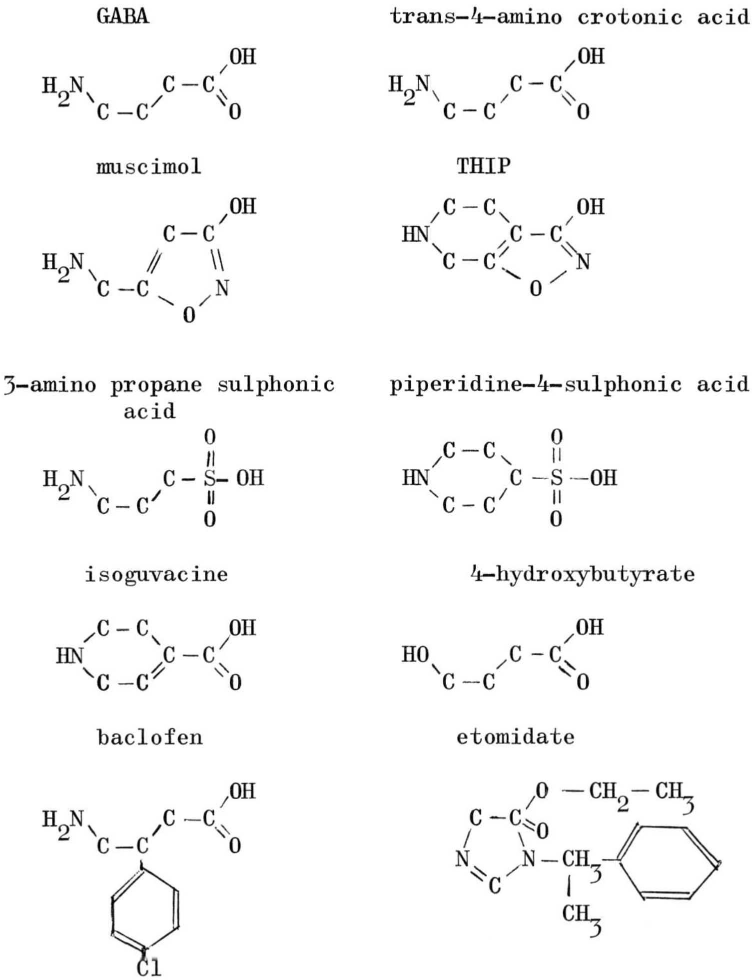

Figure 1. Molecular formulae of GABA agonists and etomidate

5-hydroxy-methylisoxazole, exacerbates the EEG abnormalities. This suggests that it is muscimol itself rather than the deaminated metabolite that is responsible for the toxic effects.

Isoguvacine (Type II)

In DBA/2 mice isoguvacine 1-32 mg/kg ip was without effect on sound-induced seizures. Intracerebroventricular administration of isoguvacine (8.0 μg in 10 μl) produced partial protection (2). In view of this evidence for exclusion by the blood brain barrier, isoguvacine has not been tested in baboons.

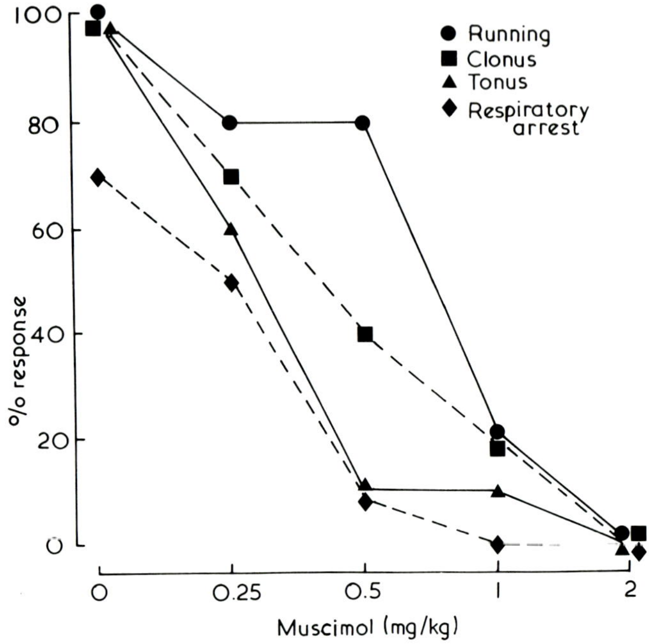

Figure 2. The effect of muscimol on audiogenic seizure responses in DBA/2 mice. Each point represents the % of 10 mice, showing the indicated phase of the seizure response ('running', 'clonus', 'tonus', 'respiratory arrest') when tested 1 hour after intraperitoneal administration of muscimol (2)

3-Amino propane sulphonic acid, 3-APS (Type II)

In DBA/2 mice 3-APS, 8-256 mg/kg ip, is without effect on sound-induced seizure responses (tested 15 min after drug injection). Because of the possibility that 3-APS cannot cross the intact blood brain barrier, we have also tested an ester that is lipid soluble. However, 3-APS benzoate, 8-256 mg/kg ip, also fails to modify sound-induced seizure responses.

In photosensitive baboons 3-APS, 25-200 mg/kg iv, does not modify myoclonic responses to photic stimulation.

These results contrast with the reported transient abolition of focal spike discharges in cats following the injection of 3-APS, 5-25 mg/kg iv (9). However, the neocortical or amygdala lesions associated with the focal discharges may facilitate the entry of 3-APS into the brain.

THIP (Type III)

In DBA/2 mice, THIP, 4,5,6,7-tetra hydroisoxazolo(5,4-C) pyridine-3-ol, 8 mg/kg ip, produces a partial protection against sound-induced seizures, but also impairs motor activity, produces a hunched posture, and a fall in rectal temperature.

In photosensitive baboons, THIP, 0.25-4.0 mg/kg iv, does not modify photically-induced myoclonic responses (23). However, THIP, 8 mg/kg, induces sustained paroxysmal abnormalities in the EEG with rhythmic spikes or spike and wave discharges, and also rhythmic or irregular myoclonus of the limb and trunk muscles.

Baclofen (Type IV)

In DBA/2 mice protection against sound-induced seizures is seen 30 minutes after baclofen, 8 mg/kg ip (25). This is associated with piloerection and reduced locomotor activity. In mice baclofen also protects against metrazol and thiosemicarbazide seizures (3).

In photosensitive baboons, (±)baclofen, 4-15 mg/kg iv, diminishes photically induced myoclonic responses (22). It provokes a sustained paroxysmal EEG activity with a rhythmic spike and wave pattern. Of the isomers only (-)baclofen acts on synaptic terminals to diminish monoamine release. In contrast, (+)baclofen enhances the release of GABA from slices of rat globus pallidus (13). In order to elucidate the mode of action of baclofen in photosensitive baboons we have compared the effects of (-)baclofen and (+)baclofen (Meldrum & Franks, unpublished). Photically-induced myoclonic responses are absent after (-)baclofen, 2 mg/kg iv, for a period of 5 hours or more. (-)Baclofen, 8 mg/kg, produces a toxic syndrome with reduced arousal, ataxia, loss of muscle tone and rhythmical limb jerks lasting for more than 10 hours. (+)Baclofen, 2-32 mg/kg, does not prevent photically-induced myoclonus or induce a toxic syndrome.

4-Hydroxybutyrate (Type IV)

In baboons photically-induced myoclonic responses are diminished or absent 5 minutes to 4 hours after iv administration of 4-hydroxybutyrate, 100-400 mg/kg. Paroxysmal EEG abnormalities, including rhythmic spike and wave discharges, become prominent on the EEG after 4-hydroxybutyrate, 200-400 mg/kg. These are associated with impaired arousal, loss of muscle tone, and some rhythmic limb jerking.

Similar paroxysmal abnormalities in the EEG have been reported previously in rats and in monkeys (10,31) and a parallel with *petit mal* attacks in man has been proposed.

GABA AGONISTS - SUMMARY

Rodent test systems often indicate that GABA agonists that act on bicuculline-sensitive post-synaptic inhibition (such as muscimol and THIP) are anticonvulsant. Effective anticonvulsant doses commonly produce locomotor impairment. GABA agonists that are without anticonvulsant, or toxic, actions, such as isoguvacine, probably do not enter the brain when administered systemically. Even active compounds, such as muscimol, show only limited entry to the brain (17).

However, when tested in a primate system that is extremely sensitive to the anticonvulsant action of barbiturates and of benzodiazepines, these GABA agonists are devoid of any anticonvulsant action, but instead induce epileptiform EEG activity and sometimes irregular spontaneous myoclonus. The occasional induction of myoclonus by muscimol has also been reported in man (6). Compounds such as (-)baclofen and 4-hydroxybutyrate, that do not act on the GABA receptor producing post-synaptic inhibition, but mimic the effect of GABA at a presynaptic receptor which influences the synaptic release of monoamine transmitter substances, also appear anticonvulsant in some rodent test systems. However, like muscimol and THIP, they produce epileptiform EEG activity.

The epileptogenic rather than anticonvulsant action of GABA agonists contrasts with the evidence that the anticonvulsant action of benzodiazepines and of barbiturates can be correlated with their ability to enhance GABA-mediated inhibition.

ETOMIDATE, BARBITURATES AND BENZODIAZEPINES

The epileptogenic action of GABA agonists has led us to look for similar actions in GABA-mimetics.

Among GABA-mimetics, etomidate is closely comparable to muscimol and THIP. In iontophoretic experiments etomidate produces post-synaptic and presynaptic inhibition, that is bicuculline-sensitive (8). It is possible that etomidate acts as a true GABA agonist. However, the molecular structure differs from the GABA agonists in that the charges relating to the N and O in the etomidate molecule are 1-1.5 Å closer together than in the extended conformation of GABA or in muscimol. Etomidate has apparent anticonvulsant action in some rodent test systems (33). However, in photosensitive baboons, etomidate 0.5-2.0 mg/kg iv, fails to block photically-induced myoclonic responses. Etomidate 2 mg/kg, leads to recurrent or sustained generalised myoclonus, with paroxysmal EEG activity. Myoclonus and epileptiform manifestations also occur in man associated with the use of etomidate as an inducing agent in anaesthesia (26).

Barbiturate anaesthetics, either during induction or the recovery phase, commonly induce myoclonic jerks and paroxysmal EEG abnormalities. Such phenomena are not normally associated with phenobarbitone therapy in epilepsy. However, some barbiturates are primarily convulsant.

Benzodiazepines do not induce comparable phenomena in therapeutic or toxic dosage.

EPILEPTOGENESIS AND TEMPOROSPATIAL PATTERNING

A theoretical framework that can explain these phenomena is provided by a consideration of the normal function of inhibitory interneurons in the cortex and elsewhere. These are activated by collaterals of excitatory inputs (i.e. synchronously with the arrival of powerful afferent volleys) and by recurrent collaterals on efferent pathways. They thus serve to restrict excitation in time and space and prevent the excessively synchronous and sustained discharges that are the basis of epilepsy. This function depends critically on the activation of GABA receptors in a temporo-spatial pattern that is tied to that of neuronal activity in input and output pathways. Benzodiazepines, in so far as they augment inhibition by increasing the affinity of the GABA receptor, enhance this process. Barbiturates will also do this if they prolong the period during which the Cl^- channel is open following GABA receptor activation. If they act indiscriminately on the Cl^- ionophore, keeping it open or shut, irrespective of events at the GABA recognition site, they will favour epileptogenesis.

GABA agonists by acting diffusely and in a sustained fashion on post-synaptic inhibitory receptors may prevent the normal functioning of GABAergic interneurons and thus facilitate excessively synchronised discharges.

An alternative explanation for the epileptogenic action of GABA agonists is that it derives from action at a site other than the post-synaptic inhibitory receptor.

CONCLUSION

GABA agonists appear to be anticonvulsant in some rodent test systems, but are epileptogenic rather than anticonvulsant in a primate model of epilepsy.

ACKNOWLEDGEMENTS

I am grateful to my colleagues, Dr.G.Anlezark and Mr.A. Franks for their collaboration and to the Medical Research Council and the British Epilepsy Association for financial support.

REFERENCES

1. Andrews,P.R. and Johnston,G.A.R. (1979): Biochem.Pharmacol., 28:2697-2702.
2. Anlezark,G.,Collins,J. and Meldrum,B. (1977):Neuroscience Lett.,7:337-340.
3. Bein,H.J. (1972): In Spasticity - a topical survey (ed. W.Birkmayer). H.Huber,Bern,pp.76-89.

4. Bowery,N.G.,Hill,D.R.,Hudson,A.L.,Doble,A.,Middlemiss,D.N., Shaw,J. and Turnbull,M. (1980):Nature,283:92-94.
5. Braestrup,C.,Nielsen,M.,Krogsgaard-Larsen,P.and Flach,E. (1979):Nature,280:331-333.
6. Chase ,T. and Tamminga,C.A. (1979): In GABA-Neurotransmitters. (ed.P.Krogsgaard-Larsen,J.Scheel-Kruger and H.Kofod) pp.283-294. Munksgaard,Copenhagen.
7. Curtis,D.R. (1979): In GABA-Neurotransmitters. (ed.P.Krogsgaard-Larsen,J.Scheel-Kruger and H.Kofod) pp.17-27,Munksgaard Copenhagen
8. Evans,R.H. and Hill,R.G. (1978): Experientia 34:1325-1326.
9. Fariello,R.G. (1979):Exper.Neurology 66:55-63.
10. Godschalk,M.,Dzoljic,M.R. and Bonta,I.L. (1977): Europ.J. Pharmacol.,44:105-111.
11. Guidotti,A.,Gale,K.,Suria,A. and Toffano,G. (1979):Brain Research 172:566-571.
12. Haefely,W.E. (1977): Agents and Actions 7:353-359.
13. Kerwin,R. and Pycock,C. (1978):J.Pharm.Pharmacol.,30:622-623.
14. Krogsgaard-Larsen,P.,Falch,E.,Schousboe,A.,Curtis,D.R. and Lodge,D. (1980):J.Neurochem.,34:756-759.
15. Krogsgaard-Larsen,P.,Hjeds,H.,Curtis,D.R.,Lodge,D. and Johnston,G.A.R. (1979):J.Neurochem.,32:1717-1724.
16. Lloyd,K.G.,Worms,P.,Depoortere,H. and Bartholinii,G. (1979): In GABA-Neurotransmitters. (ed.P.Krogsgaard-Larsen,J.Scheel-Kruger and H.Kofod) pp.308-325. Munksgaard,Copenhagen.
17. Maggi,A. and Enna,S.J. (1979): Neuropharmacology 18:361-366.
18. Matthews,W.D. and McCafferty,G.P. (1979):Neuropharmacology 18:885-889.
19. Maurer,R. (1979): Neuroscience Lett.,12:65-68.
20. Meldrum,B.S. (1975): Internat.Rev.Neurobiology 17:1-36.
21. Meldrum,B.S. (1978): J.Electroenceph.Clin.Neurophysiol.Suppl. 34:317-322.
22. Meldrum,B.S. and Horton,R.W. (1974): In Epilepsy. (ed.P. Harris and C.Mawdsley) pp.55-64.Churchill,Edinburgh.
23. Meldrum,B. and Horton,R. (1980):Europ.J.Pharmacol.,61:231-237.
24. Meldrum,B.S.,Horton,R.W. and Toseland,P. (1975):Archiv. Neurology 32:289-294.
25. Meldrum,B.,Pedley,T.,Horton,R.,Anlezark,G.and Franks,A.(1980) Brain Res.Bull.,5:Suppl.2.
26. Morgan,M.,Lunkley,J.and Whitwam,J.G. (1975):Lancet(i):955-956.
27. Naik,S.R.,Guidotti,A.and Costa,E. (1976):Neuropharmacology 15:479-484.
28. Naquet,R.and Meldrum,B.S.(1972):In Experimental Models of Epilepsy (Ed.D.P.Purpura,J.K.Penry,D.B.Tower,D.M.Woodbury and R.D.Walter) pp.373-406,Raven Press,New York.
29. Nistri,A.and Constanti,A. (1979):Progress in Neurobiology 13:117-235.
30. Pedley,T.A.,Horton,R.W.and Meldrum,B.S. (1979):Epilepsia 20:409-416.

31. Snead,O.C. (1978):Neurology 28:636-642.
32. Sloper,J.J. and Powell,T.P.S. (1979):Phil.Trans.Roy.Soc. (Lond.),285:199-226.
33. Wauquier,A.,Ashton,D.,Clincke,G.,Niemeggers,C.J.E. and Janssen,P.A.J. In Symposium über Anästhesie bei cerebralen Krampfanfällen und Intensivtherapie der Status Epilepticus (in press)

GABA and Benzodiazepine Receptors,
edited by E. Costa et al.
Raven Press, New York © 1981.

Anterior Pituitary GABA Receptors and Their Regulation of Prolactin Secretion

Lindsey Grandison

Departments of Physiology and Biophysics, College of Medicine and Dentistry of New Jersey, Rutgers Medical School, Piscataway, New Jersey 08854

The regulation of prolactin release from the anterior pituitary is a process involving the interaction of several hormonal and neuronal components. Unlike other pituitary secretions prolactin is primarily regulated through inhibition of release. Dopamine secretion into the hypophyseal portal vessels by the arcuate nucleus dopaminergic neurons provides this tonic suppression of secretion (15). Serotoninergic neurons acting through an intermediate, perhaps the unidentified prolactin releasing factor, may be the stimulus inducing the surges of prolactin secretion observed during several physiological events (1). Other neutrotransmitters also have a role in this regulatory process but their significance is not as well established (6,7,18,19). Recently GABA was observed to alter prolactin release; however, its participation in regulation has proven difficult to evaluate since both stimulatory and inhibitory effects of GABA on prolactin release have been observed. When injected into the lateral ventricle GABA was reported to stimulate prolactin release (14,15) but it was also found to block release(20). The short duration of GABA action and the large doses required to induce significant alteration of prolactin release make evaluation of these early observations difficult. This study was undertaken in order to evaluate the significance and determine the mechanism of GABA's action on prolactin release. For this purpose the effects on prolactin release of the potent and long acting GABA agonist muscimol were investigated.

ACTIONS OF MUSCIMOL *IN VIVO*

The intravenous administration of muscimol (1 mg/kg) to male rats produced only a slight decrease in serum prolactin concentration. However when a more sensitive animal model was used, the ovariectomized-estrogen-primed rat, this same dose of muscimol significantly reduced prolactin concentration by 39% from 221 ± 23 to 136 ± 26 ng/ml. Since this inhibitory activity was observed the ability of muscimol to block stimulation of prolactin release was also tested. Morphine (15 mg/kg) increased prolactin concentration from 8 ± 3 to 41 ± 3 ng/ml in male rats but when rats were given muscimol prior to morphine no increase occurred (8 ± 3 to 9 ± 2 ng/ml). Similarly when muscimol was given before haloperidol it blocked the rise in prolactin release (10 ± 3 to 48 ± 2, haloperidol vs 9 ± 1 to 7 ± 2, muscimol + haloperidol). Since both the hypothalamus and the pituitary have been proposed as the site at which GABA inhibits prolactin release (11 - 13,19,20,22), the site of muscimol action was next examined. When muscimol was injected into the lateral ventricle of male rats over the dose range of 100 to 500 ng/rat no change in basal prolactin release was noted. At a higher dose, 800 ng/rat, a significant 3 fold elevation over basal release was observed (11 ± 4 to 33 ± 8). At this dose of muscimol depression of spontaneous motor activity occurred as well. A similar elevation of basal prolactin secretion produced by high doses of GABA (5-10 micromoles/rat) has been reported for both male and female rats (14,16,19). When muscimol at 250 or 400 ng/rat was given intracerebroventricularly before morphine or haloperidol, stimulation of prolactin release was not blocked. To assure adequate stimulation of hypothalamic GABA receptors muscimol was injected directly into the basomedial hypothalamus, the final pathway regulating prolactin release. Administration of 250 or 500 ng/rat via this route produced no significant change in basal prolactin release. Moreover intrahypothalamic injection of muscimol was unable to block the morphine or haloperidol stimulation of prolactin release. Although these doses and even lower ones (100 ng/rat) can activate the hypothalamic GABA receptors involved in eating behavior (5), the concentration of muscimol in the hypothalamus following intravenous administration of 1 mg muscimol/kg was unknown.

In order to determine its resulting hypothalamic concentration 1 mg ^{3}H muscimol/kg was injected intravenously into male rats and its distribution into brain and pituitary was followed. For comparison a separate group of rats was given 100 ng ^{3}H muscimol/rat into the lateral ventricle. Table 1 shows the ratio of muscimol accumulation following intracerebroventricular compared to intravenous injection for several brain areas and the pituitary.

TABLE 1. Distribution of ^{3}H Muscimol

	Hypo	BS	Hipp	Cor	ST	AP
^{3}H muscimol IVT / ^{3}H muscimol IV	0.7	0.73	0.83	4.1	1.8	ND / 18

Rats received 1 mg muscimol/kg iv (SA = 12 μ Ci/μ mole) or 100 ng muscimol/rat intracerebroventricularly, ivt (SA 1.25 μ Ci/nmole) 30 min before decapitation, ^{3}H muscimol is in pmol/mg protein. n=3, ND= not detected, Hypo=hypothalamus, BS=brain stem, Hipp = hippocampus, Cor = cortex, ST = striatum and AP = anterior pituitary.

It can be seen from Table 1 that in most brain areas accumulation of ^{3}H muscimol was similar after injection of 100 ng intracerebroventricularly or after 1 mg/kg intravenously. The greatest difference was found in the ^{3}H muscimol content of the anterior pituitary. None was detected in those rats injected via the lateral ventricle while the highest accumulation of all areas samples occurred in rats given muscimol intravenously. These results indicated that the hypothalamus was not the locus of muscimol inhibition of prolactin release but rather suggested the pituitary as a probable site.

PITUITARY GABA RECEPTORS

To examine the effects of GABA agonists on the lactotrophs, the anterior pituitary cells secreting prolactin, GABA agonists were incubated with pituitary halves or with primary cell cultures of dispersed anterior pituitary cells. Table 2 shows that muscimol produced a dose related inhibition of prolactin release. This response is receptor-mediated since the GABA receptor blocker bicuculline methiodide at a dose which had no effect on spontaneous prolactin release, completely antagonized muscimol inhibition of secretion.

TABLE 2. Inhibition of Prolactin Release by Muscimol *In Vitro*

	% Control		
		+ bicuculline	+ sulpiride
MUSCIMOL			
10^{-7}M	76^{x}		
10^{-6}M	66^{x}	121	58^{x}
10^{-5}M	56^{x}		
APOMORPHINE			
5×18^{-9}	80^{x}		
5×10^{-8}	56^{x}	60^{x}	90
5×10^{-7}	30^{x}		

Anterior pituitaries of male rats were hemisected, preincubated for 1 hr in 2 ml of tissue culture medium 199 (TC 199) and then for 4 hrs in TC 199 without or with drug treatment. Prolactin released into the medium/mg wet ant. pituitary weight was compared between the drug treated half and the corresponding untreated half using Student's paired t test. $p < 0.05$. Bicuculline methiodide was used at a concentration of 10^{-5}M and sulpiride at 10^{-7}M.

Table 2 also shows that muscimol inhibition of prolactin release is separate from dopamine inhibition. The dopaminergic agonist apomorphine potently reduced prolactin release. This response is blocked by sulpiride; however, sulpiride is ineffective in reducing muscimol inhibition of prolactin release. Conversely bicuculline is ineffective in diminishing apomorphine inhibition of release. From this and other studies (2,18,19) it is evident that dopamine and dopaminergic agonists are much more potent than GABA and GABA agonists in reducing prolactin release. At low doses of apomorphine (5 X 10^{-8}M) the addition of muscimol (10^{-6}M) further decreased prolactin release from 47 to 33% of control. However, at higher doses addition of muscimol did not further suppress release.

To characterize the pituitary GABA receptor, the binding of ^{3}H-GABA to crude mitochrondial membrane fractions of anterior pituitary tissue was examined. ^{3}H-GABA binding to repeatedly washed membranes was saturable and occurred with a high affinity. Table 3 shows the apparent affinity constants and the binding capacity of anterior pituitary tissue from both rat and human samples.

TABLE 3. GABA Binding Sites of Pituitary Tissue

	Rat	Human
K_d (nM)	33	41
B_{max} (pmol/mg protein)	1.2	0.49

Pituitaries were prepared as previously described (8). Rat pituitaries were treated with Triton X 100 while human pituitaries were repeatedly washed to remove endogenous inhibitors of GABA binding. The binding assay involved incubating for 15 min at 4°C, 100 µl ^{3}H-GABA (5-500 nM) with 200 µg protein in 800 µl Tris citrate buffer pH 7.1 and 100 µl Tris buffer with or without GABA 10^{-3}M. The reaction was stopped by centrifugation at 48,000 X g. The resulting pellets were washed once with 1 ml H_2O and solubulized for liquid scintillation counting.

The binding of GABA by pituitary tissue was similar to binding observed to rat brain tissue. Similar high affinity constants were found; however the number of binding sites was much greater in brain tissue than in the pituitary, approximately a third for rat pituitary and a sixth for human pituitary tissue. The binding of GABA to pituitary tissue was displaced by bicuculline (IC_{50} ca. 5 X 10^{-5}M) unlabeled GABA (5 X 10^{-8}M) and unlabeled muscimol (5 X 10^{-9}M). Thus the inhibitory actions of GABA at the pituitary which previously were attributed to nonspecific effects because of the high doses required for significant inhibition may represent a receptor mediated and a physiological action of GABA. In order to examine whether these effects of muscimol measured in vitro reflect actions of GABA in vivo, serum GABA concentrations were altered by administration of amino-oxyacetic acid (AOAA) or isoniazid. Correlated with the rise in serum GABA reported to follow AOAA administration (3) is a decrease in serum prolactin concentration from 260 ± 20 to 70 ± 26 in ovariectomized-estrogen-primed rats given 25 mg AOAA/kg. Conversely the reported decrease in serum GABA produced by 450 mg isoniazid/kg (3) is associated with a rise in prolactin of ovariectomized estrogen primed rats from 238 ± 35 to 520 ± 62. Interestingly neither AOAA nor isoniazid altered prolactin release in male rats, presumably because the existing dopaminergic inhibition was producing the dominant effect under these conditions.

INTERACTIONS BETWEEN GABA AND BENZODIAZEPINES

The physiological significance of GABA in regulation of prolactin release has not been adequately evaluated. The high concentrations necessary to produce inhibition have previously been interpreted to represent nonspecific effects. These evaluations of potency are conducted in vitro using GABA agonists and pituitary cells; however, it is now recognized that the GABA receptor exists as part of a multicomponent complex of a chloride ionophore, the GABA receptor, the benzodiazepine receptor and a membrane bound protein which can alter GABA and benzodiazepine receptor sensitivity (9). Extensive electrophysiological investigation indicates that benzodiazepines can enhance GABA action (10). Therefore it was of interest to determine whether GABA inhibition of prolactin release was also enhanced by benzodiazepines. Concurrent addition of diazepam with GABA produced little enhancement of GABA inhibition. However, when diazepam was added to the medium in which anterior pituitary cells were cultured, GABA inhibition was potentiated, Table 4.

TABLE 4. Interaction Between GABA and Diazepam on Prolactin Release In Vitro

Incubation Conditions	Pretreatment Diazepam (10^{-6}M) -	+
	(Prolactin ng/dish)	
Control	182 ± 2.0	189 ± 10.7
GABA (10^{-5}M)	158 ± 6.5*	135 ± 4.5**

Rat pituitary tissue was dispersed by collagenase-hyaluronidase and then trypsin, and plated into petri dishes in Dulbecco's modified Eagle's medium supplemented with 10% horse serum and 2.5% fetal calf serum. After 72 hrs the medium was changed, one half receiving medium with diazepam and the other medium with vehicle. After 24 hrs the cells were washed 4 times and incubated without or with GABA for 2½ hrs. * $p < 0.05$ vs control ** $p < 0.05$ vs *.

The time course of exposure to diazepam for potentiation of GABA inhibition has not been extensively examined and may require much less than the 24 hrs used in this experiment. These observations suggest that pituitary GABA receptor response can be modulated and that in vitro conditions for measuring the action of GABA may not reflect the environment present in vivo.

To further examine the action of benzodiazepines on prolactin release diazepam was given to male rats. No significant alteration of prolactin release was produced in male rats. However, in haloperidol treated rats diazepam in a dose related manner reduced the stimulation of prolactin release produced by haloperidol (Table 5).

TABLE 5. Benzodiazepine Inhibition of Prolactin Release After Haloperidol

		Prolactin ng/ml		
		DIAZEPAM	CLONAZEPAM	CHLORDIAZEPOXIDE
CONTROL	11 ± 3			
HALOPERIDOL + BENZODIAZEPINE	73 ± 2			
0.1 mg/kg			30 ± 7	
0.2			10 ± 3	
0.5		61 ± 11	12 ± 3	
1				40 ± 15
2		34 ± 7	7 ± 3	
5		15 ± 4		28 ± 3
10		8 ± 2		10 ± 7

Male rats were given benzodiazepine or vehicle, 10 min later 0.1 mg haloperidol/kg ip and at 50 min were decapitated for collection of blood.

CONCLUSIONS

GABA and GABA agonists can inhibit prolactin release. This response results from the action of GABA agonists on the anterior pituitary gland. This action is both specific and receptor mediated. Blockade of the receptor with a specific receptor antagonist prevents the action on prolactin release. Moreover specific GABA binding sites have been detected on rat and human anterior pituitary tissue. This GABA inhibitory system is separate from the well established dopamine inhibition of prolactin release. Dopaminergic receptor blockade did not diminish muscimol inhibition of prolactin release nor did GABAergic receptor blockade reverse apomorphine inhibition of release. Addition of muscimol with a low dose of apomorphine produced greater inhibition of prolactin release than that produced by apomorphine alone. However by comparison dopamine inhibition of prolactin release is predominant over that produced by GABA. When the dose of apomorphine is increased to achieve maximal inhibition of release addition of muscimol produced no further decrease in release. Moreover the greatest effect of muscimol and GABA both in vitro and in vivo was observed under conditions in which the dopaminergic system is not functioning. The inhibitory effect of muscimol was most evident after administration of morphine or haloperidol both of which lead to reduced pituitary dopamine receptor stimulation.

GABA inhibition of prolactin release has not been considered of physiological significance since high concentrations of GABA (5 X 10^{-6}M - 5 X 10^{-5}M) were required to produce inhibition of release. However the in vitro conditions used to assess inhibition do not reproduce the physiological environment occurring in vivo. The correlation of changes in prolactin release with the 2 to 4 fold alteration in serum GABA induced by pharmacological treatment suggests that endogenous GABA concentration is within the range of levels that can regulate hormone release. Furthermore the ability of diazepam to potentiate the action of GABA indicates that the effectiveness of GABA inhibition of release can be modulated. Physiological conditions may exist which can mimic this action produced by the benzodiazepines. Diazepam reversal of haloperidol induced prolactin release may be interpreted to represent a GABA mediated action. Diazepam has no effect on prolactin release in vitro, yet in vivo it mimicks the action of GABA agonists. The reversal of haloperidol stimulated prolactin release by diazepam may result from potentiation of the action of endogenous GABA.

Still remaining is the determination of the source of GABA. Although GABA is present in the anterior pituitary (17,24) no glutamic acid decarboxylase (GAD) is present there (17,24). The existence of tuberoinfundibular neurons have been proposed (23). The continued presence of GAD activity in the basomedial hypothalamus after hypothalamic deafferentation suggests that a GABA neuron is located within the hypothalamus (21). Selective destruction of arcuate nucleus neurons by neonatal monosodium glutamate treatment suggests that the GABA neuron cell body is located in the arcuate nucleus (23). However the GABA content of the hypophyseal portal blood must be determined in order to demonstrate that this is indeed the source.

The contribution of GABA to hypothalamic inhibition is uncharacterized. The amount of dopamine present hypophyseal portal blood although capable of producing partial inhibition of prolactin release, does not account for all the inhibitory activity present (4,15). GABA with physiological processes modulating its receptor sensitivity may participate in the tonic inhibition of prolactin release.

ACKNOWLEDGMENTS

This work was supported in part by NIH Grant AM 26661 from the National Institute of Arthritis Metabolism and Digestive Diseases.

REFERENCES

1. Clemens, J.A., Sawyer, B.D., and Cerimele, B. (1977): Endocrinology, 100:692-698.

2. Enjalbert, A., Ruberg, M., Arancibia, S., Fiore, L., Priam, L. and Kordon, C. (1979): Endocrinology, 105:823-826.

3. Ferkany, J.W., Bulter, I.J. and Enna, S.J. (1979): J. Neurochem., 33:29-34.

4. Gibbs, D.M. and Neill, J.D. (1978): Endocrinology, 102:1895-1900.

5. Grandison, L. and Guidotti, A. (1977): Neuropharmacology, 16: 533-536.

6. Grandison, L. and Guidotti, A. (1977): Nature, 270:357-359.

7. Grandison, L. and Guidotti, A. (1979): Endocrinology, 105: 754-759.

8. Grandison, L. and Meites (1976): Endocrinology, 99:775-779.

9. Guidotti, A., Toffano, G. and Costa, E. (1978): Nature, 275: 553-555.

10. Haefely, W.E. (1978): Brit. J. Psychiat., 133:231-238.

11. Libertun, C. and McCann, S.M. (1976): IRCS Med. Sci., 4:374.

12. Locatelli, V., Cocchi, D., Frigerio, C., Betti, R., Krogsgaard-Larsen, P., Racagni, G., and Müller, E.E. (1979): Endocrinology, 105: 778-785.

13. Locatelli, V., Cocchi, D., Racagni, G., Catlabeni, F., Maggi, A., Krogsgaard-Larsen, P., and Müller, E.E. (1978): Brain Res., 145:173-179.

14. Mioduszewski, R., Grandison, L. and Meites, J. (1976): Proc. Soc. Exptl. Biol. Med., 151:44-46.

15. Neill, J.D. (1980): In: Frontiers in Neuroendocrinology, Vol. 6, edited by L. Martini and W.F. Ganong, pp 129-155. Raven Press, New York.

16. Pass, K.A., and Ondo, J.G. (1977): Endocrinology, 100:1437-1442.

17. Racagni, G., Apud, J.A., Loccatelli, V., Cocchi, D., Nistisco, G., diGiorgio, R.M. and Müller, E.E. (1979): Nature, 281: 575-578.

18. Ruberg, M., Rotsztejin, W.H., Arancibia, S. Besson, J. and Enjalbert, A. (1978): Eur. J. Pharmacol., 51:319-320.

19. Rivier, C. and Vale, W. (1977): Endocrinology, 101:506-511.

20. Schally, A.V., Redding, T.W., Arimura, A., Dupont, A. and Linthicum, C.L. (1977): Endocrinology, 100:681-691.

21. Tappaz, M.L. and Brownstein, M.J. (1977): Brain Res., 132: 95-106.

22. Vijayan, E. and McCann, S.M. (1978): Brain Res., 155:35-43.

23. Walaas, I. and Fonnum, F. (1978): Brain Res., 153:549-562.

24. Wu, J.-Y., Chude, O., Wein, J., Roberts, E., Saito, K., and Wong, E. (1978): J. Neurochem., 30:849-857.

GABA and Benzodiazepine Receptors,
edited by E. Costa et al.
Raven Press, New York © 1981.

GABA Markers in the Hypothalamic Median Eminence

M. L. Tappaz, M. Aguera, M. F. Belin, *W. H. Oertel, *D. E. Schmechel, *I. J. Kopin, and J. F. Pujol

*INSERM U 171, Groupe de Neurochemie Fonctionnelle, Université Claude Bernard, Faculté de Médecine, 69008 Lyon, France; and *Laboratory of Clinical Science, National Institute of Health, Bethesda, Maryland 20205*

The hypothalamic median eminence is the specialized structure in the medio-basal hypothalamus where the hypophysiotropic factors controlling the adenohypophysis are released : it consequently represents a privileged site for various neuroendocrine interactions including the possible GABAergic regulations reported elsewhere in this volume.

Among virtually all known CNS neurotransmitters and neuromodulators, GABA as well as GABA biosynthetic enzyme glutamate decarboxylase (GAD), were shown by us to be present in the median eminence (19) (20). In addition, by combining biochemical mapping and lesion studies, we provided data suggesting that those GABA markers in the median eminence were likely to be contained in cells intrinsic to the mediobasal hypothalamus (18) ; we thus speculated that there might be some GAD-containing componants within the tubero-infundibular pathway.

Over the last few years we have attempted a more precise description of this possible and so far largely unknown GABAergic system at the median eminence level by using GABA histological markers : GABA and GABA structural analogs autoradiography as well as more recently GAD immunohistochemistry.

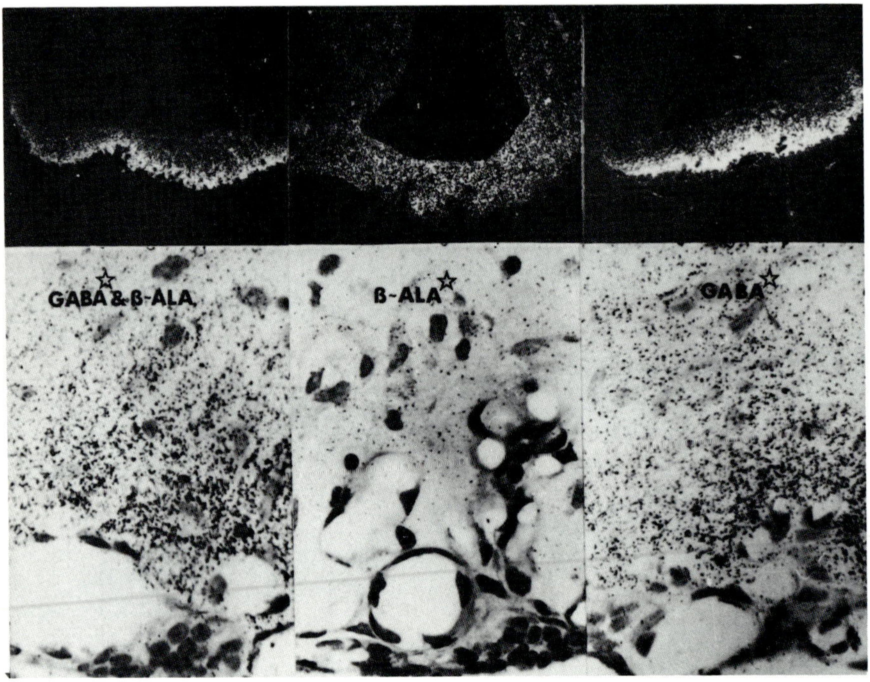

Figure 1 : Radioautogaphs of the rat median eminence following intracardiac injection of GABA and GABA analogs.

Intracardiac injection of labelled GABA led to a dense labelling over the median eminence external layer which consists of numerous silver grains concentrated in the vicinity of the perivascular space (left picture). This labelling was not significantly displaced by a 2000-fold excess of cold ß-alanine (right picture). Radiolabelled ß-alanine led to a light and even distribution of silver grains all over the entire median eminence (middle).
Above : dark field picture of the entire median eminence.
Below : enlarged medial external part from the same micrographs.
From TAPPAZ et al. 1980 (17).

GABA AUTORADIOGRAPHY

Following injection of exogenous radiolabelled GABA, a dense accumulation of silver grains could be observed by autoradiography over the external layer of the median eminence (Fig. 1). In vitro incubation with low concentration of exogenous GABA (2.5 x 10^{-7}M) led to a similar pattern of labelling (17). This labelling was not displaced by an excess a cold ß-alanine (Fig. 1) a reported specific substrate for GABA glial uptake (15). However, the labelling was at least partially reduced by a simultaneous injection of non-radioactive cis-amino-cyclohexane carboxylic acid (ACHC) (Fig. 2) a reported preferential substrate for GABA neuronal uptake (6). Thus, these findings suggested that high affinity uptake sites for GABA are present in the median eminence. They appeared to be concentrated mainly over the external layer and showed substrate specificity resembling GABA neuronal uptake characteristics as far as the effects of GABA analogs are concerned.

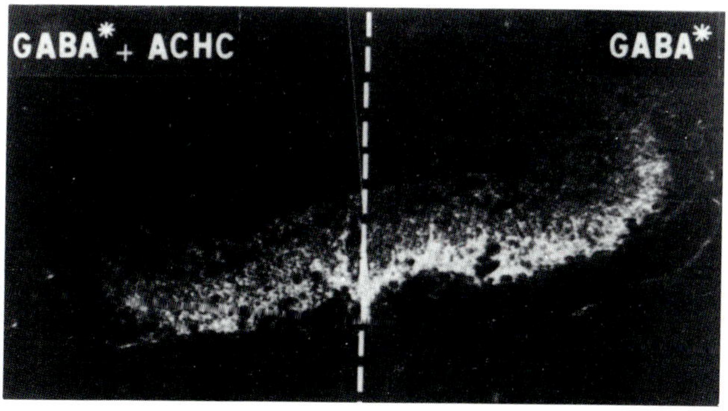

Figure 2 : Radioautographs of the rat median eminence following intracardiac injection of labelled GABA in presence of cold ACHC.

This dark field picture shows that the GABA labelling over the external layer is partially displaced by a 50-fold excess of non radioactive ACHC.
From TAPPAZ et al. 1980 (17).

GAD IMMUNOHISTOCHEMISTRY

We have recently produced an antiserum to GAD, featuring the reinjection of an antigen-antibody complexe isolated from a primary polyvalent trapping antiserum by immunological techniques (10). This second antiserum precipitated GAD activity from a partially purified GAD preparation from rat brain, detected one antigen in the same preparation by crossed immunoelectrophoresis and altered the mobility of only one antigen in brain homogenate supernatant by cross-immunoelectrophoresis with intermediate gel (10). A dense immunohistochemical staining was obtained in the substantia nigra which decreased following lesioning of the strio-nigral GABAergic descending pathway (9). In addition the staining in the cerebellum and olfactory bulb was consistant with the presumed GAD-containing cells (9). Thus, according to both its precipitating characteristics as well as to our preliminary histological checkings, this antibody seems to be specific to GAD.

Using this antibody, our preliminary investigations showed immunostaining in the median eminence which appeared more concentrated over the external layer. This dense immunoreactivity could be similarly visualized by using either the indirect immunofluoresence method (fig. 3) or the unlabeled antibody method with the peroxydase-antiperoxydase (PAP) complex (fig. 4).

EFFECT OF LESIONING OF ARCUATE NUCLEUS

A substantial portion of afferents to the median eminence are thought to originate from the neighbouring parvicellular arcuate nucleus (12) (16). A possible arcuate origin for the GAD-containing elements in the median eminence was thus investigated. Lesioning was performed by chronic parenteral injections of monosodium glutamate (MSG) in newborn rats according to Olney (11). As reported by others (21), this led to a dramatic loss of nerve cells in the arcuate nucleus (fig. 5) which was accompagnied by a decrease in GAD activity in the median eminence (table 1). While these findings are consistant with the hypothesis of a short tubero-infundibular GABAergic pathway, they cannot really prove it since trans-synaptic effects cannot be ruled out.

For example, the two peptides we measured, somatostatin (SRIF) and luteinizing-hormone releasing hormone (LH-RH), the origin of which is thought to be outside the arcuate nucleus (2) were nevertheless affected by this lesioning (table 1). It is thus conceivable that GAD decrease in the median eminence could reflect the removal of a trophic input instead of an anterograde degeneration.

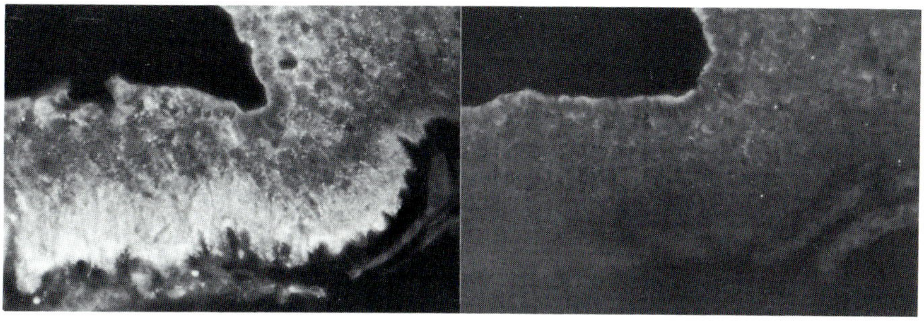

Figure 3 : Immunofluorescent micrographs of the mouse median eminence.

The sections were incubated either with the antiserum to GAD (left picture) or with the preimmune serum (right picture). A dense immunofluorescent plexus is visible over the external layer of the median eminence.
From TAPPAZ et al (unpublished).

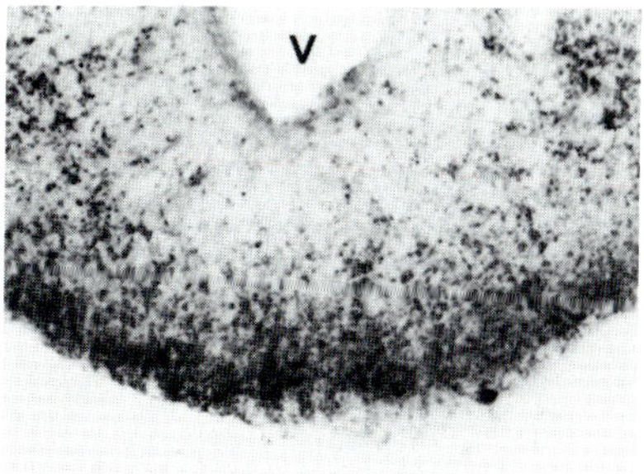

Figure 4 : PAP immunostained micrograph of the rat median eminence.

The reaction products obtained with the peroxydase- anti-peroxydase (PAP) method which visualize GAD-immunoreactivity make a dense punctuated staining over the external layer.
From TAPPAZ et al (unpublished).

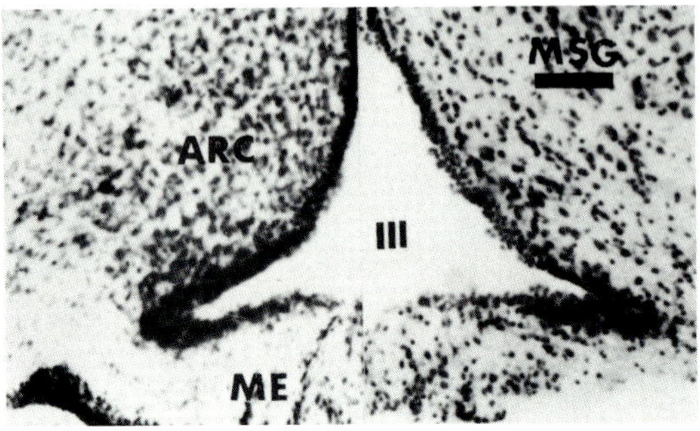

Figure 5 : Histological control of arcuate nucleus lesioning.

In monosodium glutamate (MSG) treated rats (right) an important loss of nerve cells (about 60-80 %) is visible in the arcuate nucleus (Arc).
From TAPPAZ et al (unpublished).

GAD pmoles/h/µg protein	Sham MSG-treated % change	110 ± 8 (7) 64 ± 10 (5) - 42 % p <0.01
SRIF pg/µg protein	Sham MSG treated % change	1120 ± 92 (6) 632 ± 134 (8) - 44 % p <0.01
LH-RH pg/µg protein	Sham MSG treated % change	83 ± 9 (6) 189 ± 25 (8) + 130 % p <0.01

Table 1 : Effects of arcuate lesioning through monosodium glutamate (MSG) treatment on GAD, SRIF and LH-RH content in the median eminence.
From TAPPAZ et al (unpublished).

CONCLUDING REMARKS

Thus, so far, four different GABA markers could be shown in the hypothalamic median eminence : GABA, GAD activity, GAD immunoreactivity and GABA uptake. Moreover, the two latter appeared apparently to be more concentrated over the external layer, precisely where nerve endings are mainly localized. This is suggestive of the presence of GABAergic terminals at this level which functionally could provide a possible anatomical substrate for various GABAergic regulations of hypophysiotropic hormone release reported in the literature (1) (3) (4) (5) (7) (8) (13) (14). Whether or not those GABAergic elements represent a distinctive population of GABAergic terminals or are indeed the known aminergic and/or peptidergic terminals which in addition might contain GABA markers, remains unanswered by our present findings.

Aknowledgements

This study was supported by Grant 77 5 175 6 from INSERM. The authors are indebted to Dr J. Epelbaum (Paris) for carrying out the LH-RH and SRIF radioimmunoassays.

REFERENCES

1. Enjalbert, A., Ruberg, M., Arancibia, S., Fiore, L., Priam, M., and Kordon, C. (1979). Endocrinology, 105 : 823-826.
2. Knigge, K.M., Joseph, S.A., and Hoffman, G.E. (1978). In : The hypothalamus, ed. S. Reichlin, R.J. Baldessarini and J.B. Martin, Raven Press, New York.
3. Lamberts, S.W.J., and McLeod, R. (1978). Proc. Soc. Exp. Biol. Med., 158 : 10.
4. Locatelli, V., Cocchi, D., Racagni, G., Cattabeni, F., Maggi, A., Krogsgaardlarsen, P., and Müller, E.E. (1978). Brain Res., 145 : 173-179.
5. Mioduszewski, R., Grandison, L., and Meites, J. (1976). Proc.Soc. Exp. Biol. (N.Y.), 151 : 44-46.
6. Neal, M.J., and Bowery, N.G. (1977). Brain Res., 138 : 169-174.
7. Ondo, J.G. (1974). Science, 186 : 738-739.
8. Ondo, J.G., and Pass, K.A. (1976). Endocrinology, 98 : 1248-1252.
9. Oertel, W.H., Schmechel, D.E., Tappaz, M.L., Ransom, D.H., Weise, V.K., Brownstein, M.J., Furness, J.B., and Kopin, I.J. (1980). Abstr. FASEB Meeting, Anheim (CA) U.S.A.
10. Oertel, W.H., Tappaz, M.L., Kopin, I.J., Ransom, D.H., and Schmechel, D.E. (1979). Society for Neuroscience, Satellite symposium on GABA and other inhibitory transmitter. Myrtle Beach (SC), U.S.A.

11. Olney, J.W. (1969). Science, 164 : 719-721.
12. Réthelyi, M., and Halász, B. (1970). Exp. Brain Res., 11 : 145-158.
13. Rivier, C., and Vale, W. (1977). Endocrinology, 101 : 501.
14. Schally, A.V., Redding, T.W., Arimura, A., Dupont, A., and Linthicum, G.L. (1977). Endocrinology, 100 : 681.
15. Schon, F., and Kelly, J.S. (1975). Brain Res., 86 : 243-257.
16. Szentagotai, J. (1964). In : Progress in brain research, ed. W. Bargman and J.P. Schade, Vol. 5, pp. 135-146, Elsevier, Amsterdam.
17. Tappaz, M.L., Aguera, M., Belin, M.F., and Pujol, J.F. (1980). Brain Res., 186 : 379-391.
18. Tappaz, M.L., and Brownstein, M.J. (1977). Brain Res., 132 : 95-106.
19. Tappaz, M.L., Brownstein, M.J., and Kopin, I.J. (1977). Brain Res., 125 : 109-121.
20. Tappaz, M.L., Brownstein, M.J., and Palkovits, M. (1976). Brain Res., 108 : 371-379.
21. Walaas, T., and Fonnum, F. (1978). Brain Res., 153 : 549-562.

GABA and Benzodiazepine Receptors,
edited by E. Costa et al.
Raven Press, New York © 1981.

Role of Gamma Aminobutyric Acid in Control of Anterior Pituitary Hormone Release

S. M. McCann, E. Vijayan, and A. Negro-Vilar

Department of Physiology, The University of Texas Health Science Center at Dallas, Dallas, Texas 75235

INTRODUCTION

Considerable evidence suggests the involvement of (GABA) as an inhibitory synaptic transmitter in the central nervous system (3). GABA is found in high concentrations in the hypothalamus (13), an area intimately involved in control of adenohypophyseal hormone secretion (9). Consequently, it was of interest to evaluate a possible role of GABA in control of anterior pituitary hormone secretion.

In our initial experiments we employed ovariectomized, estrogen primed rats and reported that the injection of GABA into a permanent third ventricular cannula at a dose of 150 μg/2 μl was followed by a small decrease in serum prolactin (PRL), whereas control injections of saline failed to alter levels of the hormone (7). An equivalent weight of glutamic acid also produced no significant effect and histadine similarly was ineffective in altering PRL.

At the same time, we studied the effects of intraperitoneal (ip) injection of aminooxyacetic acid (AOAA) on serum PRL titers in similarly prepared animals. This drug has been shown to induce elevations in GABA content in the CNS (15). Doses which had been effective in elevating CNS GABA lowered PRL following their ip injection, whereas saline injected similarly had no effect. Because of the relatively large dose of intraventricular GABA required to induce a reduction in PRL, we delayed publication of these results and in the meantime, Ondo (14) reported an elevation of plasma LH following injection of GABA in equally large doses.

In view of these results, we embarked on a thorough investigation of the effects of GABA on the release of anterior pituitary hormones.

METHODS

In these experiments we utilized ovariectomized (OVX) rats or

OVX animals treated with estrogen-progesterone (estradiol 50 μg, progesterone 25 mg, subcutaneously (sc) given 72 hours before use. The animals were prepared with permanent cannulae implanted into the third ventricle according to the technique of Antunes-Rodrigues and McCann (1). Furthermore, indwelling catheters were introduced into the jugular vein 24 hours before the experiment using the technique of Harms and Ojeda (6). On the day of the experiment, an extension of polyethylene tubing was attached to the distal end of the jugular cannula and the animals were left undisturbed for 30-60 min. During this time a pre-injection blood sample (0.6-0.8 ml) was withdrawn over a period of 60 seconds.

Microinjections of saline or GABA (Sigma Chemicals, Lot 32C-2210) were performed according to the following procedure. The material was prepared freshly in 0.9% NaCl adjusted to pH 7.2 and injected within 30 min. of preparation. Injections were made in a volume of 2 μl using a 10 μl Hamilton microsyringe connected by polyethylene tubing to a 30 gauge stainless steel cannula which fit within the extended lower tip of the permanent cannula. The tubing and cannula had previously been filled with the solution to be tested. To determine the specificity of the actions of GABA, a GABA antagonist, bicuculline (Sigma Chemicals, Lot 115C-0291), dissolved in 0.1 ml ethyl acetate (or equal volume of diluent), was injected ip either alone or followed 15 min. later by third ventricular injection of 4 μmoles of GABA. In all cases intraventricular injection time was about 60 seconds and all experiments were performed in the morning between 0900-1100 h. Heparinized blood samples were collected from the external jugular vein cannula at varying intervals while the animal was freely moving in the cage and the volume of samples was replaced immediately after each bleeding by an equivalent volume of saline. Plasma was separated by centrifugation and stored frozen until the day of assay. To determine if the effects of intraventricular GABA were mediated centrally, its effects after intravenous (iv) pulse injection and after incubation with hemi-pituitaries _in vitro_ were also evaluated. _In vitro_ incubation of hemipituitaries from OVX rats in tissue culture medium 199 was performed as described earlier (17). At the termination of incubation media were removed and kept frozen for later RIA of pituitary hormones.

In the final experiment, the effects of GABA on the content of catecholamines and LHRH in hypothalamus and pituitary were determined. Five to fifteen minutes after injection of GABA into the third ventricle, the rats were killed by decapitation. Blood was collected from the trunk, brains were removed and the ME, medial basal hypothalamus (MBH), and suprachiasmatic preoptic area (SCH-PO) were dissected out as previously described and homogenized in perchloric acid (10). Anterior pituitaries were also removed and similarly prepared. In all experiments pituitary hormones were assayed by RIA procedures currently in use in our laboratory. LH was measured by the procedure of Niswender et al. (11) using rat RP-1 pituitary LH reference standard but expressing results in terms of NIH-LH-S1 preparation for comparison with earlier data. Other pituitary hormones were measured by the RIA kits supplied by NIAMDD and results were expressed in terms of RP-1 reference standard provided with the kits. LHRH was measured using antiserum number 42 (generously provided by Dr. T.E. Nett, Colorado State University) at a dilution of 1-40,000 as previously described (10). Norepinephrine (NE) and dopamine (DA) were measured with a microenzymatic radioisotopic method as previously described (10).

RESULTS

Initial Plasma Concentrations of Pituitary Hormones

As expected, plasma LH and FSH titers were elevated in the OVX animals compared to basal levels in normal cycling rats in this laboratory and the values were lowered following steroid treatment. Conversely, plasma PRL was relatively low in the OVX animals and was elevated by steroid treatment. Initial levels of GH were readily detectable in the OVX animals and they were not significantly altered by treatment with estrogen and progesterone. Similarly, the readily detectable TSH levels were not altered by the steroid treatment.

Control injections

Plasma levels of pituitary hormones were not altered by intraventricular injection of 2 μl of isotonic saline in OVX or OEP rats or ip injection of 0.1 ml saline in OVX rats.

Effect of third ventricular injection of GABA in OVX rats

Intraventricular injection of 2 μl of saline containing 0.1 or 2 μmoles of GABA did not modify plasma LH at 10 and 30 min. following injection while only the 0.1 μmole dose induced a slight elevation at 60 min. (Fig. 1) (17). On the other hand, injection of 4 or 8 μmoles of GABA produced a marked elevation in plasma LH at 10 and 30 min. following injection. The response to both 4 and 8 μmole doses persisted for at least 60 min.

Bicuculline, a potent antagonist to the depressant effects of GABA (2), was injected either alone or followed by intraventricular GABA to determine the specificity of the effects of GABA. Injection of a 1 μmole dose of bicuculline alone produced a slight reduction in plasma LH at 10 and 30 min. while a dose of 2 μmole was without effect. Third ventricular injection of 4 μmoles of GABA which was clearly effective in earlier experiments, was ineffective in animals pretreated with either dose of bicuculline. There was no significant change in FSH titers induced by any of the doses of GABA and/or bicuculline employed.

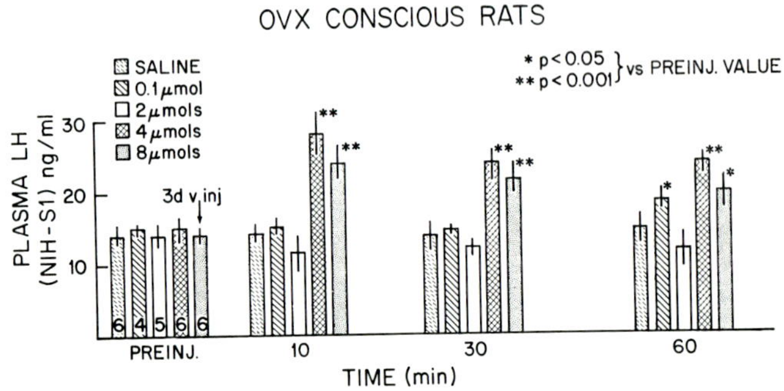

Fig. 1. Plasma LH titers in ovariectomized (OVX) conscious rats after 3rd ventricular injection of saline or different doses of GABA. In this and subsequent figures, numbers at the base of each column indicate the number of rats in each group; vertical lines above and below the mean represent the S.E.M.; arrow indicates the time of injection.

The effect on PRL release depended on the dose of GABA (10). Injection of 0.1 μmoles, the lowest dose of GABA, produced a significant reduction in plasma PRL which persisted for 60 min. (Fig. 2). There was a slight but not significant decrease in PRL levels after a 2 μmole dose of GABA. A significant increase in plasma PRL levels occurred in response to 4 and 8 μmoles of GABA and this effect was sustained over 60 min. At 10 min. after injection, plasma PRL was significantly higher in response to the 8 μmole dose than to the 4 μmole dose.

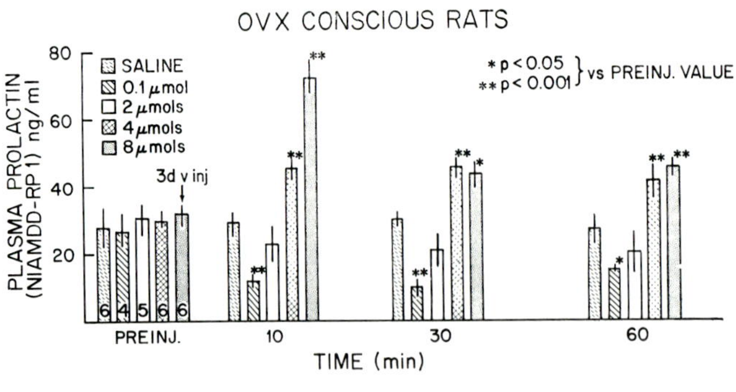

Fig. 2. The effect of 3rd ventricular injection of saline or various doses of GABA on plasma prolactin levels in OVX conscious rats.

Bicuculline at doses of either 1 or 2 µmole failed to modify plasma PRL. The 4 µmole dose of GABA was still effective in elevating PRL significantly in animals treated with 1 µmole of bicuculline while the PRL response to GABA was totally blocked by increasing the dose of bicuculline to 2 µmoles.

Plasma GH levels were significantly elevated within 10 min. of third ventricular injection of each dose of GABA (0.1-8 µmole) and the elevation persisted for the 60 min. duration of the experiment (18). The elevations obtained with the two higher doses were significantly greater than those obtained with the lower one at 10 min. but all doses were nearly equally effective at 30 min. Although bicuculline had no effect on initial levels of GH, either the 1 or 2 µmole dose ip blocked the response to the 4 µmole dose of GABA.

In sharp contrast to the effects on growth hormone, injection of GABA into the third ventricle significantly lowered plasma TSH within 10 min. and this effect persisted for 60 min. (Fig. 3). Although the suppression with higher doses was greater at all times, there was a significant dose-related effect only at 10 min. As in the case of other hormones, this reponse was blocked by bicuculline.

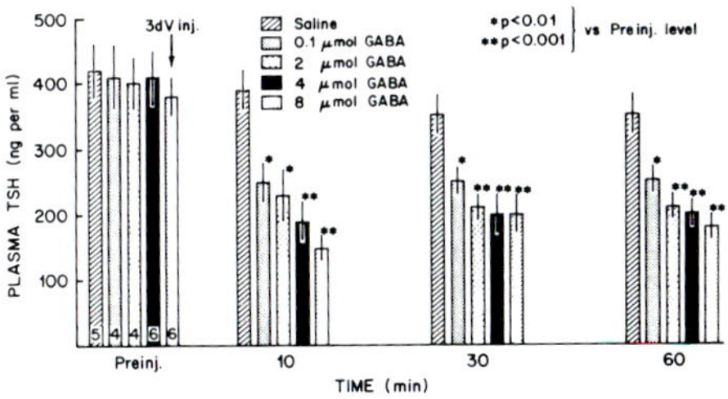

Fig. 3. The effect of 3rd ventricular injection of saline or various doses of GABA on plasma TSH levels in conscious, OVX rats.

Effect of third ventricular injection of GABA in ovariectomized, estrogen-progesterone treated rats

Steroid pretreatment did not alter the response of LH, PRL, or GH to GABA. On the other hand, GABA was less effective in lowering plasma TSH levels in steroid-primed rats. Thus 0.1 or 2 µmole doses of GABA failed to modify TSH, whereas 4 and 8 µmole doses still induced only a slight reduction.

The effects of iv GABA on pituitary hormone release

To determine if the effects of these doses of intraventricular GABA in altering pituitary hormone release were mediated centrally, a dose of 4 µmoles of GABA was injected systemically by pulse injection in OVX rats. None of the hormones were significantly altered by iv GABA.

The effect of blockade of dopamine receptors with pimozide on the response to GABA

To determine a possible role of dopamine in the action of intraventricular GABA, dopamine (DA) receptors were blocked by sc injection of pimozide (0.63 mg per kg), a dose which selectively blocks dopamine receptors (19). Ninety minutes after injection of pimozide or the tartaric acid diluent, a second blood sample was drawn and immediately thereafter 4 μmoles of GABA were injected in the third ventricle. Pimozide failed to alter the levels of LH in these ovariectomized animals and a brisk response to GABA ensued. In contrast to the lack of effect of pimozide on the response of LH to GABA, the response to PRL was altered in that instead of rising following injection of GABA, the already elevated levels, as a result of blockade of DA receptors, were significantly suppressed in the pimozide-pretreated animals. The action of GABA to elevate GH was not altered by pimozide, but the TSH-lowering action of GABA was completely blocked by the drug.

Effects of GABA (2 μmole to 4 μmole) on pituitary hormone release in vitro

When incubated with hemipituitaries in vitro, none of the doses of GABA tested had any significant effect on the release of GH TSH, FSH, LH or PRL.

Behavorial effects

Third ventricular injection of GABA or ip injection of bicuculline produced no observable behavioral effects such as altered alertness, locomotion, sniffing, licking, rearing or stereotyped movements.

Hypothalamic LHRH following intraventricular GABA

Since serum LH values were elevated at 15 min. following intraventricular injection of the 4 μmole dose of GABA, it was expected that there might be an alteration in hypothalamic LHRH content. Rather surprisingly, there were no changes in ME or MBH LHRH; however, the content in the SCH-PO was elevated at 15 min. following the higher dose of GABA (10).

Hypothalamic NE after intraventricular GABA

The content of NE in various hypothalamic areas was analyzed after intraventricular GABA. Both doses produced a rapid rise of NE in the ME at 5 min. which declined slightly at 15 min. (Fig. 4). On the other hand, there were no significant alterations in either MBH or SCH-PO.

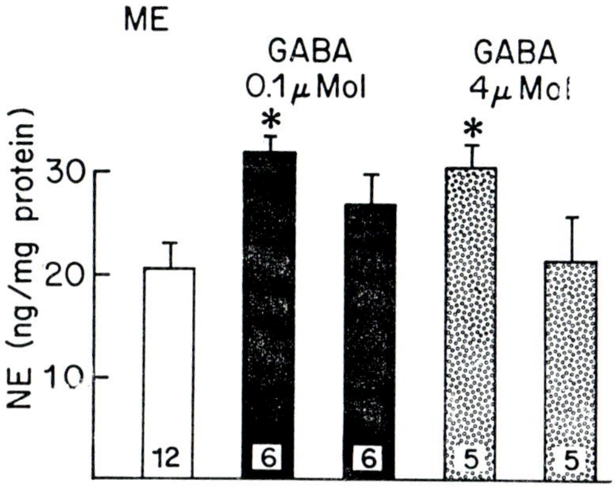

Fig. 4. Changes in norepinephrine (NE) levels in the median eminence (ME) after intraventricular GABA administration. Open bar = saline-injected controls.

Hypothalamic and pituitary DA content after intraventricular GABA

Although there were no changes in DA content in the MBH or SCH-PO following either dose of GABA, there was a rise in DA in the ME apparent at 5 min. following intraventricular injection of the lower dose of GABA. The elevation was still significant at 15 min. Surprisingly there were no alterations in DA in the ME following the higher dose of GABA. Anterior pituitary content of DA increased significantly at 15 min. following either dose of GABA (Fig. 5).

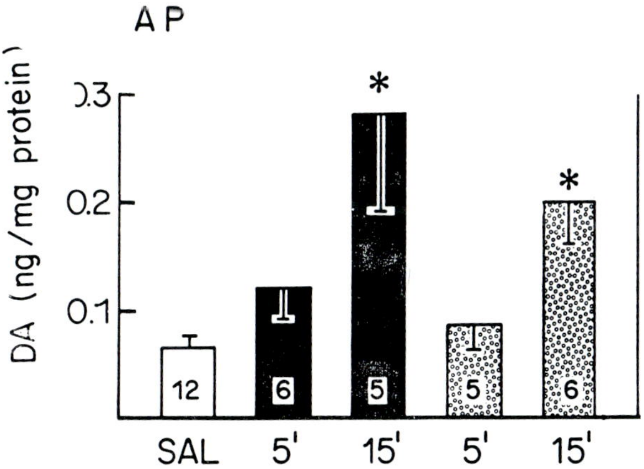

Fig. 5. Changes in anterior pituitary (AP) dopamine (DA) levels after intraventricular GABA administration. SAL = saline-injected controls.

DISCUSSION

Our results indicate that intraventricular GABA is capable of producing profound alterations in pituitary hormone release. Release of LH and GH is augmented, release of TSH is inhibited, and release of PRL exhibits different effects depending on the dose of GABA (see also 8), lower doses of GABA lowered PRL whereas higher doses of GABA elevated levels of this tropin. The effects appeared to be specific since they were blocked by the GABA antagonist, bicuculline. The physiological significance of GABA in control of anterior pituitary hormone release is not established by our experiments since we could not establish a clear dose-response relationship with bicuculline.

The results with pimozide, a selective blocker of dopamine receptors, indicate that the responses of LH and GH are not mediated via possible GABAergic stimulation of hypothalamic, dopaminergic transmission; however, since the depressant effect of GABA on TSH release was completely blocked by pimozide, it would appear that increased DA release may mediate the effects of GABA on TSH release which are presumably brought about by suppression of the release of thyrotropin-releasing hormone (TRH). This supposition is supported by the rapid elevation of DA in the median eminence within 5 minutes after injection of the lower dose of GABA. Furthermore, anterior pituitary content of DA increased significantly at 15 min. following either dose of GABA. Consequently it would appear that GABA causes release of DA from the tuberoinfundibular dopaminergic neurons. The released DA passes down the portal vessels and leads to an accumulation of the amine in the pituitary.

This stimulation of the tuberoinfundibular dopaminergic tract may also be involved in the action of GABA on PRL release since the elevation in PRL induced by higher doses of GABA was converted into a suppression in pimozide-treated animals. One could speculate that the increased DA release by the low dose of GABA could cause release of PIF which then would induce the lowering of PRL which follows this low dose of GABA. Alternatively, the suppression of PRL release induced by the lower dose of GABA could be accounted for, at least in part, by increased release of DA by this dose which then inhibited the pituitary release of PRL by direct action on the lactotrophs. This is a particularly intriguing possibility in view of the recent report that portal blood levels of DA are sufficiently high to have a direct action to inhibit prolactin release by the gland (4). The elevation of PRL induced by the higher dose of GABA appears to be associated with a smaller release of DA since ME DA failed to increase significantly and there was a smaller, albeit still significant increase in anterior pituitary DA. One could argue that this can partly account for the PRL stimulation obtained with the higher dose. Diminished inhibition by DA directly at the pituitary could contribute to the rise. Alternatively, the increased levels of DA in the anterior pituitary could be a reflection of an increased release of DA induced by the prior increment of PRL levels after GABA. The reversal of the PRL elevation induced by higher doses of GABA by the DA receptor blocker, pimozide, could be explained if there was a dopaminergic stimulation of PRL-releasing factor discharge induced by high doses of GABA.

Although we found no effects of GABA on PRL release from pituitaries incubated in vitro, others have reported such effects with very high doses of GABA (16) and more recently with lower doses of the GABA agonist muscimol (5). The recent demonstration of specific GABA receptors in the gland (5) suggests that this may be a physiological effect and that sufficient GABA may be secreted into portal vessels to play a role in directly inhibiting PRL release. It is doubtful if this is responsible for the lowering of PRL which occurs at low doses of intraventricular GABA in view of the relative ineffectiveness of GABA to alter PRL release directly.

The elevation of LH induced by GABA was associated with an elevation of LHRH in the SCH-PO after the higher dose but surprisingly ME LHRH was unaltered. This suggests that part of the action of GABA to release LH was caused by a stimulation of rostral LHRH neurons. These could have been activated by GABA acting directly at the level of LHRH perikarya. The activation of DA release at the ME may also have induced LHRH release since this catecholamine activates release of the decapeptide; however, since pimozide failed to alter LH release induced by GABA, any role of DA in GABA-induced LH release appears to be nonessential.

Associated with the GABA-induced elevation in norepinephrine in the ME was the release of GH. Norepinephrine has a stimulatory effect on release of GH and consequently it is possible that GABA acts to release GH by stimulation of NE release at the ME. This in turn could induce increased release of GH-releasing factor (GH-RF) or inhibition of somatostatin release or a combination of the two. The former possibility is the more likely in view of the very high GH levels achieved within 5-10 min. after GABA administration, which would certainly support a substantial release of GHRF.

We believe that the effects of intraventricular GABA are mediated by an action on tissue adjacent to the third ventricle, presumably in the hypothalamus. Where measured, only approximately 3% of intraventricularly injected compounds have reached the pituitary (12) and very large doses of GABA are required to inhibit PRL release by direct action on the gland. Recently, GABA receptors have been demonstrated in the anterior pituitary and the GABA antagonist muscimol, has been shown to inhibit prolactin release directly at relatively low doses (5). Therefore, the possibility that GABA may have some direct actions on the gland under physiological conditions must not be discounted. Establishing this hypothesis will require demonstration of high concentrations of GABA in portal blood or, alternatively, the demonstration of GABA levels in the anterior pituitary which fluctuate in accordance with changes in release of pituitary hormones.

In conclusion our results show that intraventricular GABA not only alters pituitary hormone release but also release of norepinephrine and dopamine from terminals in the median eminence. The released catecholamines may be important in mediating the effects of GABA on releasing factor discharge. In addition, the DA release may act directly on the pituitary to inhibit prolactin release.

REFERENCES

1. Antunes-Rodrigues, J. and McCann, S.M. (1970): Proc. Soc. Exp. Biol. 133: 1464-1470.
2. Curtis, D.R., Duggan, A.W., Felix, D. and Johnson, G.A.R. (1971): Brain Res. 32: 69-96.
3. Davidson, N. (1976): In: Neurotransmitter Amino Acids, pp. 57-108. Academic Press, New York.
4. Gibbs, D.M. and Neill, J.D. (1978): Endocr. 102: 1895.
5. Grandison, L. and Guidotti, A. (1979): Endocr. 105: 754-759.
6. Harms, P.G. and Ojeda, S.R. (1974): J. Appl. Physiol. 36: 391.
7. Libertun, C. and McCann, S.M. (1976): IRCS Med. Sci. 4: 374.
8. Locatelli, V., Cocchi, D., Frigerio, C., Betti, R., Krogsgaard-Larsen, P., Racagni, G. and Mueller, E.E. (1979): Endocr. 105: 778-785.
9. McCann, S.M., Fawcett, C.P. and Krulich, L. (1974): In: Endocrine Physiology, Vol. 5, edited by S.M. McCann, pp. 31-65. MTP Press, Lancaster.
10. Negro-Vilar, A., Vijayan, E. and McCann, S.M. (1980): Brain Res. Bull. (in press).
11. Niswender, G.D., Midgley, Jr., A.R., Monroe, S.E. and Reichert, L.E. (1968): Proc. Soc. Exp. Biol. Med. 128: 807.
12. Ojeda, S.R., Jameson, H.E. and McCann, S.M. (1978): Endocr. 102: 531.
13. Okada, Y., Nitsch-Hassler, C., Kim, J.S., Bak, I.J. and Hassler, R. (1971): Exp. Brain Res. 13: 514-518.
14. Ondo, J.G. (1974): Science 186: 738.
15. Roberts, E. (1972): Neurosci. Res. Progr. Bull. 10: 144.
16. Schally, A.V., Redding, T.W., Arimura, A., Dupont, A. and Linthicum, G.L. (1977): Endocr. 100: 681-691.
17. Vijayan, E. and McCann, S.M. (1978): Brain Res. 155: 35-43.
18. Vijayan, E. and McCann, S.M. (1978): Endocr. 103: 1888.
19. Vijayan, E. and McCann, S.M. (1979): Brain Res. 162: 69-76.

GABA and Benzodiazepine Receptors,
edited by E. Costa et al.
Raven Press, New York © 1981.

Gabergic Mechanisms in the Control of PRL and GH Release

*D. Cocchi, *F. Casanueva, *V. Locatelli, **J. Apud, *A. Martinez-Campos, **C. Civati, **G. Racagni, and † E. E. Müller

*Institute of Pharmacology and Pharmacognosy, **University of Milan and † Cagliari; and *Department of Pharmacology, University of Milan, Milan 20129, Italy*

In the last few years the concept has emerged that y-aminobutyric acid (GABA) can be added to the list of brain neurotransmitters capable of influencing the secretion of anterior pituitary (AP) hormones (22). Intraventricular (IVT) infusion of GABA blocked ACTH release in response to surgical trauma whereas GABA antagonists potentiated it (20). In both male rats(24) and ovariectomized (OVX) or OVX, estrogen (E) and progesterone-primed rats (35) (5), GABA by IVT route induced luteinizing hormone but not follicle-stimulating hormone release. In addition, evidence has been provided that the centrally-administered amino acid may stimulate growth hormone (GH) and inhibit thyrotropin (TSH) release (36). With respect to prolactin (PRL) secretion, the precise nature of the involvement of the GABAergic pathways is still controversial, both stimulatory (21,24,35) and inhibitory (19,28,35) influences having been reported.

We have presented data supporting the existence of a dual GABA ergic control of PRL secretion in the rat, one stimulatory exerted on a central nervous system (CNS) site; the other inhibitory, occurring at the level of the AP tissue (18), where receptors for GABA have been located (15).

In the present contribution, we provide new data on: 1) the mechanisms subserving the "central" stimulatory and "peripheral" inhibitory components of GABA action on PRL release, and 2) the action of the GABAergic system on the control of GH secretion.

Dual GABAergic control of PRL secretion in the rat

Most of the studies on the involvement of the GABAergic system in the control of PRL secretion were based on the use of GABA itself (21, 24, 35). The availability of muscimol (M), a rigid analog of the amino acid, with an affinity for bicuculline-sensitive GABA receptors higher than that of GABA (8), prompted the use of this compound in our investigations (18, 19). It was shown that in freely-moving male rats, administration of M (2 mg/kg ip) or central injection of ethanolamine-O-sulphate (EOS), a specific catalytic inhibitor of GABA transaminase (GABA-T) (13), resulted in a reduction of plasma PRL levels (19). The effectiveness of IVT-injected EOS to lower baseline plasma PRL was taken to indicate that EOS (and muscimol) was acting at a CNS rather than a pituitary site since GABAergic nerve terminals are apparently lacking in the AP (27). Arguing against this hypothesis was the finding that antagonists of GABAergic function, such as picrotoxin and bicuculline, which easily cross the blood brain barrier (29), did not antagonize the PRL-lowering effect of systemically-injected M or IVT-injected EOS (authors' unpublished results) but induced *per se* inhibition of baseline plasma PRL levels in both unanesthetized male rats (bicuculline) or E-primed OVX rats (bicuculline and picrotoxin) (18). These findings, together with the observation of brisk and short-lived rises in baseline PRL levels following systemic administration of M (19) and the reported ability of IVT-injected GABA to raise plasma PRL (21,24,35) led us to hypothesize a stimulatory component, likely of central origin, in the action of GABA on PRL release. Since only 0.02% of the amount of M injected peripherally in the rat is recovered in the brain (2), the stimulatory component might have been masked in the experiments in which M was injected sytemically. In this instance only the inhibitory component of M action would be evidenced.

The existence of a central GABAergic component stimulatory to PRL release was in fact demonstrated when M, injected at nanomole doses into the lateral brain ventricle of freely moving male rats, induced a short-lived but clear-cut rise in plasma PRL, which was antagonized by bicuculline (18).

In an extension of these studies, more cogent proof for the existence of the "peripheral" inhibitory GABAergic component was provided by showing that M, added directly to AP's incubated *in vitro* at 2.5×10^{-5}M but not at 0.5×10^{-5}M inhibited PRL release, an effect which was antagonized by coincubation with picrotoxin. In our experimental conditions, GABA itself (0.5 and 2.5×10^{-5} M) failed to inhibit plasma PRL release (18). In keeping with our findings, inhibition of PRL release from AP incubated *in vitro* was obtained after addition of M (10^{-6}-10^{-8} M) by Grandison and Guidotti (15), an effect which was reversed by bicuculline, and Enjalbert et al., (11) in the same AP system observed inhibition of PRL release by adding GABA (10^{-6}M), an effect which was counteracted by picrotoxin but not by the dopamine (DA) receptor blocker α-flupentixol. Demonstration of specific, high affinity binding sites for GABA and M in the rat pituitary gland (15) was the definitive proof for the "pituitary" component of GABA action, inhibitory to PRL release.

New studies on the GABAergic control of PRL secretion in the rat

The inhibitory component of GABA action on PRL release

It was apparent from the foregoing that GABA may inhibit PRL release by acting directly on specific pituitary GABA receptors. Concomitant investigations by our group had shown that GABA is present in the AP gland where is not formed locally but instead is vehicled from the CNS-where evidence has been given for a tubero-infundibular (TI) GABAergic pathway (34)-to the gland *via* the portal capillary system (see Racagni et al., this Symposium). GABA once released into the portal circulation would be competent to control in an inhibitory fashion PRL release from the AP by its interaction with the specific pituitary GABA receptors.

To substantiate the proposition that systemic administration of M lowers baseline plasma PRL through a "peripheral" mechanism of action, we studied in OVX, E-primed rats the effect of pretreatment with the specific peripheral GABA antagonist, bicuculline methiodide (BIC Met I^-) on M-induced PRL inhibition. Adult OVX rats, 15 days after surgery received a sc injection of 1.0 mg estradiol valerate and underwent the experiments 5 days later. Fig. 1 shows that a bolus injection of BIC Met I^- followed by 105 min infusion blocked the inhibitory effect of M on the E-induced PRL rise, without antagonizing the initial rise of plasma PRL induced by M.

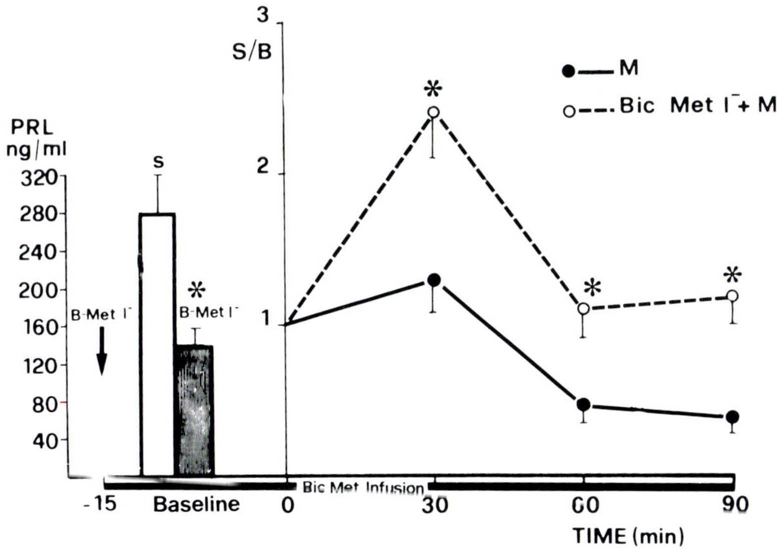

FIG. 1. Effect of bicuculline-methiodide (Bic Met I^-) on the PRL inhibitory effect of peripherally-administered Muscimol (M, 2 mg/kg iv) in Ovx rats primed with estradiol valerate. Bic Met I^- was administered as a bolus injection (1.5 mg/kg iv) at time -15' and infused (0.5 mg/kg iv) until time 90'. In the left panel of the figure, columns represent absolute PRL values at time 0 (when M was administered); in the right panel, values are expressed as the ratio suppressed to baseline (S/B). Each point represents the mean and SE of 12 determinations (pool of 2 experiments) *= $p < 0.05$ vs M alone.

This finding would indicate that the inhibition of PRL release by systemic injection of M likely results from a peripheral action of the drug, since blockade of "peripheral" GABAergic receptors by BIC Met I^-, a drug which does not penetrate the brain, fully antagonized the M-induced PRL inhibition. The presence of specific GABA receptors on pituitary cells (15), favors a "pituitary" site of action for the PRL-lowering effect of systemically-administered M. Consistent with our findings and conclusions are those of Grandison and Guidotti (15), who showed that BIC Met I^- blocked the inhibitory effect of systemically-administered M on haloperidol-induced PRL release.

We have previously shown that IVT injection of EOS (2 mg/kg) induces in male rats a lowering of baseline plasma PRL (18); this effect is coupled with a striking rise in hypothalamic and pituitary GABA concentrations (fivefold increase 4 hr post-injection and threefold increase 2 hr post-injection, respectively) (see Racagni et al., this Symposium). Since administration of a compound by IVT route precludes precise determination of its CNS site of action, we decided to instillate EOS directly into the medial basal hypothalamus (MBH). For intrahypothalamic injection, 22-gauge stainless steel guide cannulae 6.3 mm in length, were implanted at the coordinates 4.5 mm anterior and 0.5 mm lateral with the aid of a stereotaxis apparatus (9) and anchored in place with acrylic cement. The guide cannula was fitted with a wire stylet and capped to prevent clogging. After surgery, the rats were allowed 3-5 days for recovery. For injection of test solution, a 28-gauge inner cannula was inserted into the guide so that the tip projected 8.3 mm below the dorsal brain surface. Using a microsyringe, 1 µl solution was infused over a 60-sec interval. The cannula was maintained in position for 2 min to prevent back diffusion into the guide. Fig. 2 shows that direct injection of 100 µg of EOS into the MBH induced 4 hr post-injection a striking lowering of baseline PRL levels, which was accompanied by an increase in hypothalamic and pituitary GABA concentration with no rise of GABA titers in the caudate n.

In addition to hypothalamic GABAergic fibers projecting to the MBH (see also below), evidence has been provided for the existence of a TI GABA ergic pathway which projects to the median eminence (34). The finding that direct injection of EOS into the MBH increases GABA content in the hypothalamus and the AP and lowers plasma PRL strengthens the idea that the compound is inhibiting GABA-T within this pathway with ensuing GABA loading in the stalk circulation.

Mechanisms underlying the central stimulatory component of GABA action on PRL release

Intraventricular instillation of M (500 ng/rat) induces in freely-moving male rats a short-lived but clear-cut rise in plasma PRL; this effect is highly reproducible and is suppressed by previous injection of bicuculline (0.4 mg/kg iv, 1 hr before) (19). A slight stimulation of PRL release after IVT injection of muscimol (800 ng/rat) has been also reported in unanesthetized rats by Grandison and Guidotti (15). In these authors' view the response did not appear to result from the stimulation of hypothalamic GABA receptor since PRL release did not increase after basomedial hypothalamic infusion of M at high doses (100-200 ng/rat).

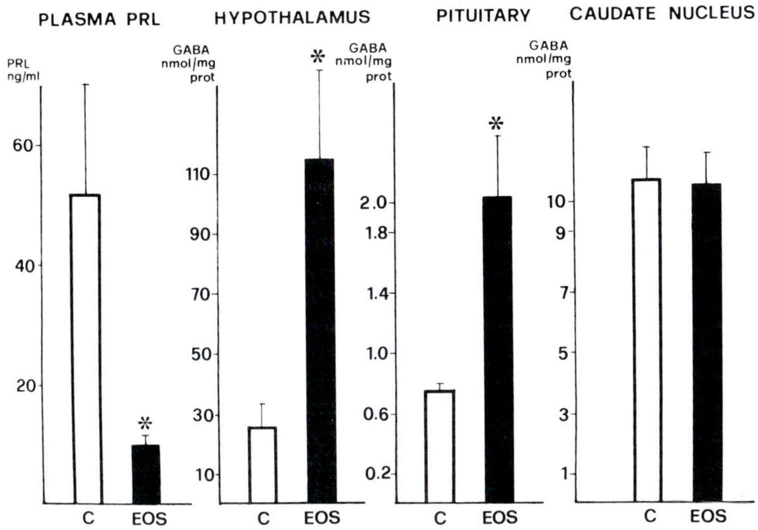

FIG. 2. Effect of EOS (100 µg) administered into the medial basal hypothalamus on plasma PRL levels and GABA concentrations in the hypothalamus, anterior pituitary and caudate n. of male rats killed 4 hr post-injection. Mean and SE of 5 determinations are reported. * = $p < 0.05$ vs control (C) group.

A nonspecific drug effect was envisioned. However, a series of observations mitigates against this view: 1) M-induced rise in plasma PRL after IVT injection is reminiscent of the increase in PRL release previously reported after IVT administration of high doses of GABA (see above); 2) the effect of both GABA and M is bicuculline-sensitive (18, 35) 3) both bicuculline and picrotoxin inhibit tonic and/or stimulated PRL release (18) 4) administration of GABAergic compounds in man invariably induces a rise in plasma PRL (31-33).

Since, based on our findings, we thought that the central component of GABA action on PRL release must not be overlooked, a series of experiments was initiated with the aim of ascertaining the mechanism(s) whereby IVT administration of M elicits in the rat PRL release. Either a direct action of the compound on hypothalamic regulatory hormones for PRL control, i.e., PRL-inhibiting (PIF) and/or releasing (PRF) factors or the involvement of other brain neurotransmitter systems relaying impulses to neurosecretory neurons, i.e., monoamines (DA and 5-HT), acetylcholine, etc., could be envisioned.

For all the experiments male S.D. rats weighing 220-250 g B.W.

were used. A small polyethylene cannula (PE-10) was implanted in the lateral brain ventricle, 3-5 days before the experiments. Rats underwent different pharmacologic manipulations and then were given M (500 ng/rat/20 µl) through the implanted cannula. Blood samples were obtained through the retroorbital venous plexus 15, 30 and 45 min after M injection.

Evidence has been presented indicating that central or systemic administration of cholinergic drugs reduces serum PRL levels in female rats (14). The same drugs are also capable of reducing in normal or estrogen-treated male rats the PRL rise present at proestrus or following 5-hydroxytryptophan administration (16).

In a first experiment the effect of pilocarpine, a stimulant of muscarinic cholinergic receptors, on the ability of IVT-injected M to release PRL was determined. Pilocarpine (10 mg/kg ip) was injected 60 min before administration of M. Control rats were given by IVT route an isotonic saline solution or M alone or systemic administration of P alone. Fig. 3 shows that P did not antagonize the rise in plasma PRL present 15 and 30 min after M administration. Pilocarpine per se decreased baseline plasma PRL (34.1 ± 5.2 vs 12.8 ± 1.4 ng/ml in saline-or pilocarpine-treated rats, respectively at time 0).

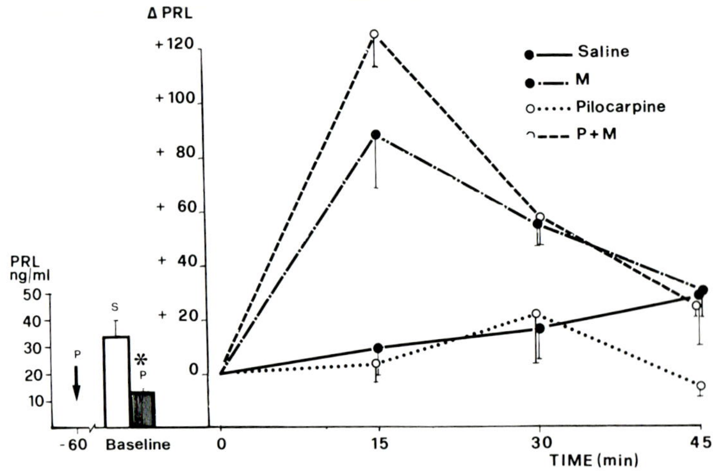

FIG. 3. Effect of pilocarpine (P, 10 mg/kg ip) on M (500 ng IVT)-induced PRL release. Values (mean ± SE of 6-8 determinations) are expressed as increments from baseline. In the left part of the figure, columns represent absolute PRL values at time 0 (when M was administered). The same description applies also to fig. 4.* = $p < 0.01$ vs Saline-pretreated group.

We have previously reported that blockade of catecholamine (CA) synthesis by α-methyl-p-tyrosine (α-MpT, 200 mg/kg ip), administered 30 min before M administration, failed to suppress the PRL-stimulatory effect of the latter. Combined administration of α-MpT and M had an additive effect in raising plasma PRL (18). Since during the first 30 min after α-MpT administration, CA biosynthesis may be only partially inhibited (10), we decided to repeat the α-MpT study using a longer time-interval between α-MpT and M administration. α-MpT was administered at the dose of 400 mg/kg ip 3 hrs before and at the dose of 200 mg/kg ip, 1 hr before IVT administration of M. Fig. 4 shows that administration of α-MpT, under these experimental conditions, significantly reduced the PRL-releasing effect of M present at 30 min. Calculation of the areas under the curves subtending the effect of M or M + α-MpT showed the existence of a significant difference ($p < 0.05$). Consistent with the results obtained by using α-MpT, are those of experiments in which depletion of monoamine stores was induced by reserpine.

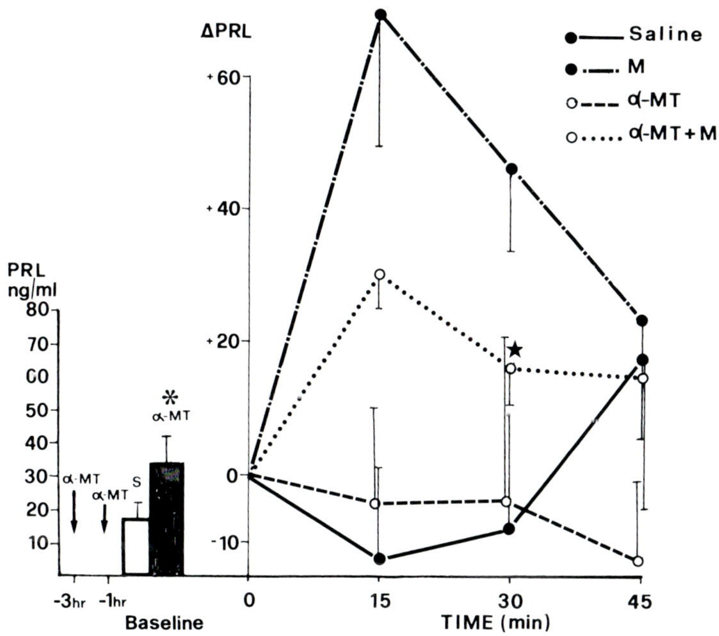

FIG. 4. Effect of α-methyl-p-tyrosine (400 mg + 200 mg/kg ip) on M (500 ng IVT)-induced PRL release. * = $p < 0.001$ vs Saline pretreated group. * = $p < 0.05$ vs M-treated group.

This drug, administered at the dose of 2.5 mg/kg ip, 18 hrs before administration of M, strikingly reduced the PRL-releasing effect of the latter at both 15 and 30 min (data not shown).

Results obtained in the above experiments with the use of α-MpT and reserpine favored the idea that the PRL-releasing effect of M was dependent, at least in part, by suppression of central CA, namely DA, function, which normally exerts a tonic inhibition over PRL secretion. More cogent demonstration of the involvement of the tuberoinfundibular DA (TIDA) pathway in the PRL-releasing effect of M was given in a subsequent experiment, in which AP concentrations of DA, a reliable indicator of TIDA function (1), were determined after IVT administration of M. It was shown that concurrent to the PRL-releasing effect of M there was a striking decrease of DA titers in the AP gland, 10 min after M administration (data not shown).

While the participation of the TIDA pathway in the effect of IVT-injected M was clearly indicated by our findings, the latter were unable to prove or disprove the involvement of additional neurotransmitter systems. Activation of 5-HT neurotransmission in the rat results in stimulation of PRL release (22) and it has been proposed that 5-HT neurons cause PRL release by stimulating the release of PRF rather than inhibiting the PIF system (6). Indications for the existence of an extradopaminergic component in the action of M on PRL release might be envisioned in the finding that pretreatment with reserpine, a depletor of both CA and 5-HT stores (3), was more effective in antagonizing the M-induced PRL rise than simple inhibition of CA biosynthesis by α-MpT.

To assess the possible participation of the 5-HT system, rats with and without pretreatment of the neurotoxic drug 5,6-dihydroxytryptamine (5, 6-DHT, 100 μg IVT, as base, 5 days before) underwent central administration of M. Pretreatment with 5, 6-DHT failed to modify the PRL-releasing effect of the GABAergic compound (data not shown). In a following experiment, also aimed to investigate the involvement of 5-HT neurotransmission, rats were pretreated with quipazine (Quip, 20 mg/kg ip) 15 min before receiving central injection of M. In Quip-pretreated rats, whose basal PRL levels had been raised by the drug, M elicited a rise in plasma PRL which at 15, 30 and 45 min was significantly lower than that elicited by this compound in rats pretreated with a placebo, though PRL values in Quip-Mus treated rats significantly outnumbered those present in the Quip + saline treated group (data not shown). Since Quip is a direct stimulant of 5-HT receptors (17, 26), blunting of the M-induced PRL rise in rats pretreated with Quip may suggest that previous activation of 5-HT receptors involved in the control of PRL secretion had generated their unavailability to a subsequent 5-HT-mediated stimulus i.e., one elicited by M. If this type of reasoning is correct, the ensuing conclusion, i.e., that M releases PRL in part via an activation of 5-HT neurotransmission, is in contrast with the inability of denervation of 5-HT system by 5,6-DHT to affect the M-induced PRL rise. Additional work is needed to assess the participation of the 5-HT system in the PRL-releasing effect of M.

GABAergic mechanisms and GH release

Third ventricular injection of μ mole doses of GABA in conscious OVX or OVX E-and progesterone-primed rats has a stimulant effect on GH release while producing a suppressive effect on TSH discharge (36).

The use of M in our experiments on PRL control led us to also investigate the effect of peripheral and central administration of the compound on GH secretion. For these experiments, OVX rats were primed 10 days after surgery with a single sc injection of 0.5 mg polyestradiol phosphate (PEP: 1 mg Estradurin, Angiolini S.p.A., Milan, Italy). Experiments were performed 6-7 days after PEP injection, at 1500 h. Rats were sampled by the retroorbital venous plexus at different time intervals after treatment. Table 1 shows that M (2 mg/ kg ip) induced a significant decrease in baseline GH levels at 30, 60 and 90 min. Bicuculline (0.4 mg/kg ip, 2 hr before M) significantly decreased baseline GH levels and enhanced M-induced GH inhibition at 30 min, though blockade after M-induced GH inhibition was present at 90 min.

TABLE 1. Effect of iv administration of Muscimol on growth hormone (GH) secretion

Treatment	Plasma GH (ng/ml)			
	T_0	T_{30min}	T_{60min}	T_{90min}
SALINE	88 ± 22.4^b	46 ± 9.1	42 ± 5.9	51 ± 7.0
MUSCIMOL	96 ± 12.7	27 ± 4.8^c	28 ± 3.7^c	4 ± 2.3^c
BICUCULLINE + MUSCIMOL	10 ± 3.4^c	8 ± 2.5^{cd}	21 ± 3.4^c	36 ± 7.1^d

[a] Muscimol 2 mg/kg ip; Bicuculline, 0.4 mg/kg, administered 120 min before Muscimol.

[b] Mean ± SE of 6-7 determinations. Ovariectomized female rats primed 5 days before with 0.5 mg polyestradiol phosphate.

[c] $p < 0.05$ vs Saline

[d] $p < 0.05$ vs Muscimol

Experiments with central administration of M were performed in freely-behaving male rats. Since the scope of these investigations was that of studying the neuroendocrine responses in an animal model which mimics Huntington's disease, a degenerative disorder of the extrapyramidal system (5), experiments were conducted in either rats injected bilaterally into the caudate n. with kainic acid (KA) (7) or in sham-operated controls. Male adult S.D. rats were given under pentobarbital anesthesia 3nmol (0.63 µg) of KA, a rigid analog of glutamate, in a volume of 1 µl saline into each striatum. Coordinates according to De Groot stereotaxic atlas (9) were: AP + 8.8 mm; ML $\pm$ 2.6 mm; and DV + 4.5 mm. The KA was infused via a 22 gauge cannula at a rate of 0.25 µl/min. After injection, the cannula was left in place for another 2 min to allow diffusion of the drug solution. Control rats underwent similar operations but received microinjections of the vehicle alone. After the initial aphagia and adipsia had subsided and KA-injected rats had regained the original weight, rats were prepared with chronic indwelling jugular cannulae which were inserted into the right atrium, and underwent experiments 2 days later. Administration of M (500 ng) induced in sham-operated controls a clear-cut rise in plasma GH with peak levels at 30 min (from 33.0 $\pm$ 11.4 to 117.5 $\pm$ 44.8 ng/ml); in the lesioned rats, M induced a more prompt and striking rise in plasma GH with peak levels occurring at 15 min (from 33.3 $\pm$ 18.9 to 377.6 $\pm$ 96.6 ng/ml, $p < 0.05$). A significant difference in GH levels was present between KA-lesioned and sham-operated rats at 15 min ($p < 0.05$) (data not shown). These findings are only preliminary and their corroboration is needed before a dual role of GABAergic system on GH release, analogous to that disclosed for PRL control, may be envisioned. Certainly, inhibition of GH release by peripherally-administered M and failure of bicuculline to antagonize the M-induced GH inhibition, but instead its potentiating effect, call forth a similar pattern evidenced in the PRL studies. Studies performed so far in laboratory animals on the GABAergic system and GH regulation have been confined to the investigation of the effect of centrally administered compounds. In addition to GABA in µ mole doses (36), IVT administration of adminoxyacetic acid, a blocker of GABA transaminase, and of y-hydroxybutyric acid, a physiological metabolite of GABA, induced an increase in plasma GH and hypothalamic concentrations of GH-inhibiting factor (30). Similarly, in man administration of GABA or GABA-mimetic drugs induces a rise in plasma GH(4,12,30,32,33). The possible existence of a "peripheral" component of GABA action inhibitory to GH release warrants further investigation.

COMMENTS

Further studies aimed at deepening present knowledge on the role of GABAergic mechanisms in the control of PRL secretion have brought new information on both the inhibitory and the stimulatory components of GABA action. Use of the specific peripheral GABA antagonist BIC Met I^- blocked the inhibition of PRL release induced by systemic administration of M, thus providing *in vivo* evidence that peripheral GABA receptors play a major role in this endocrine response.

Failure of BIC Met I^- to counteract the initial M-induced PRL rise substantiates the view that the latter is due to activation of central GABA receptor sites. In fact, IVT administration of M stimulates PRL release, an effect which is antagonized by administration of bicuculline. The M-induced PRL rise appears to be mainly mediated by inhibition of TIDA neurons, standing: 1) its counteraction by pretreatment with both α -MpT and reserpine and 2) direct demonstration of decreased pituitary DA concentrations after IVT administration of the amino acid analog. Neuroanatomical substrate for this central GABAergic component involved in PRL secretion is provided by the detection of GABAergic terminals on the arcuate and ventromedial n. (34), areas which give rise to the TIDA pathway.

Like peripherally-injected M, administration of EOS into the MBH lowers baseline plasma PRL, an indication that blockade of GABA-T effected by EOS at the level of a TI GABAergic pathway (34) increases GABA in the portal capillary system (25) and results in a final activation of pituitary GABA receptors. Failure of bicuculline to antagonize EOS-induced inhibition of PRL release and, conversely, its ability to suppress the M-induced PRL rise support the concept that the mechanism(s) (and, site of actions), subserving the two drugs' action are quite dissimilar. Further studies are needed to ascertain the existence of possible functional interactions between the central and the "peripheral" components of GABA action on PRL release.

Preliminary experiments on the involvement of the GABAergic mechanisms in the control of GH secretion, would suggest that, similar to PRL control, there exists, in addition to a central GABAergic component stimulatory to GH release (36), a peripheral (pituitary?) inhibitory component.

Stressful stimuli are inhibitory to GH release in the rat (22). However, arguing against the possibility that the GH-lowering effect of systemically-administered M and bicuculline was due to a nonspecific stress effect is the finding that in the same experimental conditions the two drugs lowered plasma levels of PRL (18, 19) which, unlike GH, does respond positively to the stressful events in the rat (23).

Injection of KA into the caudate n., a procedure which induces a marked diminution of GABA concentrations in this area (7) but not in the hypothalamus (authors' unpublished results), greatly enhanced, through a still unknown mechanism, the central stimulatory component of GABA action on GH release, suggesting the existence of a functional interaction between the extrapyramidal system and the endocrine hypothalamus.

ACKNOWLEDGEMENT

These studies were supported in part by the project Biology of Reproduction of C.N.R. and by C.N.R. grant C.T. 78.02055.04. The participation in the initial stages of the research of Dr. P. Krogsgaard-Larsen is gratefully acknowledged as well as the work of Dr. Paola Zanardi and Miss Isabella Zago in preparing the manuscript.

REFERENCES

1. Apud, J., Cocchi, D., Iuliano, E., Casanueva, F., Müller, E.E. and Racagni, G. (1980): Brain Res. 186: 226-231.
2. Baraldi, M., Grandison, L. and Guidotti, A. (1979): Neuropharmacology 18: 57-62.
3. Brodie, B.B., Tomich, E.G., Kuntzman, R. and Shore, P.A. (1957): J. Pharmacol. Exp. Ther. 119: 461-467.
4. Cavagnini, P., Invitti, C., Di Landro, A., Tenconi, L., Maraschini, C. and Girotti, G. (1977): J. Clin. Endocrinol. Metab. 45: 579-584.
5. Chase, T.N., Wexler, N.S. and Barbeau, A. (Eds.) (1979): Huntington's Disease, Adv. Neurol. vol. 23, Raven Press, New York.
6. Clemens, J.A., Roush, M.E. and Füller, R.W. (1978): Life Sci. 22: 2209-2214.
7. Coyle, J.T. and Schwartz, R. (1976): Nature (Lond.) 263: 244-246.
8. Curtis, D.R., Duggan, A.V., Felix, D. and Johnston, C.A.R. (1971): Brain Res. 32: 69-96.
9. De Groot, J. (1967): The rat forebrain in stereotaxic coordinates, North-Holland, Amsterdam.
10. Doteuchi, M., Wang, C. and Costa, E. (1974): Molec. Pharmacol. 10: 225-234.
11. Enjalbert, A., Ruberg, M., Fiore, L. and Kordon, C. (1978): Ann. Endoc. (Paris) 39: 237-238.
12. Fioretti, P., Melis, G.B., Paoletti, A.M., Parodo, G., Caminiti, F., Corsini, P.G. and Martini, L. (1978): J. Clin. Endocrinol. Metab. 47: 1336-1340.
13. Fowler, L.J. and John, R.A. (1972): Biochem. J. 130: 569-573.
14. Grandison, L., Gelato, M. and Meites, J. (1974): Proc. Soc. Exp. Biol. Med. 145: 1263.
15. Grandison, L. and Guidotti, A. (1979): Endocrinology 105: 754-759.
16. Grandison, L. and Meites, J. (1975): Fed. Proc. Fed. Am. Soc. Exp. Biol. 35: Abs. 356.
17. Honing, E., Sancilio, F.L., Vargas, R. and Pardo, E.G. (1969): Europ. J. Pharmacol. 6: 274-280.
18. Locatelli, V., Cocchi, D., Frigerio, C., Betti, R., Krosgaard-Larsen, P. Racagni, G. and Müller, E.E. (1979): Endocrinology 105: 778-783.
19. Locatelli, V., Cocchi, D., Racagni, G., Cattabeni, F., Maggi, A., Krosgaard-Larsen, P. and Müller, E.E. (1978): Brain Res. 145: 173-179.
20. Makara, G.B. and Stark, E. (1974): Neuroendocrinology 16: 178-190.
21. Mioduszewski, R., Grandison, L. and Meites, J. (1976): Proc. Soc. Exp. Biol. Med. 151: 44-46.
22. Müller, E.E., Nisticò, G. and Scapagnini, U. (1978): Neurotransmitters and Anterior Pituitary Function. Academic Press, New York.

23. Neill, J.D. (1970): Endocrinology 87: 1192.
24. Ondo, J.G. and Pass, K.A. (1976): Endocrinology 98: 1248-1252.
25. Racagni, G., Apud, J.A., Locatelli, V., Cocchi, D., Nisticò, G., di Giorgio, R.M. and Müller, E.E. (1979): Nature 281:575-578.
26. Rodriguez, R., Rojas-Ramirez, A. and Drucker-Colin, R.R. (1973): Europ. J. Pharmacol. 24: 164-171.
27. Saavedra, J.M., Palkovits, M., Kizer, J.S., Brownstein, M.J. and Zivin, J.A. (1975): J. Neurochem. 25: 257-260.
28. Schally, A.V., Redding, T.W., Arimura, A., Dupont, A. and Linthicum, G.L. (1977): Endocrinology 100: 681-691.
29. Straughan, D.W., Neal, M.J., Simmonds, M.A., Collins, G.G.S. and Hill, R.G. (1971): Nature 233: 352-354.
30. Takahara, J., Yunoki, S., Hosogi, H., Yakushiji, J., Kageyama, J. and Ofuji, T. (1980a): Endocrinology 106: 343-347.
31. Takahara, J., Yunoki, S., Yakushiji, W., Hosogi, H. and Ofuji, T. (1980b): Horm. Met. Res. 12: 31-34.
32. Takahara, J., Yunoki, S., Yakushiji, W., Yamauchi, J., Jamara, Y. and Ofuji, T. (1977): J. Clin. Endocrinol. Metab. 44: 1014-1019.
33. Tamminga, C.A., Neophytides, A., Chase, T.N. and Frohman, L.A. (1978): J. Clin. Endocrinol. Metab. 47: 1348-1351.
34. Tappaz, M.L. and Brownstein, M.J. (1977): Brain Res. 132: 95-106.
35. Vijayan, E. and McCann, S.M. (1978a): Brain Res. 155: 35-43.
36. Vijayan, E. and McCann, S.M. (1978b): Endocrinology 103: 1888-1893.

GABA and Benzodiazepine Receptors,
edited by E. Costa et al.
Raven Press, New York © 1981.

Neurochemical Aspects of GABA and Glutamate in the Hypothalamo-Pituitary System

G. Racagni, J. A. Apud, C. Civati, *D. Cocchi, *F. Casanueva, *V. Locatelli, **G. Nisticò, and †E. E. Müller

*Institute of Pharmacology and Pharmacognosy, University of Milan and Cagliari †; Department of Pharmacology, University of Milan *; and Institute of Pharmacology, University of Messina **, Italy*

There are many candidates for functional neurotransmitters in the tubero-infundibular region of the hypothalamus. Biochemical studies using the punching technique to localize putative neurotransmitters have demonstrated relatively high concentrations of dopamine (DA), norepinephrine (27), serotonin (32), histamine (2) and acetylcholine (4) in this region. Recently, evidence has accumulated that, in addition to classic hypothalamic neurohormones (17,18,41), other peptide molecules such as enkephalins (20), endorphins (15) and substance P (19) can subserve a transmitter or modulator role within the medio-basal hypothalamus (MBH).

With respect to γ-aminobutyric acid (GABA), neither the exact tracing of its neural paths in the MBH nor its precise function have been determined. However, recently, data have been provided on the neuroanatomical organization of GABA in the MBH. In fact, an uneven distribution of glutamic acid decarboxylase (GAD), the enzyme responsible for GABA synthesis (31), has been reported within discrete hypothalamic nuclei (37) and very dense networks of GAD-positive nerve terminals observed within the external layer of the median eminence (ME) (12). Moreover, cell elements in this area in close vicinity to the portal vessels are capable of accumulating exogenous GABA according to its neuronal uptake characteristics (38).

Hypothalamic deafferentation studies and measurements of GAD activity have indicated that in several hypothalamic nuclei GABA nerve terminals arise from cell bodies located outside the hypothalamus (3), though GABA nerve terminals in the ME appear to have an hypothalamic origin (36). In all, these data would suggest that an intrinsic GABAergic ventrobasal pathway exists in the rat hypothalamus. Such an organization of the GABAergic fibers could provide the anatomical substrate for GABAergic regulation of pituitary hormone release (8,22,26,34,35,39) through an action exerted either at the level of the hypothalamus or directly on the anterior pituitary (AP).

In addition to GABA, its precursor molecule glutamic acid (GLU) seems also to act as a neurotransmitter in several central nervous system (CNS) areas (7,21,28). GLU, administered to rodents causes lesions in selective hypothalamic nuclei (25), thus implying the existence of glutamatergic inputs to these areas.

The aim of the present investigation is that of providing evidence on the biochemical organization of GABA and GLU in the MBH-AP system and correlating particular aspects of GABAergic and glutamatergic function with the secretion of AP hormones.

DISTRIBUTION OF GABA AND GLUTAMATE IN THE HYPOTHALAMO-PITUITARY SYSTEM.

Table 1 shows the concentrations of GABA and GLU and GAD activity in the hypothalamus and the anterior and posterior (PP) lobes of the pituitary. It is evident that in all tissues investigated absolute concentrations of GLU are consistently higher than those of GABA. While GABA content in the AP is strikingly lower than in the PP and the hypothalamus, the concentrations of GLU are slightly higher in the PP and almost doubled in the hypothalamus. The absence of GAD activity in the AP demonstrates that in this portion of the gland GLU is not a precursor of GABA and, thus, the latter must derive from other body compartments. The AP gland is anatomically linked to the MBH via the portal capillary system and, in addition, it receives a blood supply from the systemic circulation. Hence, an attempt has been made to investigate the possible source of GABA present in the AP.

HYPOTHALAMIC ORIGIN OF GABA PRESENT IN THE ANTERIOR PITUITARY.

A wide series of experiments support the possibility that GABA in AP may derive from CNS areas. As shown in Table 2 the intracerebroventricular (IVT) injection of ethanolamine-O-sulphate (EOS) (2 mg/kg), a specific GABA-transaminase (GABA-T) blocker (11), induces at 2,4 and 8 hrs post-treatment a striking

TABLE 1. GABA and Glutamic acid (GLU) concentrations and Glutamic acid decarboxylase (GAD) activity in the hypothalamo-pituitary system.

TISSUE	GABA (nmol/mg protein)	GAD (pmol CO_2/mg protein/h)	GLU (nmol/mg protein)
ANTERIOR LOBE	0.76 ± 0.07	None	61.59 ± 4.20
POSTERIOR LOBE	5.53 ± 0.60	0.547 ± 0.017	96.41 ± 6.30
HYPOTHALAMUS	40.11 ± 3.81	6.320 ± 450	115.94 ± 13.84

- The values for GABA and GLU represent the mean ± SEM of at least 15 determinations (3 experiments). Both amino acids were determined by mass fragmentographic technique (5) in rats sacrificed by microwave radiation (14).
- GAD was determined by radioenzymatic assay (30). Values represent the mean ± SEM of five determinations obtained from a pool of 10 glands or 4 hypothalamic fragments, respectively.

rise in both hypothalamic and AP GABA concentrations, which is concomitant to a clear-cut decline of baseline PRL titers in the plasma. The likelihood that the above changes are caused by an effect of EOS on GABA catabolism exerted at the level of the gland is denied by the finding that the IVT administration of the enzyme inhibitor does not block GABA-T activity in the AP (Table 3). Proof that GABA changes in the AP actually reflect primarily alterations occurring in the CNS is given inferentially with the demonstration that EOS administered systemically at doses 25-200 times higher than the IVT-injected dose does alter neither GABA content in the gland nor plasma PRL levels (1,29).

More careful determination of the CNS source responsible for supplying GABA to the AP is achieved with the demonstration that direct administration of 100 μg of EOS into the MBH is able to increase GABA in the hypothalamus and AP and induces the usual decline of plasma PRL concentrations (Table 4). No change of GABA have been detected in the striatum of the same animals suggesting that EOS had not diffused. In keeping with the last findings, surgical deafferentation of the MBH does not alter the concentrations of GABA in the hypothalamic island, though

TABLE 2. Hypothalamic (HYP) and Anterior Pituitary (AP) GABA concentrations and plasma prolactin (PRL) titers at different times after intraventricular (IVT) injection of ethanolamine-O-sulphate (EOS).

	GABA		PROLACTIN
TIME (h)	HYP (nmol/mg protein)	AP (nmol/mg protein)	PLASMA (ng/ml)
0	40.42 ± 7..52	0.61 ± 0.20	31.11 ± 4.40
2	91.18 ± 15.5*	3.11 ± 0.87*	11.66 ± 1.36*
4	235.94 ± 48.88*	2.00 ± 0.70*	11.23 ± 3.16*
8	175.70 ± 31.25*	1.20 ± 0.20*	5.51 ± 1.53*

- Plasma PRL was measured by radioimmunoassay (24).
- For GABA and PRL, values represent the mean ± SEM of at least 5 determinations.
- EOS was injected at the dose of 2 mg/kg, in the lateral ventricle of unanesthetized male rats through an implanted cannula.

* $p < 0.01$ vs. baseline values (Dunnett's test).

TABLE 3. GABA concentrations and GABA-Transaminase (GABA-T) activity in the hypothalamo-pituitary system after intraventricular (IVT) injection of ethanolamine-O-sulphate (EOS).

	Anterior Pituitary		Posterior Pituitary		Hypothalamus	
	GABA	GABA-T	GABA	GABA-T	GABA	GABA-T
CONTROL	0.73 ± 0.056	37.1 ± 1.2	8.6 ± 0.4	37.6 ± 0.68	51.2 ± 1.5	24.2 ± 1.8
EOS	1.38 ± 0.16*	35.2 ± 1.3	15.7 ± 0.5*	24.5 ± 0.78*	161.4 ± 14.6*	12.8 ± 1.5*

- GABA is expressed as nmol/mg protein.
- GABA-T, determined by radiometric assay, is expressed as µmol of succinic semialdehyde per 100 mg of protein per hour.
- IVT injected EOS (2 mg/kg) was administered in the lateral ventricle through an implanted cannula 3 hours before sacrifice.

* $p < 0.01$ (Student's "t" test).

TABLE 4. Hypothalamic (HYP), Anterior Pituitary (AP) and Striatal (ST) GABA concentrations and plasma prolactin (PRL) titers after intramedio-basal hypothalamic administration of ethanolamine-O-sulphate (EOS).

	GABA (nmol/mg protein)			PLASMA PROLACTIN (ng/ml)
	HYP	AP	ST	
CONTROL	20.60 ± 6.38	0.76 ± 0.08	10.68 ± 1.11	49.30 ± 18.0
EOS	105.10 ± 28.4*	2.04 ± 0.40*	10.62 ± 1.00	9.36 ± 1.34*

- Animals were sacrificed by microwave radiation 4 hours after administration of EOS (100 ug).
- For GABA and PRL, values represent the mean ± SEM of at least 5 determinations.

*p 0.05 (Student's "t" test).

it induces a slight decrease in GAD activity (Table 5). Similarly, GABA concentrations are not modified in the AP and PP lobes of the gland nor is plasma PRL modified (Table 5).

GLUTAMIC ACID IN THE HYPOTHALAMO-PITUITARY AXIS.

Administration of sodium glutamate to rodents induces lesions preferentially located in the arcuate nucleus of the hypothalamus and decreases choline acetyltransferase and GAD in the ME (40). This indicates that likely glutamatergic fibers abut on neuronal cells present in the MBH. Proof that this is the case is presented in Table 5. In fact, the deafferentation of the MBH elicits a marked decrease of GLU in the hypothalamic island and the pituitary.

That GABA and GLU have a different biochemical and functional organization in the hypothalamic and pituitary system is suggested by the observation that 1) transplantation of the gland in a site far remote from central connections, while induces a decrease of GABA concentrations, does not alter GLU content (Table 6); 2) unlike GABA, which is capable of affecting PRL secretion from "in vitro" AP (23), GLU at molar doses does not affect the release of luteinizing hormone (LH), growth hormone (GH) and PRL in the same AP system (Table 7).

TABLE 5. GABA and Glutamic acid (GLU) concentrations in the hypothalamo-pituitary system and plasma prolactin (PRL) titers after medio-basal hypothalamus (MBH) deafferentation.

	GABA (nmol/mg protein)		GLUTAMIC ACID (nmol/mg protein)		PLASMA PRL (ng/ml)	
	Control	Deaff.	Control	Deaff.	Control	Deaff.
MBH	30.52 ± 7.90	29.74 ± 6.80	115.94 ± 13.84	52.28 ± 9.90**		
Anterior Pituitary	0.51 ± 0.03	0.60 ± 0.07	61.59 ± 4.20	37.23 ± 3.86*	12.9 ± 3.6	15.0 ± 2.9
Posterior Pituitary	6.04 ± 0.24	8.01 ± 1.03	97.41 ± 5.30	37.56 ± 5.83**		

- Values represent the mean ± SEM of at least 5 determinations.
- GABA and GLU were determined by mass fragmentographic technique (5).
- Animals were sacrificed by microwave radiation 7 days after deafferentation of the MBH (16).

* $p < 0.05$ (Student's "t" test)

** $p < 0.01$ (Student's "t" test)

TABLE 6. GABA and Glutamic acid (GLU) concentrations in "in situ" and ectopic anterior pituitaries (AP).

	GABA (nmol/mg protein)	GLUTAMIC ACID (nmol/mg protein)
AP "in situ"	0.65 ± 0.13	67.78 ± 7.24
AP ectopic	0.24 ± 0.057*	97.90 ± 11.84

Sprague Dawley rats were hypophysectomized by transauricular route (10) and received 15 days later implants of one AP, obtained from an intact female littermate, under the kidney capsule. GABA and GLU concentrations were determined in the ectopic gland ten days after transplantation.

- Values represent the mean ± SEM of at least 5 determinations.

* $p < 0.01$ (Student's "t" test)

TABLE 7. Effect of monosodium glutamate on growth hormone (GH) prolactin (PRL) and luteinizing hormone (LH) release from "in vitro" pituitaries (pit).

	GH (μg/ml/mg pit)	PRL (ng/ml/mg pit)	LH (ng/ml/mg pit)
CONTROL	9.8 ± 2.2	126.4 ± 10.2	13.7 ± 0.9
Glutamate (10^{-4} M)	9.9 ± 1.6	128.2 ± 27.8	13.4 ± 0.5
Glutamate (10^{-3} M)	9.6 ± 1.9	126.1 ± 14.8	12.2 ± 1.1

- 4 hemipituitaries from male Sprague-Dawley rats for each tube (2 ml medium) were incubated during 4 hours after 1 hour of preincubation (for details see reference 6). Hormones were determined by radioimmunoassay techniques (24).

DISCUSSION

The results presented suggest the following considerations:

1. Detection of GABA and GLU at AP level extends the list of neurotransmitters which have been identified in the gland (33).

2. The AP, though equipped with biochemical machinery for GABA degradation, is apparently unable to synthesize the amino acid, suggesting that the function of GABA-T at the AP would be mainly to catabolize GABA released from CNS and then transported thorugh the hypophyseal portal circulation. The time-related rise in hypothalamus-and AP-GABA concentration after blockade of GABA-T and the decrease of GABA levels in the ectopic pituitaries strongly suggest this mechanism.

3. MBH seems to be the area from which GABA is transported to the AP. Experiments based on direct injection of EOS into the MBH and on the lack of changes in GABA concentrations in the hypothalamic island after MBH deafferentation support this contention.

4. GABA in MBH subserves the function of controlling in an inhibitory fashion PRL release from the AP, acting at the level of specific GABAergic receptors identified in the gland (13). This mechanisms most likly operates via release of the amino acid from terminals of a tubero-infundibular GABAergic pathway (29,38, and this study).

5. GLU present in the AP seems to have no role as a precursor for GABA synthesis "in situ", since GAD activity is lacking in the AP gland. The study of this excitatory amino acid in the AP, thus, might be used a suitable model to ascertain a role of GLU as transmitter independent of its conversion to GABA.

6. The decrease of GLU after MBH deafferentation suggests the existence of fibers projecting from other portions of the hypothalamus or, alternatively, of extra-hypothalamic pathways terminating in the MBH. Consistent with this view is the finding that a severing of the fimbria-fornix tract results in a decrease of GLU levels in the MBH (Fonnum et al., in this volume).

7. A functional role of GLU on LH, GH, and PRL secretion exerted directly on putative pituitary glutamatergic receptors appears to be negated by its failure to affect hormone secretion when added in molar concentrations to AP glands "in vitro". The possibility cannot be excluded that GLU may affect the secretion of other pituitary hormones via a direct pituitary action or through modulation of neurotransmitter or neuro-

secretory neurons in the hypothalamus.

In conclusion, from the data herein presented, it appears that a functional analogy exists between DA and GABA at the level of the hypothalamo-pituitary system since both transmitters are carried from the ME through the hypophyseal portal vessels to reach specific receptor sites located in the AP. Data have previously been presented by us (23,29) and other groups (9), which indicate that the two systems function independently. While the physiological role of DA on PRL secretion has been unequivocally ascertained, the physiological role of GABA on PRL secretion has yet to be elucidated.

REFERENCES

1. Apud, J.A., Racagni, G., Iuliano, E., Cocchi, D., Casanueva, F., and Muller, E.E. (1980): Endocrinology, in press.
2. Brownstein, M.J., Saavedra, J.M., Palkovits, M., and Axelrod, J. (1974): Brain Research, 77:151-156.
3. Brownstein, M.J., Palkovits, M., Tappaz, M.L., Saavedra, J., and Kizer, S. (1976): Brain Research, 117:287-295.
4. Carson, K.A., Nemeroff, C.B., Rone, M.S., Young-Blood, W.W., Prange, A.J.Jr., Hanker, J.S., and Kizer, J.S. (1977): Brain Research, 129:169-173.
5. Cattabeni, F., Galli, C.L., and Eros, T. (1976): Anal. Biochemistry, 72:1-7.
6. Cocchi, D., Locatelli, D., Carminati, R., and Muller, E.E. (1978): Life Sciences, 23:927-936.
7. Curtis, D.R., and Watkins, J.C. (1960): J. Neurochem., 6: 117-141.
8. Enjalbert, A., Ruberg, M., Fiore, L., and Kordon, C. (1978): Ann. Endocr., 39:237-238.
9. Enjalbert, A., Ruberg, M., Arancibia, S., Fiore, L., Priam, M., and Kordon, C. (1979): Endocrinology, 105:823-826.
10. Falconi, G., and Rossi, G. (1964): Endocrinology, 74:301-303
11. Fowler, L.J., and John, R.A. (1972): Biochem. J., 130:569-573.
12. Fuxe, K., Andersson, K., Ogren, S.O., Perez De La Mora, M., Schwarcz, R., Hokfelt, T., Eneroth, P., Gustafsson, J.A., and Skett, P. (1979) In: GABA-Neurotransmitters edited by P. Krogsgaard-Larsen, J. Scheel-Kruger and H. Kofold, pp. 74-94, Munksgaard, Copenhagen.
13. Grandison, L., and Guidotti, A. (1979): Endocrinology, 105: 754-759.

14. Guidotti, A., Cheney, D.L., Trabucchi, M., Doteuchi, M., Wang, C.T., and Hawkins, R.A. (1974): Neuropharmacol., 13: 1115-1122.
15. Guillemin, R. (1978) In: The Hypothalamus, edited by S. Reichlin, R.J. Baldessarini and J.B. Martin, pp. 155-194, Raven Press, New York.
16. Halaz, B., and Pupp, L. (1965): Endocrinology, 77:553.
17. Hökfelt, T., Efendic, S., Hellerstrom, C., Johansson, O., Luft, R., and Arimura, A. (1975): Acta Endocrinol., Suppl. 200:5-41.
18. Hökfelt, T., Fuxe, K., Johansson, O., Jeffcoate, S.L., and White, N. (1975): Europ. J. Pharmacol., 34:389-392.
19. Hökfelt, T., Kellerth, J.O., Nilsson, B. (1975): Science, 190:889-890.
20. Hökfelt, T., Elde, B., Johansson, O., Terenius, L., and Stein, L. (1977): Neurosci. Lett. 5:25-33.
21. Krnjevic, K. (1965): Br. med. Bull., 21:10-14.
22. Locatelli, V., Cocchi, D., Racagni, G., Cattabeni, F., Maggi, A., Krogsgaard-Larsen, P., and Müller, E.E. (1978): Brain Research, 145:173-179.
23. Locatelli, V., Cocchi, D., Frigerio, C., Betti, R., Krogsgaard-Larsen, P., Racagni, G., and Müller, E.E. (1979): Endocrinology, 105:778-783.
24. Niswender, G.D., Chen, C.L., Midgley, A.R., Meites, J., and Ellis, S. (1969): Proc. Soc. Exp. Biol. Med., 130:793-797.
25. Olney, J.W., and Ho, O.L. (1970): Science, 195:1356-1358.
26. Ondo, J.G., and Pass, K.A. (1976): Endocrinology, 98:1248-1252.
27. Palkovits, M., Brownstein, M., Saavedra, J.M., and Axelrod, J. (1974): Brain Research, 77:137-149.
28. Prusiner, S., and Stadtman, E.R. (1973) In: The Enzymes of Glutamine Metabolism, Academic Press, New York.
29. Racagni, G., Apud, J.A., Locatelli, V., Cocchi, D., Nisticò, G., Di Giorgio, R.M., and Müller, E.E. (1979): Nature (Lond) 281:575-578.
30. Roberts, E., and Simonsen, D.G. (1963): Biochem. Pharmac., 12:113-116.
31. Roberts, E., Chase, T.N., and Tower, D.B. (1975): GABA in Nervous System Function, Raven Press, New York.
32. Saavedra, J.M., Palkovits, M., Brownstein, M., and Axelrod, J. (1974): Brain Research, 77:157-165.
33. Saavedra, J.M., Palkovits, M., Kizer, J.S., Brownstein, M.J. and Zivin, J.A. (1975): J. Neurochem., 25:257-260.
34. Schally, A.V., Redding, T.W., Arimura, A., Dupont, A., and Linthicum, G.L. (1977): Endocrinology, 100:681-691.

35. Takahara, J., Yunoki, S., Hosogi, H., Yakushiji, W., Kageyama, J., and Ofuji, T. (1980): Endocrinology, 106:343-347.

36. Tappaz, M.L., and Brownstein, M.J. (1977): Brain Research, 132:95-106.

37. Tappaz, M.L., Brownstein, M.J., and Kopin, I.J. (1977): Brain Research, 125:109-121.

38. Tappaz, M., Aguera, M., Belin, M.F., and Pujol, J.F. (1980): Brain Research, 186:379-391.

39. Vijayan, E., and McCann, S.M. (1978): Brain Research, 155: 35-43.

40. Walaas, I., and Fonnum, G. (1978): Brain Research, 153:549-562.

41. Zimmerman, E.A. (1976) In: Frontiers in Neuroendocrinology, edited by L. Martini and W.F. Ganong, pp. 25-62, Raven Press, New York.

GABA and Benzodiazepine Receptors,
edited by E. Costa et al.
Raven Press, New York © 1981.

Positron Tomography. A New Method for *In Vivo* Brain Studies of Benzodiazepine, in Animal and in Man

M. Mazière, J. M. Godot, G. Berger, J. C. Baron, D. Comar,
†*C. Cepeda, Ch. Menini, and*R. Naquet

*Service Hospitalier F. Joliot, Départemement de Biologie, CEA-Saclay; and*Département de Neurophysiologie Appliquée—Laboratoire de Physiologie Nerveuse, C.N.R.S., 91190 Gif-sur-Yvette, France*

INTRODUCTION

The specific binding sites of benzodiazepines have been described in various experiments, in which generally:

- the binding and binding measurements were carried out "*in vitro*" on brain samples or
- the binding was carried out "*in vivo*" after labelled benzodiazepine administration to the animal, but, in most cases, measurements were taken by counting the organ sampled after the death of the animal.

These methods, naturally, cannot be used in humans.

Since, significant changes in benzodiazepine receptors, relating to their affinity or their density, have been reported in certain diseases such as Huntington's chorea (11) ; we have attempted to develop a method in which the study of benzodiazepine in brain, is designed to facilitate medical diagnosis and is totally non invasive and hence applicable in humans.

Two tools were necessary to achieve this: an adequately labelled ligand and an effective means of external detection.

Based on various investigations (3, 14), flunitrazepam, among currently available benzodiazepines, appeared to have the most interesting features for use as a labelled benzodiazepine receptor ligand.

Carbon 11 was selected for labelling because it is a carbon radioisotope, cyclotron produced, with a short half life (20.33 min.) and a high specific activity (10^4 Ci/µmole theoretically) ; it can be used to label, isotopically, molecules at high specific activity which can therefore be utilized for receptor study and safely administered to humans.

† Fellow of the French Government.

The positrons and associated annihilation gamma rays emitted by carbon 11 make possible external visualization of the intra-cerebral localization, and quantitative measurement by positron emission tomography of the flunitrazepam labelled by carbon 11

First, we will briefly describe the method used to label flunitrazepam with carbon 11.

Then, the "*in vivo*" study of ^{11}C-flunitrazepam in the brain of the baboon using a positron emission tomographic camera and the observation of its "*in vivo*" displacement from brain receptors by various benzodiazepines will be presented.

In conclusion, we will discuss the value and limits of the method as well as its application to humans.

EXPERIMENTAL

Preparation of ^{11}C-flunitrazepam

The ^{11}C-flunitrazepam was prepared by the methylation of nor-flunitrazepam (1 μM) (figure 1) by ^{11}C-methyl iodide in acetone (200 μℓ) in basic medium (10 μℓ NaOH 10N). The reaction takes place in a hermetically-sealed tube heated at 90°C for 8 minutes (yield 90 %) (9).

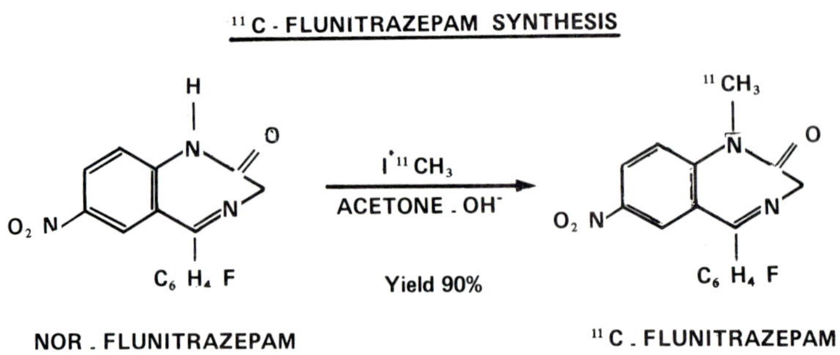

FIG. 1.

The ^{11}C-methyl iodide was prepared from $^{11}CO_2$ (7) obtained by transmutation of nitrogen by 20 MeV protons accelerated in a cyclotron (figure 2).

^{11}C - METHYL IODIDE PREPARATION

1) **^{11}C - CARBON DIOXIDE**

$$^{14}N\,(p,\alpha)\,^{11}C \longrightarrow {}^{11}CO_2$$

2) **^{11}C - METHANOL**

$$4\,{}^{11}CO_2 + 3\,Al\,Li\,H_4 \longrightarrow 2\,Al\,Li\,O_2 + Al\,Li\,(O\,{}^{11}C\,H_3)_4.$$

$$Al\,Li\,(O\,{}^{11}C\,H_3)_4 + 4\,H_2\,O \longrightarrow Al\,(O\,H)_3 + Li\,O\,H + 4\,{}^{11}C\,H_3\,O\,H$$

3) **^{11}C - METHYL IODIDE**

$$^{11}C\,H_3O\,H + I\,H \longrightarrow {}^{11}C\,H_3\,I + H_2\,O$$

FIG. 2.

The ^{11}C carbon dioxide was then reduced to ^{11}C methanol by the action of lithium aluminum hydride and subsequent hydrolysis of the intermediate compound formed. ^{11}C-methyl iodide was prepared instantaneously by the action of the ^{11}C-methanol on hydriodic acid, under reflux. In view of the very high levels of radioactivity involved throughout this preparation, all the required handling operations were carried out semi-automatically in a lead-shielded hood. After purification by high performance liquid chromatography, (identity and stability of the labelled product were checked by H.P.L.C and mass spectra), about 100 mCi of chemically and radiochemically pure labelled flunitrazepam were obtained with a specific activity of around 800 mCi/μmole ; this means that for a radioactivity of 10 to 30 mCi sufficient for the examination of an animal by the positron camera for one hour, the mass of flunitrazepam injected was in the range of nanomoles.

Brain Distribution in the Animal

The "*in vivo*" study of benzodiazepines was carried out on the baboon Papio-papio 10-12 Kg of weight by a positron emission tomograph using ^{11}C-flunitrazepam as the benzodiazepine receptor ligand.

The positron detection system (ECAT-ORTEC) consists of six banks of detectors in hexagonal array, each composed of 11 crystals of Na I (Tℓ) ; at the centre of this array the head of the animal is placed. The radioactivity emitted by a slice 2 cm in thickness is recorded by the detectors in coincidence mode. Rotation of these detectors around the animal allows multivue detection which, after mathematical reconstruction, gives a tomographic picture showing the distribution of the radioactivity in the slice with a resolution of 15 mm. Only one slice can be measured at a time ; longitudinal movement of the bed on which the animal lies is necessary to obtain successive slices. The counting time for one slice is of the order of 2 minutes (13). The animal was anesthetized with ketamine (150 mg I.M , five hours before beginning the experiment), and then intubated, installed on the positron camera bed, in a painless position, placed under artificial respiration and curarized by alloferine (3 mg I.V). The head was positioned so that a laser ray indicating the centre of the 2 cm thick brain slice was superimposed on the axis determined by the inion-orbital line of the animal. Two successive slices overlapping by 1 cm were made at approximately 3 minute intervals.

The cerebral and extracerebral radioactivity after thorough standardization were quantified from regions of interest demarcated on the image of each slice. Blood radioactivity was measured throughout the experiment by counting of samples taken after catheterization, under local anesthesia, of the femoral artery.

After the end of the experiment, the animal is decurarized by prostigmine (0.5 mg I.V) desintubated, the artery sutured under local anesthesia ; then, the baboon is transferred to his cage and not used again for 15 days.

Some twenty experiments were conducted on a limited number of different animals.

On each baboon, the experiment consisted of the following :

First, determination of the cerebral, extracerebral, and blood kinetics of ^{11}C-flunitrazepam after intravenous administration of 25 mCi.

Then, to examine the specific hence saturable character of this brain uptake, the cerebral radioactivity was displaced by cold benzodiazepines of different pharmacological potencies, administered in therapeutic doses. On the basis of the work of Braestrup and Squires on the inhibition of the specific binding of tritiated diazepam in the cells of human brain membranes (1) : first we selected lorazepam, then two stereoisomers : Ro 11.6896(+), which is pharmacologically active, and Ro11.6893(-), which is pharmacologically inactive (10), as well as chlordiazepoxide, which only displays activity in high doses (15).

The cold benzodiazepine load was injected intravenously in a dose of 5 mg 29 minutes after administration of the radioactive ligand. This time was chosen because it is the place at which the cerebral ^{11}C-flunitrazepam curve changes to a less steep slope and a displacement could thus be more easily detected.

In some experiments, $^{68}GaCl_3$, a protein label, was injected intravenously after complete disappearance of the carbon 11 radioactivity, in order to measure the brain blood pool (8).

RESULTS

The cerebral, extracerebral and blood kinetics of ^{11}C-flunitrazepam are shown in Figure 3.

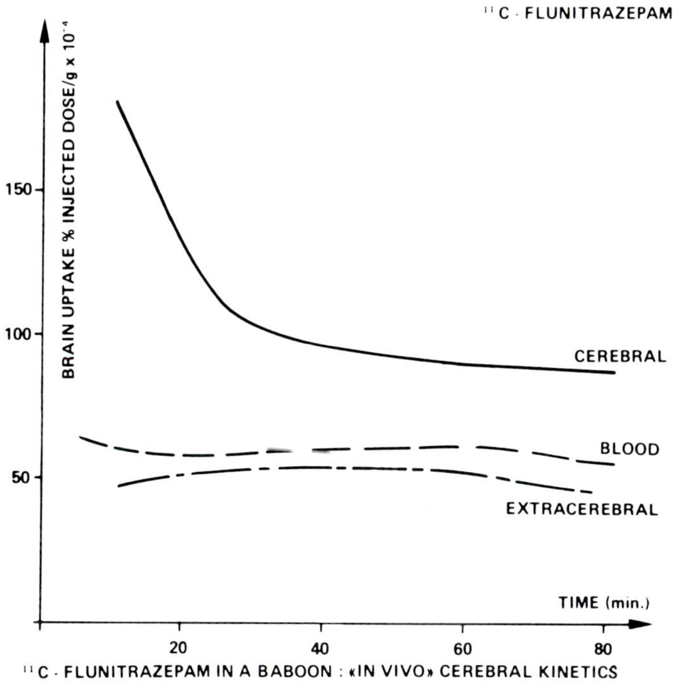

FIG. 3.

The abscissa shows the time in minutes, and the ordinate shows the radioactivity expressed as percentage of the injected dose per gm of tissue. A few minutes after the injection, brain radioactivity peaks and then drops very rapidly for about 30 minutes, after which the slope of the curve becomes more gentle until the end of the experiment.

Comparatively, the radioactivity of the extracerebral zone, as well as blood radioactivity, remain fairly low throughout the experiment.

When lorazepam was administered to the baboon (4) 29 minutes after ^{11}C-flunitrazepam, as soon as the injection was terminated, a marked decrease was observed in brain radioactivity, which was to some extent expelled by the influx of cold benzodiazepine (figure 4). On the other hand, the extracerebral tissue and blood radioactivity curves changed only slightly.

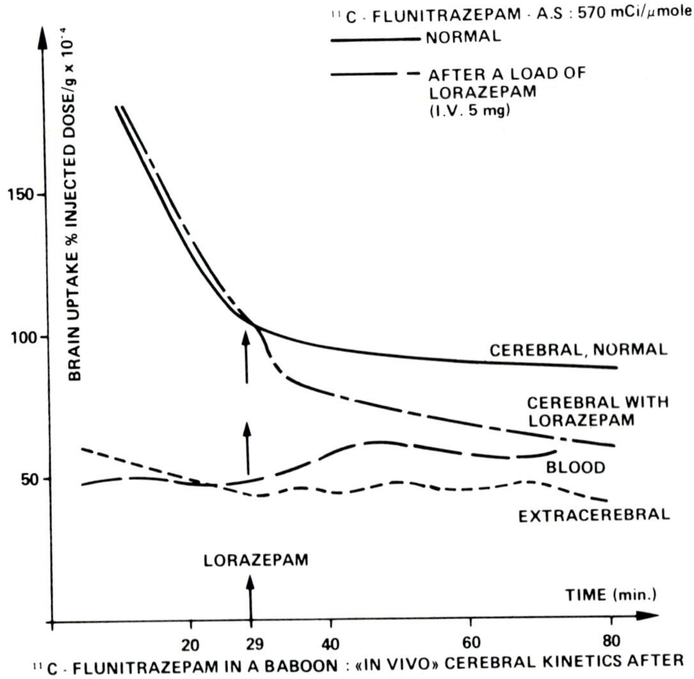

^{11}C - FLUNITRAZEPAM IN A BABOON : «IN VIVO» CEREBRAL KINETICS AFTER A LOAD OF LORAZEPAM (5 mg)

FIG. 4.

Figure 5 groups the images illustrating the foregoing experiment, on a baboon, 17 and 53 minutes after the administration of 25 mCi ^{11}C-flunitrazepam. The upper images were obtained during an experiment without displacement; the lower images were obtained in the same conditions and substantially in the same time intervals, but the baboon was administered a 5 mg lorazepam load intravenously between the times of the two images

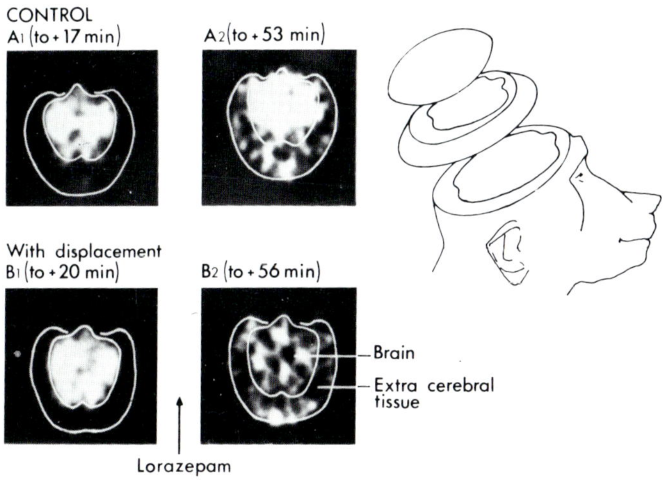

FIG. 5. ^{11}C-FLUNITRAZEPAM IN A BABOON. CEREBRAL DISTRIBUTION AFTER I.V. INJECTION OF 25 mCi.
UPPER PICTURES : WITHOUT LOAD.
LOWER PICTURES : AFTER A LOAD OF 5 mg LORAZEPAM.

In the top left image, taken 17 minutes after ^{11}C-flunitrazepam administration, only brain radioactivity appears (brighter region) while in the right-hand image, taken 35 minutes later, the brain radioactivity was much lower and thus the extracerebral radioactivity is comparatively more visible. The two left-hand images naturally are perfectly superimposable. However, the image taken after the lorazepam load (bottom right) shows a sharp drop in brain radioactivity, in comparison with the top image taken in the same conditions but without lorazepam load. The radioactivity of the extracerebral zone remained identical in both cases.

The results obtained after administration of the two stereoisomers and chlordiazepoxide 29 minutes after ^{11}C-flunitrazepam administration were initially surprising. In fact, instead of observing a drop in brain radioactivity as in the case of lorazepam, we observed an increase in radioactivity (by 10 to 50 %) during the 10 minutes following the administration of Ro 11.6893 (-) (figure 6) ; thereafter, the curve declines with a sometimes steeper slope than that of the reference curve obtained with ^{11}C-flunitrazepam. Blood radioactivity also rises in the 10 minutes after the load administration, simultaneously with the brain curve but always greater (40 to 50 %). Subsequently, in the 10 minutes following the radioactivity peak, the two curves are parallel with identical slopes, and the blood radioactivity then declines more slowly until the experiment is over. It nevertheless always remains greater than the blood curve obtained without load.

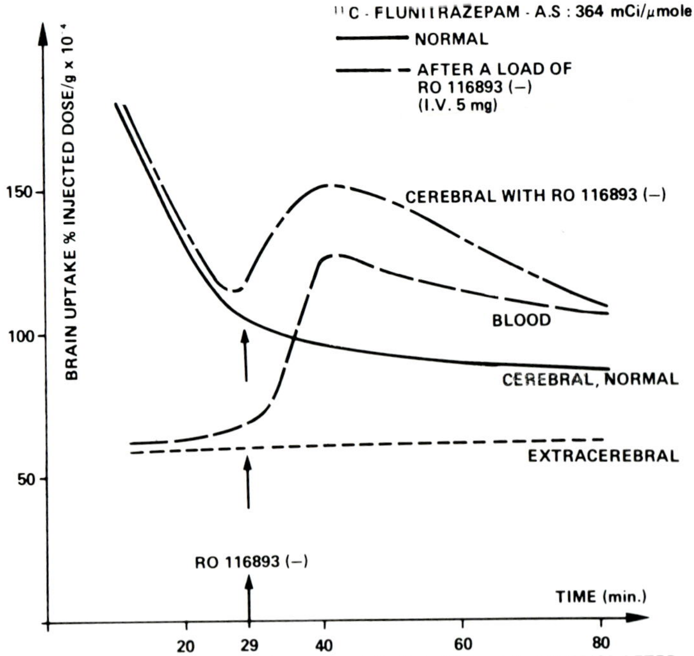

^{11}C - FLUNITRAZEPAM IN A BABOON : «IN VIVO» CEREBRAL KINETICS AFTER A LOAD OF RO 116893 (–)

FIG. 6.

Following the intravenous administration of chlordiazepoxide (5 mg) (Figure 7) 29 minutes after ^{11}C-flunitrazepam, the blood radioactivity curve rises slowly but steadily until the end of the experiment (∿ 20 %). The brain curve after load exhibits a very slight increase in radioactivity ; this radioactivity remains always greater than that of the control curve obtained without load, at the end of the experiment.

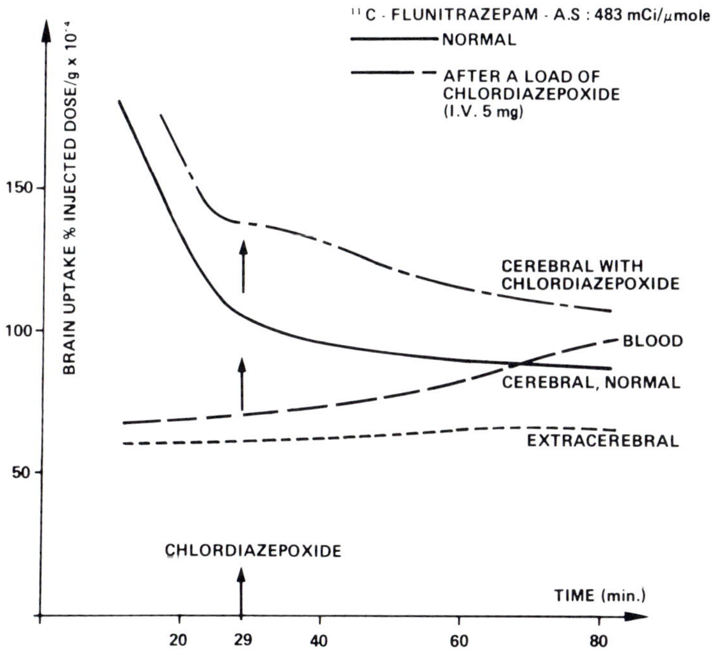

¹¹C - FLUNITRAZEPAM IN A BABOON : «IN VIVO» CEREBRAL KINETICS AFTER A LOAD OF CHLORDIAZEPOXIDE

FIG. 7.

DISCUSSION

The method employed here has enabled us to investigate the cerebral, extracerebral and blood kinetics of ^{11}C-flunitrazepam "*in vivo*" in the baboon ; we succeeded in demonstrating *in vivo* the strong affinity of ^{11}C-flunitrazepam for brain tissue, as well as its weak affinity for extracerebral tissue and blood.

In the baboon *in vivo*, it was also possible to observe the displacement of the brain radioactivity by lorazepam 29 minutes after the administration of ^{11}C-flunitrazepam. However, in the same experimental conditions, when lorazepam was replaced by other benzodiazepines, Roll.6896(+), Roll.6893(-) and chlordiazepoxide, instead of observing a drop in brain radioactivity, we observed an increase in radioactivity which varied according to the benzodiazepine employed. This observation leads us to discuss the various problems encountered in a study conducted entirely on a living animal. Different aspects may be considered ...

We selected the baboon because this animal, owing to its size, conformation and similarity to man appeared to be ideal for a preliminary study of this type. However its brain is quite small and since most previous studies of benzodiazepines were conducted on the rat and mouse, we lack accurate information concerning the distribution, metabolism, pharmacokinetics and mode of binding of most benzodiazepines in the baboon during the earliest period (i.e: 30 seconds to 60 minutes) after intravenous administration.

Only one animal can be studied in each experiment so the statistical accuracy is very low in regard to the total number of animals,but this is compensated by the fact that all data points were obtained in a single animal rather than in a series of sequentially sacrificed animals.

During "*in vitro*" investigations, measurements are generally taken after washing all or certain parts of the isolated brain, thus allowing a separation of the brain radioactivity bound specifically to the receptors, not only from non-specifically bound radioactivity, but also from the free radioactivity and blood radioactivity. In an "*in vivo*" study, it is not possible to isolate the brain receptors ; during external detection, the camera accounts for total brain and blood radioactivity in the tomographic slice of brain investigated whether it is specifically bound or not.

These receptors are temperature-sensitive. The amount of bound benzodiazepine is far less at 37°C than at 4°C: temperature at which "*in vitro*" studies are often carried out (17). Moreover, it is unlikely that a single chemical type of benzodiazepine receptor exists but, on the whole, a group of different benzodiazepine receptor complexes (16).

The ^{11}C-flunitrazepam used as a ligand easily penetrates the blood brain barrier so that variations in the concentration in the blood would have an immediate effect upon its brain uptake. So, returning to the previous curves, the increase in brain radioactivity observed after the administration of the stereoisomere (fig.6) may result from an increase of the radioactivity in the blood which itself results from the displacement of the radioactivity due to ^{11}C-flunitrazepam by the cold benzodiazepine load, from the peripheral organs (kidney, liver, etc (2). This major increase in total brain radioactivity can thus mask a possible displacement of the radioactivity of the brain receptors.

After administration of chlordiazepoxide (fig.7) the blood curve rises slowly until the end of the experiment and the brain curve displays very slight variations. In the case of Lorazepam (fig.4) since blood radioactivity only increases slightly during the experiment, the increase in total brain radioactivity was not large enough to mask the entire displacement and could thus be demonstrated clearly by the positron camera.

However, if we examine figure 8 where the upper pictures represent images of brain slices (1 cm and 2 cm above the inion-orbital line) obtained 2 and 4 minutes after I.V. administration of the labelled ligand (8 mCi) and the two lower pictures represent the same slice 3 hours later, 10 minutes after injection of 3 mCi $^{68}GaCl_3$, it is clear that after ^{11}C-flunitrazepam injection the radioactivity is very high in the cerebral tissue (upper pictures) while the radioactivity representing the cerebral blood distribution (lower pictures) is very low, and is distributed differently (extracerebral regions - venous sinus).

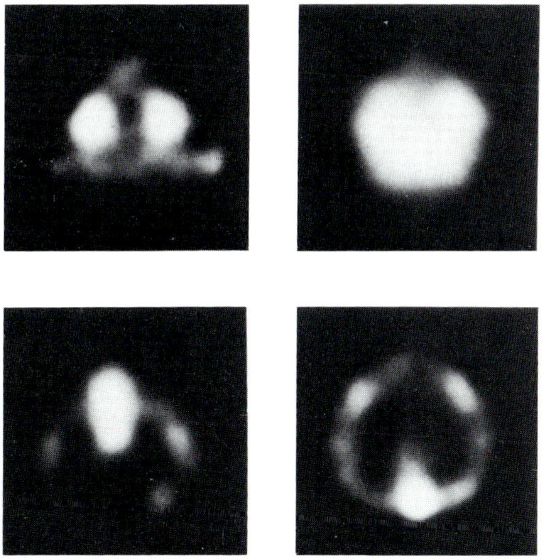

BRAIN DISTRIBUTION OF ^{11}C - FLUNITRAZEPAM (UPPER PICTURES)
AND $^{68}GaCl_3$ (LOWER PICTURES)
AFTER I.V. ADMINISTRATION IN A BABOON

FIG. 8.

Therefore, the fraction of the radioactivity due to the cerebral blood compared to that of the total brain radioactivity is quite negligible. Radioactivity arising from peripheral organs brought by the blood to the brain, thus crosses the blood-brain barrier and is taken up again by cerebral tissue (specifically or non specifically).

^{11}C-flunitrazepam appears to be a satisfactory ligand for "*in vivo*" studies of benzodiazepine receptors as it easily crosses the blood-brain barrier and displays high affinity and specificity for brain receptors. However, it is slightly metabolized during the hour following its administration (12) and a small but significant part of the radioactivity measured at the brain level is not in the form of unchanged ^{11}C-flunitrazepam. Its high pharmacological potency and low solubility in painless injectable solvents make its use in man rather difficult.

It is nearly impossible to make labelled flunitrazepam at a specific radioactivity which is at the same time constant and as high as possible ; the consequent variations in specific activity have an effect on the cerebral uptake of ^{11}C-flunitrazepam especially during the initial period (6).

Problems also arise concerning the benzodiazepines employed to achieve the "*in vivo*" displacements relating to their solubility, toxicity, metabolism, distribution and the appropriate dose and time for administration. The detection device (positron emission tomograph) used in these experiments does not allow sufficient differentiation of brain structure in relation to the size of the baboon brain.

As we have shown previously (5) and as is demonstrated in figure 9, positron emission tomography is better adaptated to human brain studies ; this picture represents 3 transverse sections

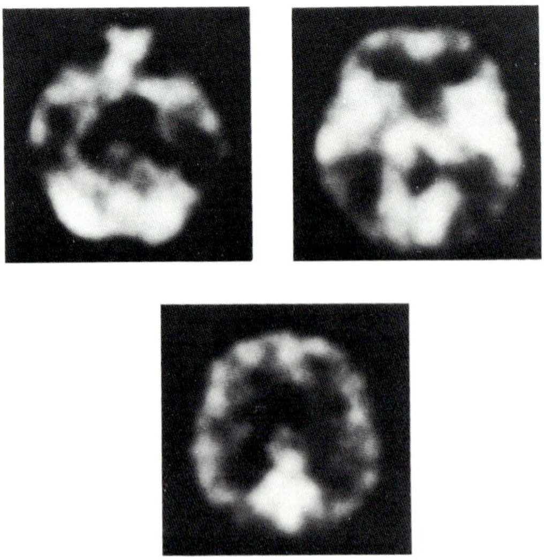

^{11}C - FLUNITRAZEPAM : CEREBRAL DISTRIBUTION AFTER I.V. ADMINISTRATION OF 20 mCi, IN MAN

FIG. 9.

of a normal human brain taken at 2,4, and 6 cm above the orbito-meatal line obtained within 10 minutes after I.V. injection of 20 mCi of ^{11}C-flunitrazepam corresponding to 15 nanomoles of the drug. Grey and white matter are clearly separated and we expect that displacement studies will be better visualized in human brain than in the small brain of the baboon.

CONCLUSION

With the use of carbon 11 as a tracer and the positron camera as an external detection device it has been possible to study, in a living baboon, with a non invasive method, the cerebral and extracerebral kinetics of flunitrazepam and its "in vivo" interactions with other benzodiazepines. In spite of its limits we thaink that this method useful in man, should be helpful in the field of medical applications.

ACKNOWLEDGMENTS

This study was partially supported by grants from C.N.R.S. (ATP 4170) and INSERM (C.R.L. 5213).

We thank Miss J. Sastre, Mrs. M. Crouzel, MM Guibert and Guillon for technical assistance, Hoffman-La Roche, and Wyeth-Byla Laboratories for providing Flunitrazepam, Ro11.6893, Ro11.6896, Chlordiazepoxide and Lorazepam, and the GRCD Laboratory, Radioagronomy Service, CEN Cadarache for mass spectrum determina - tion.

REFERENCES

1. Braestrup, C., Albrechtsen, R., Squires, R.F. (1977): Nature, 269, pp. 702-704.
2. Braestrup, C., Squires, R.F. (1977): Proc. Natl. Acad. Sci. U.S.A. 74 no. 9, pp. 3805-3809.
3. Chang, R.S.L., and Snyder, S.H. (1978): European J. Pharmacol. 48, pp. 213-218.
4. Comar, D., Maziere, M., Godot, J.M., Berger, G., Soussaline, F., Menini, C., Arfel, G., and Naquet, R. (1979): Nature, 280 no.5720, pp. 329-331.
5. Comar, D., Zarifian, M., Verhas, M., Soussaline, F., Maziere, M. Berger, G., Loo, H., Cuche, H., Kellershohn, C., and Deniker, P. (1979): Psychiatry Research 1, pp. 23-29.
6. Duka, T., Höllt, V., and Herz, A. (1979): Brain Research 179 pp. 147-156.
7. Marazano, C., Maziere, M., Berger, G., and Comar, D. (1977): Inter. J. of Appl. Rad. Isotopes, 28, pp. 49-52.
8. Maziere, B., Loc'h, C., Comar, D. (1980): Third international Symposoium on Radiopharmaceutical Chemistry, St.Louis U.S.A. June 16-20.
9. Maziere, M., Godot, J.M., Berger, G., Prenant, C., and Comar, D. J. Radioanal. Chem. (1980) 56, no.1-2, pp. 229-235.

10. Möhler, H., Okata, T. (1977): Science 198, pp. 849-851.
11. Reisine, T.D., Wastek, G.J., Speth, R.C., Bird, E.D., and Yamamura, H.I. (1979): Brain Research 165, pp. 183-187.
12. Singlas, E. (1979): La nouvelle presse medicale 8, pp.2519-23.
13. Soussaline, F., Todd-Pokropek, A.E., Plummer, D., Comar D., Loc'h, C., Houle, S., and Kellershohn, C. (1979): Eur. J. Nucl. Med. 4, pp. 237-249.
14. Speth, R.C., Wastek, G.J., Johnson, P.C., and Yamamura, H.I. (1978): Life Sciences 22 no.10, pp. 859-866.
15. Squires, R.F., Braestrup, C. (1977): Nature 266, pp. 732-734.
16. Squires, R.F., Benson, D.I., Braestrup, C., Coupet, C., Klepner, A., Myers, V., Beer, B. (1979): Pharmacol. Biochem. Behav. 10, pp. 825.
17. Williamson, M.J., Paul, S.M., Kolnick, P. (1978): Nature 275 pp. 551-553.

GABA and Benzodiazepine Receptors,
edited by E. Costa et al.
Raven Press, New York © 1981.

On a Possible Role of GABA in Mania. Therapeutic Efficacy of Sodium Valproate

*H. M. Emrich, D. v. Zerssen, W. Kissling, and H.-J. Möller

Max-Planck-Institut für Psychiatrie, D-8000 München 40, Germany

A crucial role of GABA, acting in a predominantly inhibitory fashion, in regulatory processes in the CNS has been established in recent years and possible clinical aspects of its action evaluated in patients suffering from hyperkinetic syndromes (e.g. Huntington's disease, tardive dyskinesia) or epilepsy (summaries: 12, 16, 26). However, a consideration of the possible clinical implications of the functions of GABA has not been confined to the problem of neurological disorders but also encompassed neurobiochemical questions as to the pathogenesis of endogenous psychoses. Based on the fact that GABA acts as a presynaptic modulator of dopaminergic neurons (28, 29) the hypothesis of a possible defect in the GABA system as a causative factor in schizophrenia has been developed (25). Van Kammen (15) in a summarizing paper, speculatively extends this idea to manic psychoses suggesting that the dopamine hypothesis of schizophrenia and mania could implicate a GABA defect as involved in these psychiatric disorders, since GABA and dopamine appeared to mutually regulate each others functional activity. However, any convincing experimental evidence supportative of these hypotheses is, as yet, lacking. In a single-blind study Frederiksen (11) administered para-chlor-phenyl GABA (baclophen) to chronic schizophrenic patients and observed an amelioration in psychotic symptoms, in several cases within a few days. However, Beckmann et al. (2), using baclophen in 21 schizophrenic patients, could not reproduce these results and discussed several reasons for this lack of success. Besides the possibility that baclophen penetrates the blood-brain barrier

*Supported by a grant (Heisenberg-program) of the Deutsche Forschungsgemeinschaft

very poorly (10), it is possible that baclophen does not act via GABA-ergic receptors (5, 6). Interestingly, there are some preliminary results pointing to a possible curative action of the GABA-ergic (14) weak anticonvulsant valproate in schizophrenic patients, observed in a single-blind pilot study (13). In this context the results obtained recently by Beckmann (1) concerning the effect of high-dosage treatment of schizophrenic patients with diazepam, which may possess GABA-ergic properties, are of importance.

The following reasons led us to postulate a possible therapeutic value of valproate. Firstly, we have made the observation that the antimanic property of the ß-receptor blocking agent propranolol is not confined to its l-stereoisomer but is also - although to a lower extent - possessed by the d-isomer which exerts no ß-receptor blocking activity (9, 21). Since there are some indications for a GABA-ergic action of propranolol, derived from studies using an animal model of monoamine-induced excitation (8) a GABA-ergic mechanism may underly the antimanic action of propranolol. The observation that GABA-turnover, in vitro, is reduced by d- and l-propranolol to approximately the same extent (8) is consonant with this hypothesis.

Another source of evidence suggestive of a possible antimanic action of valproate came from the clinical findings of Lambert et al. (18) who used dipropylacetamide for treatment of manic depressive psychoses. Since dipropylacetamide is rapidly metabolized to valproate, a similar therapeutic mode of action could be occurent. However, the work of Lambert et al. (18) was performed without the use of either rating scales for psychopathological evaluation or placebo controls. Therefore, their publication represents only a clinical impression. Nevertheless, a noteworthy finding of these authors was that lithium non-responders showed a marked improvement if a combination of lithium with dipropylacetamide was given.

Hypothetical consideration as to a possible role of GABA in the pharmacotherapy of manic syndromes can furthermore be based upon the GABA-ergic mode of action of several antiepileptic compounds which have also turned out to be effective antimanic agents. Diphenylhydantoine (DPH), for example, which has been shown, in the crayfish-stretch-receptor preparation, to modulate postsynaptic chloride currents via a GABA-ergic mechanism (7) has been shown to be more suitable, therapeutically, in manic psychoses than in schizophrenia (17). Another antiepileptic drug which apparently possesses antimanic properties is carbamazepine (tegretol). This substance has been found to be effective in acute, in addition to prophylactic treatments (23, 24), an observation which has recently been replicated in the NIMH (3). Although the mechanism of action of carbamazepine has not, as yet, been established, it is possible that it acts indirectly via a GABA-ergic mechanism (8). Another important finding is the demonstration by Costa's group (20) that GABA-turnover in the n.accumbens and globus pallidus is increased by neuroleptic drugs which fail to cause extrapyramidal side effects or tardive dyskinesia.

The present paper constitutes an investigation as to the therapeutic value of sodium valproate in manic psychoses, and has been performed employing the following two designs. Firstly, by use of a double-blind placebo-controlled ABA-design with acutely manic inpatients, and secondly, in an open trial, with prophylactic long-term treatment of lithium non-responders (outpatients).

METHODS

Acute Treatments: Five inpatients* with pure maniform psychoses (ICD 296.3) were treated with valproate using a double-blind ABA-design with placebo control. Prior to inition of the trial, informed consent was obtained from both the patients themselves and their close relatives. 300 mg tablets of valproate were given 3 times daily (at 7:45, 12:15, and 18:15) up to a dosage in one case, of a total of 3.8 g/d. Psychopathological evaluation was performed by a physician using the Inpatient Multidimensional Psychiatric Scale (19) Five of the twelve IMPS-factors (EXC, HOS, GRN, MTR, CNP) were summed in order to give a score reflecting the pationt's manic symptomatology (cf. 30). In three patients the mania rating scale (MS-M, 22) was also used. In all patients an extensive physical and neurological examination was performed prior to commencement of the trial. The laboratory tests performed prior to starting the trial included a X-ray examination of the chest, ECG, EEG and routine chemical measurements, particularly liver function tests. Thrombocyte-count and bleeding time, in particular, were controlled both before and during valproate medication.

Chronic Prophylactic Treatments: Prophylactic long-term medication with valproate was performed in seven lithium non-responders, in six of them in combination with low doses of lithium and in one case without

---

*One patient was treated in the Bezirkskrankenhaus Haar. We are greatly indebted to director Dr.Dr.Ch. Schulz and Dr. R. Oechsner for their very valuable cooperation.

lithium owing to the severity of lithium side effects. Also in these patients laboratory routine, including liver function tests, was performed.

The clinical time-course of recovery or otherwise of these outpatients was assessed by a physician (open study) by use of the VBS (Verlaufs-Beurteilungs-Skala), a self-constructed scale with 8 degrees of intensity, adapted here to relate to the global impression of 'manic behavior' and 'depression'.

RESULTS

The time-course of the psychopathological data obtained during the five acute trials is represented in figs. 1-3. In patient VL an immediate response to

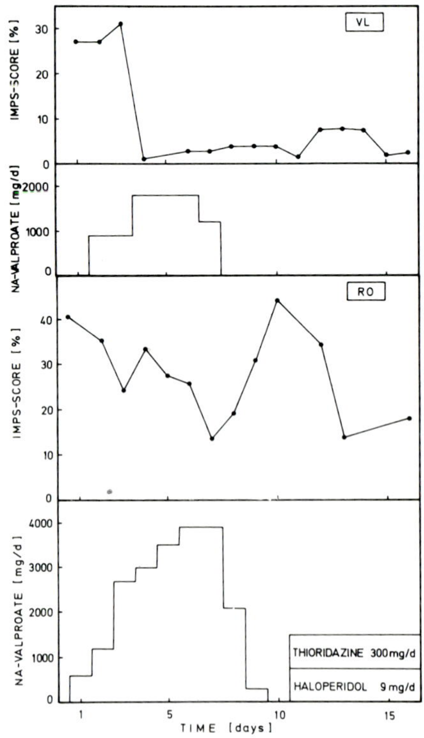

FIG. 1. Time-course of psychopathological data (mean IMPS-scores: EXC, HOS, GRN, MTR, CNP) and of valproate dosage in two patients with maniform psychoses.

valproate medication occurred, and, after discontinuation of this treatment, there was only a slight relapse in manic symptomatology. In patient RO the response to valproate was very pronounced. In the second placebo phase, administration of neuroleptics proved necessary. The side effects of these neuroleptics were estimated by the patient to be very uncomfortable in comparison with those of valproate. In patient RA a pronounced response to valproate occurred which - during the second placebo phase - was followed by an immediate relapse. Patient MO also showed, during treatment with valproate, a significant response, whilst after discontinuation of medication the relapse in manic symptoms

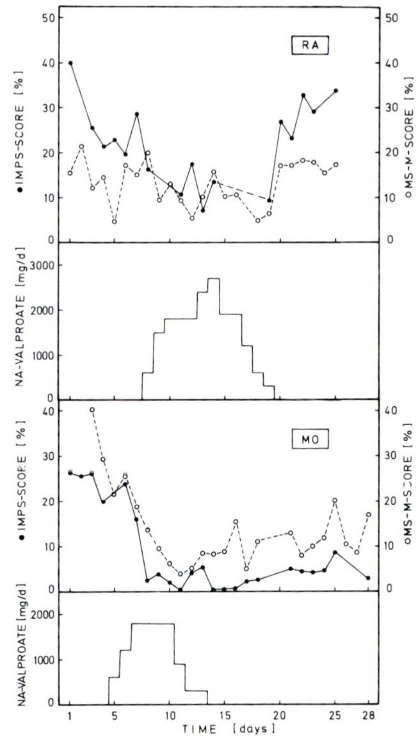

FIG. 2. Time-course of psychopathological data (mean IMPS-scores: EXC, HOS, GRN, MTR, CNP; MS-M-scores = mania-scale by Murphy) and of valproate dosage in two patients with maniform psychoses.

was only very slight. In patient FI, two treatment schedules with valproate were ineffective: However, this patient also did not respond to neuroleptic therapy and was released from the clinic eight weeks later after spontaneous remission.

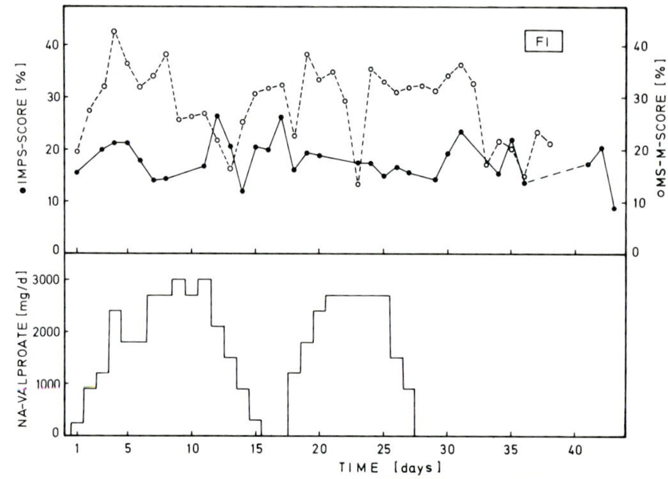

FIG. 3. Time-course of psychopathological data (mean IMPS-scores: EXC, HOS, GRN, MTR, CNP; MS-M-scores = mania-scale by Murphy) and of valproate dosage in a patient with maniform psychosis.

Prophylactic Treatment: Five of the seven patients, included in this study have been treated over a period of one year and the other two (S.W., S.A.) for 2 1/2 and 1 3/4 years respectively. The clinical time-course of these two patients is shown in figs. 4 and 5. In none of the seven patients was it necessary to withdraw the drug or to reduce the dosage owing to medication side effects. By a careful anamnestic examination of the patients and comparison with the different hospital reports the time-course was documented retrospectively by using an eight degrees rating scale (VBS) for mania (upwards in figs. 4 and 5) and for depression (downwards in figs. 4 and 5). Further evaluation was performed by rating the state of the patient monthly in the same way (dots in figs. 4 and 5). These patients are practically free of affective symptoms since they are treated with a combination of low doses of lithium and valproate. The other five patients have shown, as yet, no signs of relapse. The dosage used in the chronic treatment ranges from 800 - 1800 mg/d. In one case some hair-loss occurred and in another there were slight abdominal cramps. No other adverse reactions or side effects and particularly no pathological liver tests have been observed.

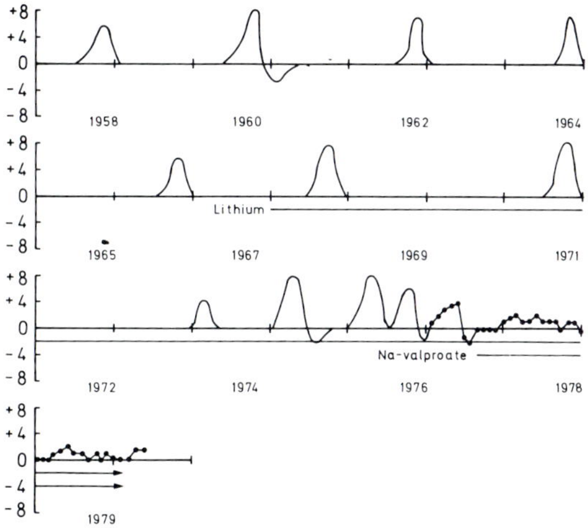

FIG. 4. Course of the affective state of a patient with monopolar endogenous mania, represented by use of the VBS.

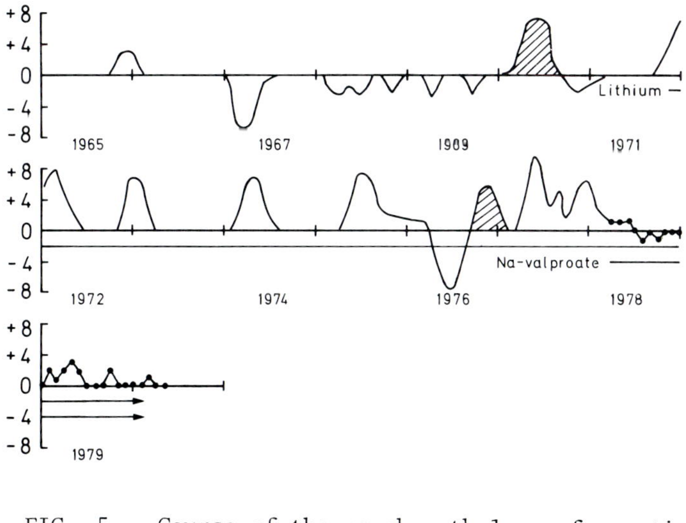

FIG. 5. Course of the psychopathology of a patient with a schizoaffective psychosis, represented by use of the VBS. Cross-hatched areas represent admixture of schizophrenic symptoms.

DISCUSSION

The following two main reasons constitute the rationale underlying the performance of the present study. Firstly, our experience with high-dosage propranolol treatment in manic syndromes was - as concerning the specificity of the effect - so encouraging as to suggest the desirability of finding a substance with a similar profile of action usable in a normal range and possessing less side effects. Secondly, the aim of the present study was to provide empirical support for the hypothesis of a GABA-dysfunction in mania. The findings documented here represent a preliminary report - the study is, as yet, incomplete. However, the present data strongly suggest that valproate is a promising candidate for use in the treatment of manic syndromes, since the dosage range required for its prophylactic and acute effects upon mania is in the same range as in the pharmacotherapy of epileptic disorders and, also, since side effects are rare. In this respect, however, the possible hepatotoxic effects of valproate require careful attention (27). Our results are consistent with the assumption that an activation of the GABA-system may produce antimanic effects. Such an hypothesis is also favored by the recent data of Zimmer (31), who observed lower CSF levels of GABA in patients with schizoaffective psychoses - compared with other patient groups - who had a predominantly manic psychopathology. Our data also represent a confirmation of the results of Lambert et al. (18).

The observation in lithium non-responders that long-term treatment with a combination of low doses of lithium and valproate has prophylactic properties appears valuable in two respects. On the one hand, it fills a therapeutic gap for those patients who receive no benefit from lithium therapy. Moreover, the nephrotoxic properties of lithium (4) necessitate the development of a new class of substances with which to substitute lithium therapy or some type of an 'adjuvant' which enables us to use lower lithium doses than those used at present.

ACKNOWLEDGEMENTS

For the kind supply of valproate thankful appreciation is given to Dr. F. Hahn, Labaz GmbH, Düsseldorf. Furthermore, we wish to thank Miss A. Wendl and the nurses of our wards for excellent technical assistance.

REFERENCES

1. Beckmann, H.: Personal communication
2. Beckmann, H., Frische, M., Rüther, E., and Zimmer, R. (1977): Pharmakopsychiat., 10: 26-31.
3. Bunney, W.E., jr.: Personal communication
4. Cooper, T.B., Gershon, S., Kline, N.S., and Schou, M. (1979): Lithium - Controversies and Unresolved Problems. Excerpta Medica, Amsterdam-Oxford-Princeton.
5. Curtis, D.R., Game, C.J.A., Johnston, G.A.R., and McCulloch, R.M. (1974): Brain Res., 70: 493-499.
6. Davies, J., and Watkins, J.C. (1974): Brain Res., 70: 501-505.
7. Deisz, R.A., and Lux, H.D. (1977): Neurosci. Lett., 5: 199-203.
8. Delini-Stula, A.: Personal communication
9. Emrich, H.M., v. Zerssen, D., Möller, H.-J., Kissling, W., Cording, C., Schietsch, H.J., and Riedel, E. (1979): Pharmakopsychiat., 12: 295-304.
10. Faigle, J.W., and Keberle, H. (1972): In: Aspekte der Muskelspastik, edited by W. Birkmayer, pp. 94-100. Huber, Bern-Stuttgart-Wien.
11. Frederiksen, P.K. (1975): Lancet, I: 702.
12. Garattini, S., Pujol, J.F., and Samanin, R., editors (1978): Interactions Between Putative Neurotransmitters in the Brain. Raven Press, New York.
13. Gündürewa, M., Beckmann, H., Zimmer, R., and Rüther, E. (1980): Arzneim.-Forsch./Drug. Res. (in press).
14. Harvey, P.K.P., Bradford, H.F., and Davison, A.N. (1975): FEBS Letters, 52: 251-254.
15. Kammen, D.P. van (1977): Amer. J. Psychiat., 134: 138-143.
16. Krogsgaard-Larsen, P., Scheel-Krüger, J., and Koford, H., editors (1979): GABA-Neurotransmitters. Pharmacochemical, Biochemical and Pharmacological Aspects. Munksgaard, Copenhagen.
17. Kubanek, J.L., and Rowell, R.C. (1946): Dis. nerv. Syst., 7: 1-4.
18. Lambert, P.-A., Carraz, G., Borselli, S., and Bouchardy, M. (1975): L'Encéphale, I: 25-31.
19. Lorr, M., Klett, C.J., McNair, D.M., and Lasky, J.J. (1962): Inpatient Multidimensional Psychiatric Scale. Consulting Psychologists Press, Palo Alto/Calif.
20. Mao, C.C., Marco, E., Revuelta, A., and Costa, E. (1978): In: Interactions Between Putative Neurotransmitters in the Brain, edited by S.Garattini,

J.F. Pujol, and R. Samanin, pp. 151-160. Raven Press, New York.

21. Möller, H.-J., v. Zerssen, D., Emrich, H.M., Kissling, W., Cording, C., Schietsch, H.J., and Riedel, E. (1979): Arch. Psychiat. Nervenkr., 227: 301-317.
22. Murphy, D.L., Beigel, A., Weinbartner, H., and Bunney, W.E. (1974): In: Psychological Measurements in Psychopharmacology, edited by P. Pichot, pp. 203-220. Karger, Basel.
23. Okuma, T., Inanaga, K., Otsuki, S., Sarai, K., Takahashi, R., Hazama, H., Mori, A., and Watanabe, M. (1979): Psychopharmacology, 66: 211-217.
24. Okuma, T., Kishimoto, A., and Inone, K. (1973): Folia Psychiat. Neurol. Jpn., 27: 283-297.
25. Roberts, E. (1972): Neurosci. Res. Program Bull., 10: 468-481.
26. Roberts, E., Chase, T.N., and Towert, D.B., editors (1976): GABA in Nervous System Function. Raven Press, New York.
27. Suchy, F.J., Balistreri, W.F., Buchino, J.J., Sondheimer, J.M., Bates, S.R., Kearns, G.L., Stull, J.D., and Bove, K.E. (1979): New Engl. J. Med., 300: 962-966.
28. Tapia, R. (1974): In: Neurohumoral Coding of Brain Function, edited by R.D. Myers, and R.R. Drucker-Colin, pp. 3-26. Plenum Press, New York.
29. Wu, J.Y., and Roberts, E. (1974): J. Neurochem., 23: 759-767.
30. Zerssen, D. v., and Cording, C. (1978): Arch. Psychiat. Nervenkr., 226: 95-112.
31. Zimmer, R.: Personal communication

Subject Index